OXFORD MEDICAL PUBLICATIONS

International Surgical Practice

International Surgical Practice

Edited by

David J. Leaper
University Department of Surgery
Southmead Hospital
Bristol, UK

and

Frank J. Branicki
University of Queensland Department of Surgery
Royal Brisbane Hospital
Queensland, Australia

Oxford New York Tokyo
OXFORD UNIVERSITY PRESS
1992

Oxford University Press, Walton Street, Oxford OX2 6DP
Oxford New York Toronto
Delhi Bombay Calcutta Madras Karachi
Petaling Jaya Singapore Hong Kong Tokyo
Nairobi Dar es Salaam Cape Town
Melbourne Auckland
and associated companies in
Berlin Ibadan

Oxford is a trade mark of Oxford University Press

Published in the United States
by Oxford University Press, New York

A catalogue record for this book is available from the British Library

Library of Congress Cataloging-in-Publication Data
International surgical practice / edited by David J. Leaper and Frank J. Branicki.
(Oxford medical publications)
Includes bibliographical references.
1. Surgery. I. Leaper, David J. II. Branicki, Frank J. III. Series.
[DNLM: 1. Surgery, Operative — methods. WO 500 1594]
RD11.I58 1922 617 — dc20 92-5914
ISBN 0-19-261999-3 (hbk.)
ISBN 0-19-262252-8 (pbk.)

Typeset by Graphicraft Typesetters Ltd, Hong Kong
Printed in Great Britain by
Bookcraft Ltd, Midsomer Norton, Avon

Preface

The concept of a text to cover several aspects of international surgical practice was conceived in 1989 during a joint period of service which we undertook with the University of Hong Kong. Originally our goal was to provide a reference work for surgical practice in Asia. A variety of disorders, some largely peculiar to the region and often given scant attention in standard texts from the western world, we felt required better definition of management guidelines. These have been sadly lacking for bedside decision-making in many instances. It was envisaged that such a text be of value both to surgical trainees and consultant practitioners alike. Subsequently, the nature of the text was expanded considerably to include contributions from other distinguished authors in Europe, Africa, Australia, and North America. In this regard we have drawn on the expertise of leading surgeons, each with particular views to espouse in an area of special interest. Consequently, the product has undergone something of a metamorphosis to appeal to greater numbers of surgeons with diverse world-wide interests in general surgery.

The purpose of these reviews is to provide a current overview of some areas of controversy in management. Despite the desire to ensure that articles conform to house style, each contributor has documented personal views and literature evaluation according to individual preference. This has facilitated comprehensive reviews based on an evaluation of current surgical practice and opinion. The different styles of approach have also proved to be enlightening.

This book also provides an opportunity for surgeons of varied geographical background to collaborate in a text with both western and oriental flavours. International surgical meetings in many disciplines provide a regular forum for the presentation of new innovations on management and open debate of controversial surgical procedures. It is more than fortuitous that our contributors are no strangers to such surgical arenas. It is to be hoped that, to some extent, this text will bear the same stamp of freedom of expression and help to consolidate such intercontinental co-operation. In this way the surgical fraternity may be enriched with the exchange of ideas which may have far wider than national implications.

Not every trainee has the opportunity early in his or her career to participate in overseas conferences. If this text can help to kindle such interest and promote closer liaisons between individuals and institutions then it will have served its purpose.

Bristol, UK
Queensland, Australia
August 1991

David J. Leaper
Frank J. Branicki

Contents

Contributors

Anne C. Bayley

Formerly Professor of Surgery, University of Zambia, Lusaka, Zambia.

Sven-Erik Bergentz

Professor of Surgery, University of Lund, Malmo General Hospital, Malmo, Sweden.

Roger W. Blamey

Professor of Surgical Science, Nottingham City Hospital, Nottingham, UK.

Murray F. Brennan

Chairman, Department of Surgery, Memorial Sloan-Kettering Cancer Center, New York, USA.

Sira Bunyaratavej

Professor of Neurosurgery, Ramathibodi Hospital, Mahidol University, Bangkok, Thailand.

Brian R. Davidson

Lecturer in Surgery, The Royal Free Hospital, London, UK.

David C. Gotley

Senior Lecturer in Surgery, Princess Alexandra Hospital, The University of Queensland, Australia.

Finn Gottrup

Professor of Surgical Gastroenterology, Hvidovre University Hospital, Denmark.

Nagy A. Habib

Consultant Senior Lecturer, Department of Surgery, Hammersmith Hospital, London, UK.

Jack D. Hardcastle

Professor of Surgery, Department of Surgery, Queens Medical Centre, Nottingham, UK.

Ulla Hedner

Professor of Coagulation Research, Goteborg University, Bagsvaerd, Denmark.

Guo Jun Huang

Professor of Thoracic Surgery, Cancer Institute and Hospital, Chinese Academy of Medical Sciences, Beijing, People's Republic of China.

John E. Jellis

Orthopaedic Surgeon, Department of Surgery, University of Zambia, Lusaka, Zambia.

Jin-Pok Kim

Professor of Surgery, Seoul National University Hospital, Seoul, Korea.

Chue-Shue Lee

Professor of Surgery, National Taiwan University, Taipei, Taiwan.

Stephen T.K. Lim

Consultant Urologist, Mount Elizabeth Medical Centre, Singapore.

Carlos M. Magsanoc

Assistant Chairman, Department of Surgery, College of Medicine and Philippine General Hospital, Manila, Philippines.

Naofumi Nagasue

Associate Professor, Second Department of Surgery, Shimane Medical University, Izumo, Japan.

Na'il Al-Naqeeb

Undersecretary, Ministry of Public Health, Kuwait, Arabian Gulf.

Arun Pausawasdi

Chairman, Department of Surgery, Siriraj Hospital, Manhidol University, Bangkok, Thailand.

John H. Pemberton

Associate Professor of Surgery, Mayo Medical School, Rochester, USA.

Man Hei Shiu

Consultant Surgeon, Hong Kong.

Eric W. Taylor

Consultant Surgeon, Vale of Leven District General Hospital, Alexandria, UK.

Irving Taylor

Professor of Surgery, University Surgical Unit, Southampton General Hospital, Southampton, UK.

W.M. Thomas

Research Fellow and Surgical Registrar, Department of Surgery, Queens Medical Centre, Nottingham, UK.

James Toouli

Head of Gastrointestinal Surgical and Liver Transplant Unit, Flinders Medical Centre, South Australia.

David K. Watters

Senior Lecturer, Department of Surgery, University of Zambia, Lusaka, Zambia.

Robin C.N. Williamson

Director of Surgery, Royal Postgraduate Medical School, London, UK.

Riad N. Younes

Consultant Surgeon, Sao Paulo, Brazil.

1. Surgical complications of tropical diseases in South-East Asia

Arun Pausawasdi and Robin C.N. Williamson

The disadvantage of living and working in a developing country, especially within the tropics, is the scarcity of the amenities required to lead a healthy life. Besides lack of the four basic needs of human beings — home, clothing, food, and medicine — these regions are rife with infectious diseases. Fortunately some tropical diseases are self-limiting, being confined to certain areas. In Thailand, for example, more than half of the north-east population is infested with liver flukes (*Opisthorchis viverrini*). This condition only affects people in the north, the north-east, and parts of the east of Thailand, while those outside these areas are virtually free of the disease. Likewise, distribution of the malarial parasite is patchy.

The acquired immune deficiency syndrome (AIDS), which originated some years ago from developing countries in Africa, has become a modern-day scourge. Yet tuberculosis, amoebiasis, liver abscess, and typhoid are still causing death with regularity. Medical practitioners in tropical countries, especially surgeons, must always be aware of these diseases and the complications that necessitate surgical management. Such awareness can bring about early diagnosis, which in turn improves the results of treatment. The surgical aspects of these conditions include pathogenesis, diagnosis, treatment, and prognosis.

Tropical acute acalculous cholecystitis

As stated above, opisthorchiasis is prevalent in parts of north-east Thailand, where up to 70 per cent of the population is infested (Fig. 1.1). Chronic infestation with the liver fluke *Opisthorchis viverrini* can lead to cholangiocarcinoma in the fourth and fifth decades of life. Males are affected between two and four times as often as females.

A serious complication of the liver fluke is acute inflammation of the gallbladder, which develops in the absence of gallstones. In western countries, acute acalculous cholecystitis (AAC) shows a more rapid progression than acute calculous cholecystitis, with a higher incidence of gangrene, perforation, and death; in postoperative or post-traumatic cases gangrene of the gallbladder is found in up to 60 per cent of cases. Similarly, tropical

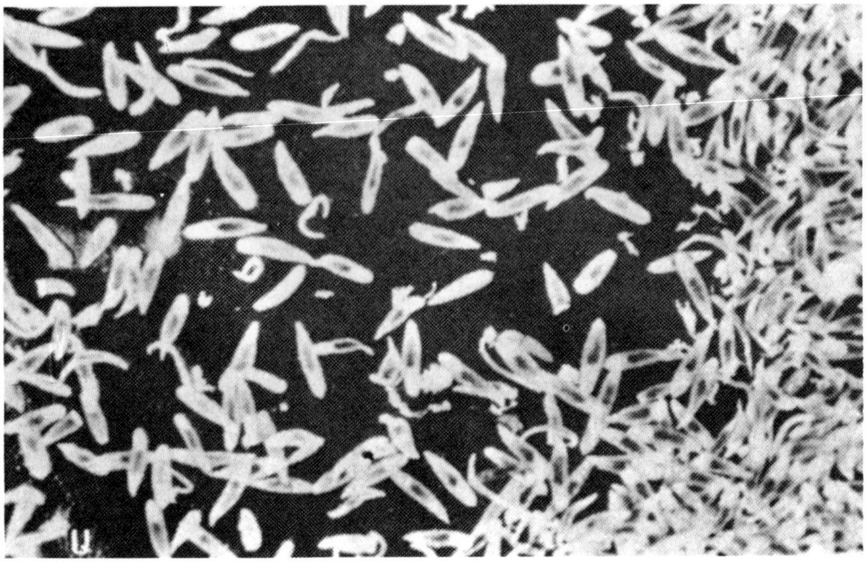

Fig. 1.1. More than 10 000 liver flukes (*Opisthorchis viverrini*) were found in the intrahepatic biliary tree of a patient who died from cholangiocarcinoma.

AAC is a rapidly progressive disease. In more than 80 per cent of cases associated with opisthorchiasis the gallbladder shows patchy gangrene, and calculi are seldom present. The wall of the gallbladder is thick and fibrotic, and the cystic duct lumen is obliterated by fibrosis. Typically the gallbladder contains mucus and biliary sludge (Fig. 1.2), and bacteriological cultures grow both aerobes and anaerobes. The difference between 'western' AAC and 'tropical' AAC is that nearly always the tropical variety affects young patients who are otherwise fit, whereas the western variety often affects the elderly (except in post-traumatic cases); indeed atherosclerosis of the cystic artery may predispose to the condition.

In approximately 10 per cent of tropical cases there is concomitant carcinoma of the cystic duct. The gallbladder becomes markedly distended, containing as much as 300–500 ml of fluid; parasitic ova can be found within the lumen (Fig. 1.3).

Diagnosis

The symptoms and signs of tropical AAC are similar to those of acute calculous cholecystitis, except that constitutional upset is generally greater and develops quite quickly. In most cases palpation reveals a tender mass in the right hypochondrium, and mild jaundice is common. Ultrasonography

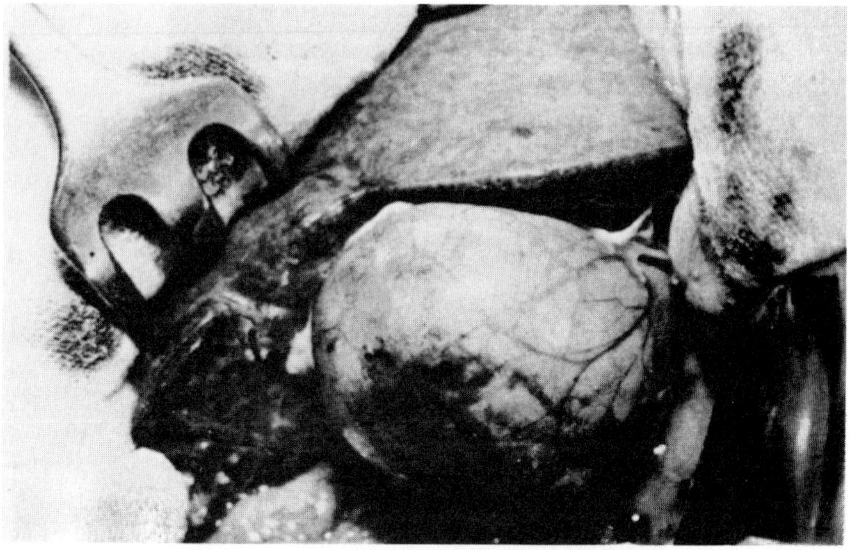

Fig. 1.2. Gallbladder specimen showing marked distension with focal gangrene of the wall in a case of tropical acute acalculous cholecystitis.

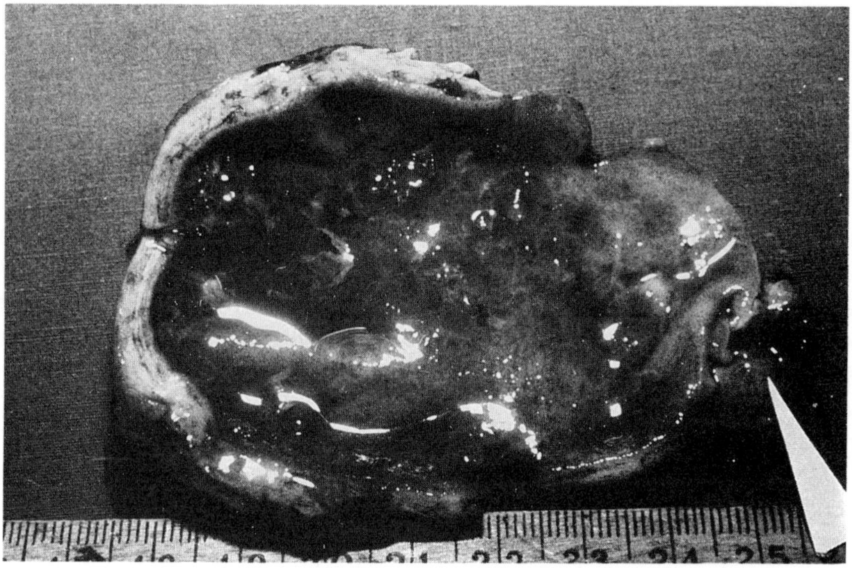

Fig. 1.3. Example of carcinoma of the cystic duct as found in approximately 10 per cent of patients with tropical acute acalculous cholecystitis.

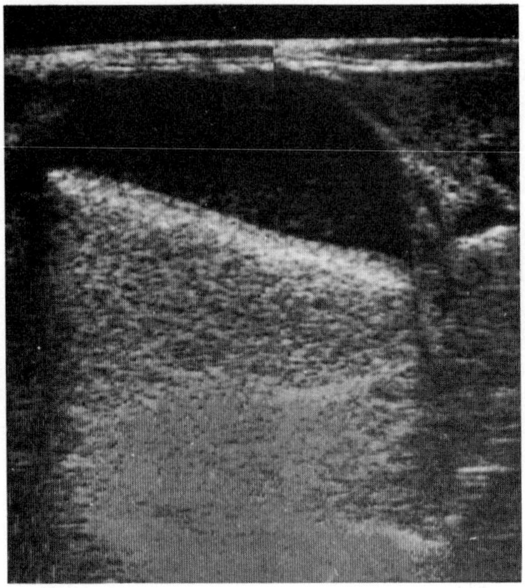

Fig. 1.4. Ultrasonographic scan of the gallbladder in tropical acute acalculous cholecystitis, showing a markedly distended gallbladder with a thickened wall, containing sludge but no stone.

of the gallbladder and liver is of great benefit (Fig. 1.4). Scans show a markedly distended gallbladder, full of sludge but devoid of stones. There is thickening of the wall and in some cases (with perforation) a pericholecystic collection of fluid.

Treatment

As for other types of AAC, emergency cholecystectomy is recommended for the tropical variety. Conservative treatment and delayed operation increase the mortality rate. In the future percutaneous cholecystostomy under ultrasonographic control may prove to be of value in some cases.

Prognosis

Among 345 patients undergoing cholecystectomy in Siriraj Hospital, Bangkok, there have been 43 (12 per cent) with AAC, and 60 per cent of these were associated with opisthorchiasis. This 12 per cent proportion of acalculous disease in acute cholecystitis is similar to the proportion seen in Europe and North America. Emergency cholecystectomy without drainage was performed in every case of ours, and there were no postoperative deaths. The overall mortality rate of AAC in western countries is about 15 per cent.

Abdominal tuberculosis

Although pulmonary tuberculosis still represents a common health problem in many tropical countries, abdominal tuberculosis seems to be declining in incidence. Before 1970 abdominal tuberculosis was quite a common diagnostic challenge, especially since it can mimic many other abdominal conditions, including carcinoma. Exploratory laparotomy was usually needed to establish the diagnosis.

Tuberculosis is a systemic disease caused by infection with two strains of *Mycobacterium tuberculosis*, either human or bovine. Logically, abdominal tuberculosis should be caused by the bovine strain (following ingestion of infected milk), but in practice it is more often due to the human bacillus even in geographical areas in which the bovine strain coexists. Abdominal tuberculosis can affect every part of the gastrointestinal tract from the oropharynx to the anus, as well as other intra-abdominal structures, such as the peritoneum, lymph nodes, mesentery, liver, spleen, pancreas, gallbladder, and even the common bile duct. The small intestine and caecum are the most frequently involved sites.

Patients with abdominal tuberculosis are usually young adults, and females are affected two to three times more often than males. Only a minority of patients have a history of previous pulmonary tuberculosis or an abnormal chest radiograph. Nevertheless, autopsy findings show that 50–70 per cent of patients have concomitant pulmonary tuberculosis. Although the bacteria may infect the bowel through the bloodstream, lymphatics, or by direct extension from pelvic organs, tuberculous enteritis usually results from swallowing infected sputum.

Diagnosis

There are no pathognomonic symptoms or signs of abdominal tuberculosis. Typically the history is insidious: loss of weight, abdominal pain, malaise, and fever. Pyrexia, ascites, superficial lymphadenopathy, and abdominal tenderness are the commonest physical findings. In some cases there is hepatosplenomegaly and jaundice.

Abdominal tuberculosis usually presents in one of three forms: generalized or localized peritonitis, intestinal obstruction, or an abdominal mass. These types may coexist. Differential diagnosis includes other causes of visceral perforation, carcinoma, and Crohn's disease.

The absolute diagnosis of abdominal tuberculosis requires either positive histological or bacteriological proof. Histological diagnosis is generally much simpler. The best and safest way of obtaining the tissue for histology is by needle biopsy under direct vision via laparoscopy (Fig. 1.5). The radiological appearances are non-specific but may include distended loops of bowel and multiple air–fluid levels in obstruction. An intubated small bowel meal may

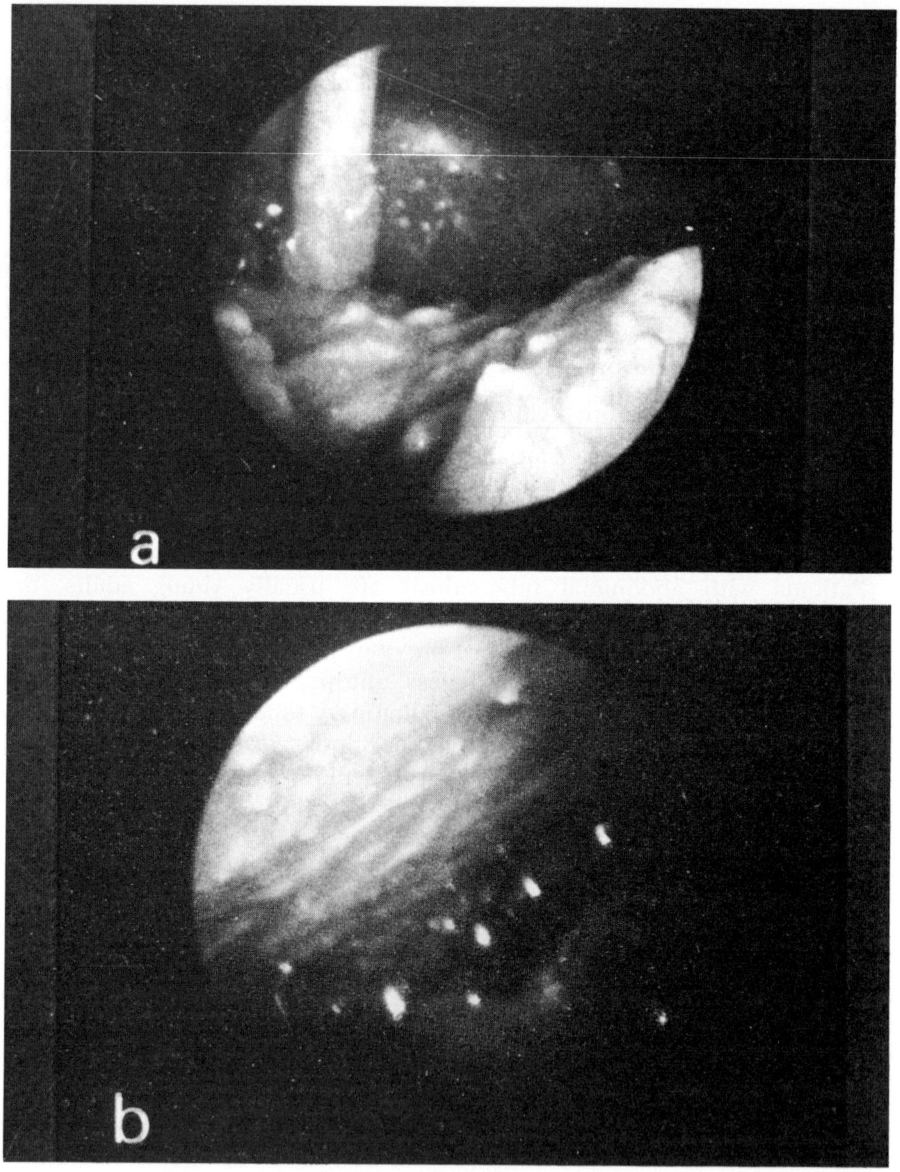

Fig. 1.5. Laparoscopic picture in tuberculous peritonitis. (a) Diffuse, small tubercles of the same size are seen on the surface of liver (above), falciform ligament (on the left), and omentum (below). In some areas the tubercles are coalescent, resembling carcinomatosis peritonei. (b) Similar tubercles are seen on the surface of the peritoneum covering the liver. Some thin fibrous strands can be seen between the surface of the liver and the parietal peritoneum.

show mucosal oedema and an ileal stricture in chronic partial obstruction of the small intestine, or a contracted caecum and ascending colon if the large bowel is involved. Endoscopy and tissue biopsy are very helpful, whereas staining for acid-fast bacilli and culture of tuberculous ascitic fluid are of very limited value.

Treatment

Contrary to typhoid peritonitis, tuberculous peritonitis is mainly treated conservatively with standard anti-tuberculous chemotherapy. Operation should be reserved for the following indications: (1) peritonitis from bowel perforation; (2) combination of bowel perforation and intestinal obstruction; (3) complete intestinal obstruction; and (4) abdominal mass of unknown origin.

In most cases, perforation of the small bowel is solitary and occurs within or proximal to an area of stricture formation. Simple suture of the perforation is insufficient. Resection of the involved segment with end-to-end anastomosis is required. If resection is not possible because of the extent of disease, a bypass procedure is necessary. When an abdominal mass is found, frozen section must be performed. If the mass proves to be tuberculous, total removal is not indicated.

Prognosis

In the past 8 years 33 patients with abdominal tuberculosis have been explored in our unit. Of these, 18 cases were tuberculosis of the gastrointestinal tract, 13 cases involved the peritoneum, one case involved the liver, and one the common bile duct. Surgical procedures for the patients with tuberculosis of the gastrointestinal tract included right hemicolectomy in three, ileal resection in one and enteroenterostomy in two. The 13 patients with peritoneal involvement had an exploratory laparotomy and biopsy of tubercles from peritoneum and mesentery. There were no operative deaths and no serious complications. All patients received appropriate antituberculous therapy for 18–24 months after operation.

Amoebiasis

Although amoebiasis is probably the third leading parasitic cause of death world-wide, in an endemic area such as Thailand it is not an important national health problem. The incidence of the disease has remained constant over 10 years, but the morbidity and mortality rates have decreased. The reasons for this decrease are complex, including better diagnostic procedures, specific antimicrobials, and improvements in anaesthetic technique, pre- and post-operative care and nutritional support.

Amoebiasis is classically defined as infection with *Entamoeba histolytica*. It presents in two distinct clinical forms, intestinal and extra-intestinal. The intestinal form involves the caecum, ascending colon, sigmoid colon, transverse colon, and rectum. The terminal ileum is very rarely affected. The extra-intestinal form involves the liver, lung, brain, and skin. The commonest tissue complication is liver abscess, which causes problems to both physicians and surgeons.

Reported complications of intestinal amoebiasis are colonic perforation, rectal bleeding, amoeboma, toxic megacolon, and fulminating colitis, each of which is potentially fatal. Fortunately, at the present time, each of these complications is very uncommon, and the mortality rate is less than 15 per cent.

Diagnosis

The clinical manifestations of amoebiasis, whether intestinal or hepatic, are at best only suggestive of the disease. In most patients with intestinal disease, microscopic examination of the stool specimen is positive for amoebic trophozoites. In the extra-intestinal form, serological tests are positive in about 90 per cent of cases.

Increasingly during the past 10 years we have used ultrasonography for examination of the abdomen at Siriraj Hospital, and the total experience now exceeds 10 000 patients. Of these, about 70 per cent had a hepato-biliary examination. Liver abscess ranks third among the diseases of the liver, behind diffuse parenchymal diseases and carcinoma.

We have diagnosed 364 cases of liver abscess by means of ultrasonography. In 53 of these the clinical diagnosis was made before ultrasonic examination, 258 cases were suspicious, but in 53 cases the clinician did not suspect liver abscess.

Ninety-eight per cent of amoebic liver abscesses show hypo-echoic resonance on the ultrasonogram, which is opposite to the picture of hepatoma (Fig 1.6). In 2 per cent of cases the ultrasonogram is hyper-echoic. In equivocal cases, clinical evaluation, serological tests, and tissue biopsy under ultrasonic guidance (for histopathology) are helpful. The ultrasonographic pattern is not of much benefit in differentiating amoebic from pyogenic liver abscess. However, in approximately 90 per cent of amoebic liver abscesses the cavity is unilocular, situated in the postero-superior part of the right liver and contains homogeneous contents. Ultrasonography can demonstrate progression of the lesion from early formation to rupture of the abscess (Fig. 1.7).

Thus, an experienced operator can diagnose liver abscess with a sensitivity of 98 per cent, a specificity of 99 per cent, and an accuracy of 99 per cent. These results compare favourably with those of computed tomographic scanning. General surgeons should learn to use the ultrasonic probe themselves as effectively as physicians use the stethoscope or vascular surgeons the Doppler probe.

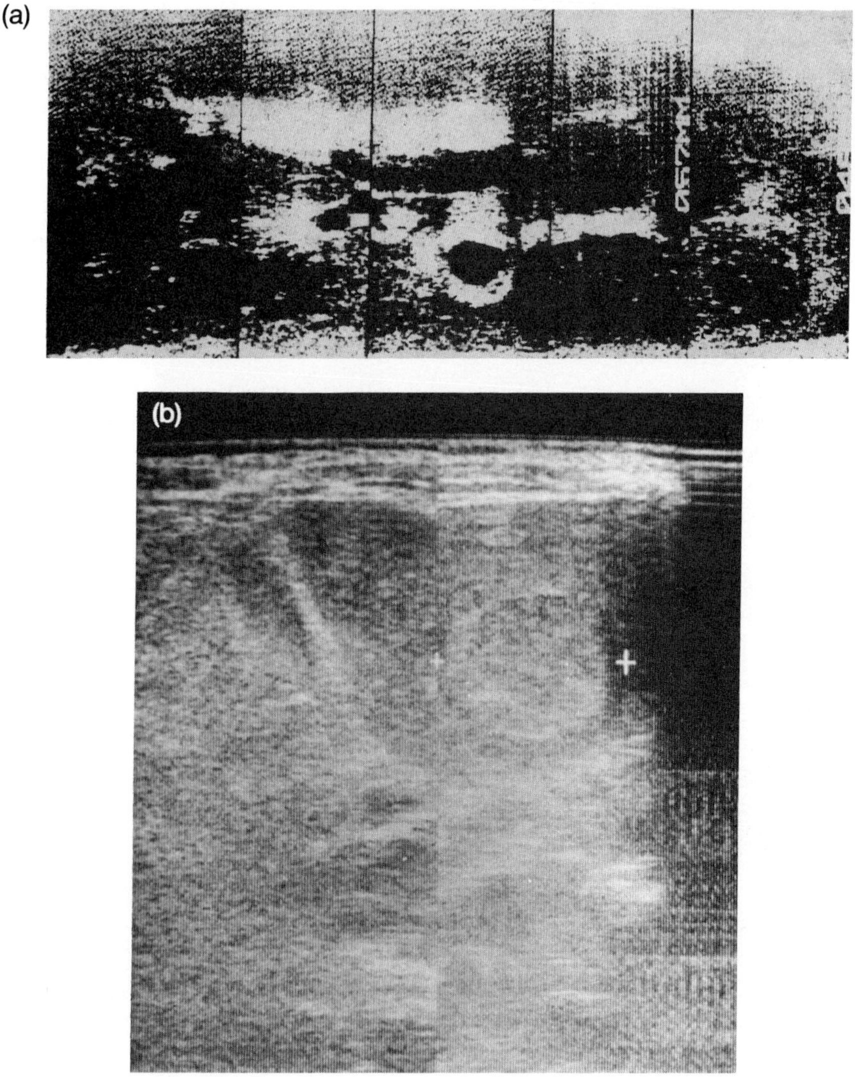

Fig. 1.6. Ultrasonographic picture of abscess in both lobes of the liver (a) and hepatoma (b). GB, gallbladder.

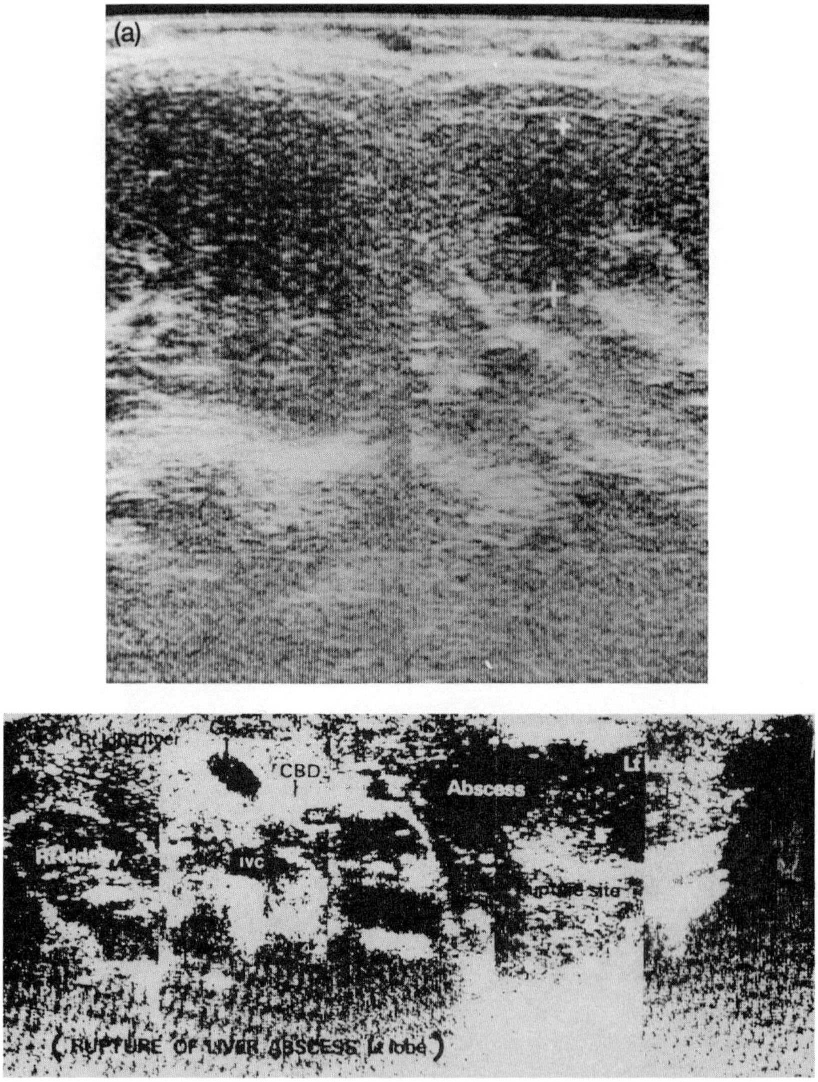

Fig. 1.7. (a) Ultrasonogram of the liver showing an area of hypo-echoic resonance, compatible with early formation of an abscess. (b) Ultrasonogram showing rupture of an amoebic liver abscess (left lobe) with localized peritonitis. CBD, common bile duct; GB, gallbladder, IVC, (inferior vena cava); PV, (portal vein).

Treatment

Standard amoebicidal therapy comprises oral metronidazole 400 mg three times daily for 5 days in acute amoebic colitis and for 10–12 days in the chronic form of the disease. More than 90 per cent of patients respond to this regimen, but the remainder require a second course of treatment; emetine is no longer needed for intestinal amoebiasis. In hepatic amoebiasis (liver abscess) 97 per cent of patients respond to metronidazole 600 mg four times daily for 10 days. In those who cannot tolerate oral fluids, parenteral therapy is needed. For the 3 per cent who fail to respond, dihydroemetine, emetine hydrochloride, and diodoquine may be efficacious.

Operation is still necessary for the intestinal complications of intestinal amoebiasis, such as peritonitis from colonic perforation or severe bleeding. Resection of the affected segment will sometimes necessitate panproctocolectomy. Appropriate amoebicidal drugs and antibiotics should be used to cover the operation. Simple suture of a perforation or primary anastomosis is not recommended. It is safer to exteriorize the bowel ends and restore colonic continuity at a later date rather than proceed to primary anastomosis. Nutritional support is essential in malnourished patients with severe disease.

For amoebic liver abscess, operation is now seldom required, even in some established case of ruptured abscess. Needle aspiration is required only if the cavity of the abscess is larger than 5 cm in diameter and there is no response to amoebicidal agents within 24–48 hours. For a ruptured abscess with generalized peritonitis or a liver abscess with associated intestinal complications (e.g. toxic megacolon, colonic perforation, fulminating colitis), operation remains essential.

Prognosis

Most deaths arise when the diagnosis is missed. There were no deaths among our 364 cases of amoebic liver abscess treated after diagnosis with ultrasonography.

Surgical complications of typhoid fever

Typhoid fever is a systemic illness caused by infection with *Salmonella typhi*. Humans are the only known reservoir for this Gram-negative bacillus. Typhoid fever has been almost eliminated from developed countries, but it remains a common disease and a major public health problem in many developing countries. The principal vehicles for spread of this disease are contaminated water and food. Despite the widespread use of antibiotics nowadays in most developing countries, typhoid fever can still carry a mortality rate (about 10 per cent) similar to that in the pre-antibiotic era. One reason for this high mortality rate is the risk of serious complications, such as intestinal perforation, intestinal haemorrhage, myocarditis, and pneumonia. Other complications of typhoid fever are arthritis and psoas abscess.

Diagnosis

Typhoid usually affects young adults, especially men. The diagnosis of bowel perforation rests mainly on the history and clinical features. The Widal test is positive in about 70 per cent of cases. In most cases the average duration of fever is 2 weeks. Patients often present 2–4 days after perforation, but some as late as 10 days. The important clinical features are fever, headache, abdominal pain, constipation, a dry and coated tongue, abdominal tenderness, guarding, and rigidity with or without loss of liver dullness. Patients are malnourished, toxaemic, and dehydrated. In nearly 80 per cent of cases free air is observed under the dome of the right diaphragm on an erect chest or abdominal radiograph.

The typical perforation(s) of the bowel in typhoid fever lie within the terminal ileum, with their long axis in the longitudinal plane of the bowel (as opposed to the circular ulceration of tuberculosis). In some patients Peyer's patches can be palpated in this area.

Treatment

It is now generally accepted that operation combined with broad-spectrum antibiotics is the most appropriate treatment for typhoid bowel perforation and/or massive lower gastrointestinal haemorrhage. The problems that remain are when to operate and what to do at operation.

Immediately after admission chloramphenicol should be administered, and operation deferred until the patient's general condition improves. Dehydration, fluid–electrolyte imbalance, and anaemia must be corrected. Intravenous hyperalimentation is often advantageous in the post-operative period. Variations in operative technique have been recommended for typhoid bowel perforations. Our experience over the past 10 years includes about 20 cases of typhoid bowel perforation with generalized peritonitis requiring operation. Simple closure of the perforated bowel by means of a single layer of sutures was used. Lavage of the abdominal cavity with normal saline solution was followed by closure of the abdominal cavity in layers without drainage. Post-operative recovery was smooth and uncomplicated. For massive bleeding in typhoid fever (10 cases), segmental resection of the affected bowel was performed with end-to-end anastomosis, again without a death. Thus, improvements in pre- and post-operative care plus a simple operative technique can prevent fatalities in complicated typhoid fever.

Prognosis

For reasons that are obscure, lower gastrointestinal haemorrhage has become commoner than ileal perforation in typhoid fever in Thailand over the past 10 years. Thanks to improvements in pre- and post-operative surgical care, we have had no deaths during this period.

References

Tropical acute acalculous cholecystitis

Bhamarapravati, N. and Viranuvatti, V. (1966). Liver diseases in Thailand. An analysis of liver biopsies. *Am. J. Gastroenterol.* **45**, 267–75.

Chainuvatti, T., Pausawasdi, A., Sripranoth, M., Manasatith, S., and Viranuvatti, V. (1976). Carcinoma of the cystic duct associated with opisthorchiasis. *Southeast Asian J. Trop. Med. Public Health* **7**, 482–6.

Kang, J.-Y. and Williamson, R.C.N. (1990). Cholecystitis without gallstones. *HPB Surgery* **2**, 83–103.

Koompairochana, C., Sonakul, D., Chinda, K., and Stithimarnkarn, T., (1976). Opisthorchis: a clinico-pathologic study of 154 autopsy cases. *Southeast Asian J. Trop. Med. Public Health* **9**, 60–4.

Pausawasdi, A. (1986). Liver flukes. In *Biliary tract surgery* (ed.) A. Pausawasdi pp. 401–20. Bangkok Medical Publisher, Bankok (in Thai).

Ujjin P. (1961) Retention cyst of liver hydrops of gallbladder due to opisthorchiasis, *J. Med. Assoc. Thai.* **44**, 151–9.

Viranuvatti, V. and Stitrimankarn, T. (1972). Liver fluke infection and infestation in southeast Asia. *Prog. Liver Dis.* **4**, 537–47.

Abdominal tuberculosis

Archampong, E.Q. (1985). Tropical diseases of the small bowel. *World. J. Surg.* **9**, 887–96.

Aston, N.O. and de Costa, A.M. (1986). Tuberculous perforation of the small bowel. *Postgrad. Med. J.* **61**, 251–2.

Homan, W.P., Grafe, W.R., and Dineen, P. (1977). A 44-year experience with tuberculosis enterocolitis. *World J. Surg.* **1**, 245–50.

Ibrahim, E.M., Amin, J.T., Al-Idrissi, H., AlMohaya, S., Al Dorsary, J., and Grant, G.S. (1985). Abdominal tuberculosis: a frequent diagnostic challenge. *J. Trop. Med. Parasitol.* **79**, 163–7.

Kasulke, R.J., Anderson, W.J., Glota, S.K., and Gliedman, M.L. (1981). Primary tuberculous enterocolitis. Report of three cases and review of literature. *Arch. Surg.* **116**, 110–13.

Lambrianides, A., Ackroyd, D.N., and Shorey, B. (1980). Abdominal tuberculosis. *Br. J. Surg.* **67**, 887–9.

Plengvanich, U. and Chinapak, O. (1983). Intra-abdominal tuberculosis. In *Gastroenterology* (ed. U. Plengnich and O. Chinapak) pp. 197–210. Bangkok Medical Publisher, Bankok (in Thai).

Sherman, S., Rohwedder, J.J., Ravikrishvan, K.P., and Weg, J.G. (1980). Tuberculous enteritis and peritonitis. *Arch. Intern. Med.* **140**, 506–8.

Wells, A.D., Northover, J.M.A., and Howard, E.R. (1986). Abdominal tuberculosis, still a problem today. *J. R. Soc. Med.* **79**, 149–53.

Amoebiasis

Adams, E.B. and MacLeod, I.N. (1977) Invasive amoebic dysentery and its complications. *Medicine.* **56**, 315–23.

Archampong, E.Q. (1972). Peritonitis from amoebic liver abscess. *Br. J. Surg.* **59**, 179–81.

Greaney, G.C., Reynolds, T.B., and Donovan, A.J. (1985). Ruptured amoebic liver abscess. *Arch. Surg.* **120**, 551–61.

Greenstein, A.J., Barth, J., Dicker, A., Bottone, E.J., and Aufses, A.H. (1985). Amoebic liver abscess: a study of 11 cases compared with a series of 38 patients with pyogenic liver abscess. *Am. J. Gastroenterol.* **80**, 472–8.

Guerrant, R.L. (1986). Amoebiasis: introduction, current status and research questions. *Rev. Infect. Dis.* **8**, 218–27.

Powell, S.J., Wilmot, A.J., and Elsdon-Dew, R. (1967). Further trials of metronidazole in amoebic dysentery and amoeic liver abscess. *Ann. Trop. Med. Parasitol.* **51**, 511–20.

Rally, P.W., Collectti, P.M., Quinn, M.F., *et al.* (1982). Sonographic findings in hepatic amoebic abscess. *Radiology* **145**, 123–6.

Thompson, J.E., Forlenza, S., and Verna, R. (1985). Amoebic liver abscess: a therapeutic approach. *Rev. Infect. Dis.* **7**, 171–9.

Typhoid fever

Archampong, E.Q. (1985). Tropical diseases of the small bowel. *World J. Surg.* **9**, 887–96.

Bitar, R. and Tarpley, J. (1985). Intestinal perforation in typhoid fever: a historical and state-of-the-art review. *Rev. Infect. Dis.* **7**, 257–71.

Butler, T., Knight, J., Nath, S.K., Spedwan, P., Roy, S.K., and Azad, M.A.K. (1985). Typhoid fever complicated by intestinal perforation: a persisting fatal disease requiring surgical management. *Rev. Infect. Dis.* **7**, 244–55.

Eggleston, F.C. and Santoshi, B. (1981). Typhoid perforation: choice of operation. *Br. J. Surg.* **243**, 341–2

Eustache, J.M. and Kries, D.J. (1983). Typhoid perforation of the intestine. *Arch. Surg.* **6**, 523–9.

Kumar, N.B., Nostrant, T.T., and Appleman, H.D. (1982). The histopathologic spectrum of acute self-limited colitis (acute infectious-type colitis). *Am. J. Surg. Pathol.* **6**, 523–9.

Maurya, S.D., Gupta, H.C., Tiwari, A., and Sharma R.D. (1984). Typhoid bowel perforation: a review of 264 cases. *Int. Surg.* **69**, 155–8.

Reyes, E., Hernandez, J., and Gonzales, A. (1986). Typhoid colitis with massive lower gastrointestinal bleeding. An unexpected behaviour of *Salmonella typhi*. *Dis. Colon Rectum* **29**, 511–14.

2. Measurement and evaluation of tissue perfusion in surgery
(to optimize wound healing and resistance to infection)

Finn Gottrup

Mortality statistics for the last 30 years show that the peri-operative mortality rate has not changed significantly in spite of new advances in observation and treatment of patients in intensive care patients (Ahnefeld and Heinrich 1983). In patients undergoing general, thoracic, and vascular surgery, Mayr and Hannemann (1989) reported an overall mortality rate of 5 per cent, whereas 15 per cent of patients treated in the intensive care unit after operation succumbed. Sixty per cent of the patients died from sepsis with multiple organ failure. To improve these mortality figures, the full use of available monitoring systems must be considered. This goal can be fulfilled by: (a) pre-operative assessment and monitoring of immune status and peri-operative risk factors; and (b) per- and post-operative monitoring of the status of cell function in both central and peripheral tissues.

Recently, our knowledge of pre-operative risk factors has increased and many of these can be corrected before elective surgery. Our knowledge of assessment and modulation of the immune system is still, however, incomplete, and the sensitivity and specificity of known parameters are too low to consider these criteria for routine clinical use. For many years cardiopulmonary monitoring systems have been used during and after operation for all patients considered to be in a higher risk group before operation. In Denmark, about 4 per cent of all surgical patients are considered to be in this category and are monitored haemodynamically during and after operation (Sorensen 1986). Despite this approach, however, their overall mortality rate remains unchanged. One of the fundamental reasons for this is that available methods of haemodynamic monitoring (blood pressure, heart rate, pulmonary artery pressure, cardiac output, mixed venous blood oxygenation, and pulse oximetry) all assess the central haemodynamic situation, whereas little is known of the extent to which requirements of peripheral cells are fulfilled. Monitoring of both central and peripheral perfusion and oxygenation is necessary to achieve optimal function of both central and peripheral cells. In this way it may be a possible to improve morbidity and mortality rates.

This chapter summarizes the theory, applications, advantages, and disadvantages of new and currently employed methods for measurement of tissue perfusion in surgery. There are a variety of techniques available for these measurements, but to date very few are suitable for routine clinical use, and only those techniques shown to be of value in clinical practice are described.

Background for measuring tissue perfusion and oxygenation in surgery

The primary goal for all types of surgery is a successful operation with safe healing of the injured tissues and no post-operative complications. Especially important are optimal collagen synthesis, neovascularization, epithelialization, and resistance to infection. In addition to surgical expertise, the type of operation, and suture materials, the major contributing biological factor is sufficient nutrition of all tissues during and after operation.

Each living cell in the body requires energy to maintain its structure and functional capacities. This energy is acquired primarily by the oxidation of nutrients. For energy to be obtained by aerobic metabolism a substrate, such as carbohydrate, protein, or fat, and molecular oxygen must be present in the cell in adequate concentrations. Anaerobic metabolism is much less economic and can maintain cell function for a shorter period. For these reasons a principal goal is preservation of optimal oxygen perfusion. In most surgical patients the main difficulty is to secure sufficient continuous delivery of oxygen to the cell to maintain normal aerobic metabolism. Patient monitoring systems consequently focus on oxygen delivery from inspired gas to the cell.

Cell function and oxygenation

Most tissues have no oxygen store apart from that in physical solution, and a reduction in oxygen supply leads to oxygen deficiency as soon as momentary oxygen requirements are not completely met. After surgery, local hypoxia due to tissue injury and vascular damage rapidly develops, with oxygen tensions ranging approximately from 0 to 30 mmHg in the wound space (Hunt 1988). Thus, in some cells, the minimal oxygen partial pressure is less than 1 mmHg in the region of the mitochondria, lower than the so-called critical mitochondrial oxygen partial pressure (Grote 1989). Below this level, reduced cytochrome oxidase can no longer be completely oxidized, and as a result energy metabolism cannot continue at the normal rate. In many cases, however, measured local tissue oxygen is far from being as low as the critical mitochondrial oxygen pressure, which implies that mitochondrial function, which accounts for 85–90 per cent of the resting whole-body oxygen consumption through a single exzyme, cytochrome a_3 oxidase (Denison 1989), will continue unaffected.

Unfortunately other enzymes, important for wound healing and development of infection, need much higher oxygen tension in order to function optimally. Prolyl hydroxylase, a dioxygenase, is a key enzyme in collagen synthesis and has a K_m for oxygen (concentration of substrate at which the rate of reaction is 50 per cent of maximal) of approximately 20 mmHg (Myllyla, Tuderman, and Kivirikko 1977) and a V_{max} of 50–100 mmHg. The structure of collagen, especially cross-linking which is important for development of strength, is also influenced by a dioxygenase, prolyl-3-hydroxylase, and an oxidase, lysyl oxidase. Their K_ms for oxygen are also more than 20 mmHg and when oxygen tension falls below 40 mmHg their maximal function rates starts to fall. Dysfunction of lysyl oxidase leads to weak, poorly cross-linked collagen and it is therefore possible that hypoxia will have the same effect (Prockop, Kivirikko, Tuderman, and Guzman 1979). This implies that both the quantity of collagen produced and its qualitative structure are decreased. The biomechanical strength of all types of surgical wounds are directly related to collagen deposition and cross-linking (Viidik and Gottrup 1986) and it has also been shown that oxygen tension is directly related to both collagen deposition (Hunt and Pai 1972) and tensile strength of wounds (Niinikoski 1977).

Neovascularization and oxygenation

Neovascularization is also influenced by perfusion and oxygenation of the tissues. Angiogenesis is enhanced with raised arterial oxygen tension even though the central space oxygen tension is only minimally changed (Knighton, Silver, and Hunt 1981). Both the rate of new vessel migration and the number of vessels per unit tissue volume are increased by arterial hyperoxia. On the contrary, arterial hypoxia slows angiogenesis. Recent investigations have shown that angiogenesis is initiated by macrophages lining the wound space which have been stimulated by increased lactate concentration and hypoxia (Jensen, Hunt, Scheuenstuhl, and Banda 1986; Knighton, Hunt, Scheuenstuhl, Halliday, Werb, and Banda 1983). The growth of new vessels is, however, directly proportional to arterial oxygen tension and therefore also to tissue perfusion and oxygenation.

Epithelialization and oxygenation

The relationship between perfusion/oxygenation and epithelialization is not fully understood. Epithelial healing consists of replication of epithelial cells and production of a basement membrane of collagen. The mitotic rate of regenerating epidermal cells has been found to be oxygen dependent (Winter 1972). However, because oxygen diffuses poorly through exudate, eschar and in desiccated tissues, oxygen for replication (as well as collagen formation of the basement membrane) must come from the circulation.

Infection and oxygenation

If wound edges during surgery show any sign of ischaemia there is a risk of impaired wound healing with wound leakage and infection. The fact that perfusion is the major factor for resistance to infection is obvious from our knowledge of healing of wounds of the face and anus. In spite of massive contamination of the latter, both types of wounds nearly always heal without infection if the patient has normal function of the immune system. The difference between these wounds and other wounds is not an improved local immunity, but an increased perfusion and oxygenation. Increased oxygen tension improves resistance to infection through leukocyte function. When leukocytes ingest bacteria, an oxidase in the phagosomal membrane is activated and converts dissolved molecular oxygen to superoxide radicals. This process increases oxygen consumption by phagocytic cells several-fold. Together with other radicals, superoxide accounts for about half of the capacity of granulocytes to kill *Staphylococcus aureus* (Hunt, *et al.* 1991). The rate of superoxide production in leukocytes depends on oxygen tension, and bactericidal activity of human leukocytes begins to fail as oxygen tension falls below about 30–40 mmHg. The clinical relevance of flow and oxygen supply to healing and infection has been shown in experiments on skin flaps in dogs (Gottrup, Firmin, Hunt, and Mathes 1984*a*; Gottrup, Orredsson, Price, Mathes, and Hohn 1984*b*; Jonsson, Hunt, and Mathes 1988). In flaps with a high flow the tissue oxygen tension was also high and no infection was documented after injection of bacteria. Invasive, necrotizing infections were found only in flap areas in which oxygen tension was less than about 40 mmHg. When oxygen tension in inspired gas and in arterial blood was raised or lowered the infection rate correlated with tissue oxygen tension, not with oxygen carrying capacity.

Tissue perfusion and oxygenation

Adequate peripheral perfusion and delivery of oxygen to the cells at operation relates to the end-results of surgery. Peripheral tissue perfusion is influenced by multiple cardiovascular regulatory mechanisms. In response to haemorrhage these mechanisms maintain blood flow to vital organs such as heart and brain, while most other tissues have a decrease in blood flow. Circulatory adjustments are effected by local as well as systemic mechanisms that change the calibre of the arterioles and other resistance vessels and alter hydrostatic pressures in the capillaries. The systemic mechanisms act in surgery with local mechanisms and adjust vascular responses throughout the body.

Detection of poor tissue perfusion, and especially tissue oxygenation, is crucial in post-operative care. Monitoring systems can evaluate the adequacy of central haemodynamics, the oxygen uptake by the lungs, the microcirculation, and oxygen transport to the tissues. Prevention of tissue ischaemia secondary to flow-limited oxygen delivery (D_{O_2}) has been the rationale for haemodynamic monitoring in the intensive care unit (Fink 1989). The presumption has been that monitoring haemodynamic variables enables the clinician to intervene appropriately so that adequate oxygen delivery to vital organs and tissues may be ensured. Thus, sophisticated and often invasive haemodynamic monitoring devices have routinely been used in the intensive care unit. These methods include pulmonary arterial (Swan–Ganz) catheterization (enabling measurements of stroke volume), systolic, diastolic, and mean pulmonary pressures, pulmonary artery wedge pressure (PAWP), systemic vascular resistance, mixed venous oxygen content, systemic D_{O_2}, and oxygen consumption (V_{O_2}). In addition, non-invasive techniques such as thoracic electrical impedance plethysmography, Doppler flowmetry, trans-oesophageal echocardiography, and indicator dilution techniques have used for assessing cardiac output.

Evaluation of cardiac output and related parameters assess the central haemodynamic situation and perfusion. Little is known of the extent to which peripheral tissue oxygenation is fulfilling the demand for oxygen in the peripheral tissues, which may be of particular importance in surgery. Evaluation of adequate perfusion has, for most surgeons, primarily been based on assessment of parameters such as skin temperature, urine output, blood pressure, and pulse. Maintenance of intravascular volume to assure sufficient tissue perfusion is, however, a far more complex process. Urine output and blood pressure are maintained until hypovolaemia is quite severe (Jensen, Riggs, Vasconez, Goodson, Rabkin, and Hunt 1987; Jonsson, Jensen, Goodson, West, and Hunt 1987). Mild hypovolaemia releases catecholamines and peripheral tissue perfusion decreases, but this will not be reflected in urine output and blood pressure, and, unfortunately, even major vasoconstriction will not be detected by standard clinical methods. In the case of non-optimal functioning haemostatic mechanisms, the surgical patient may be underperfused post-operatively and have decreased tissue oxygenation in an area of wounded tissue. Consequently, healing and resistance to infection may be impaired.

Hunt (1988) has indicated that concepts of tissue perfusion and tissue oxygenation have been difficult to incorporate into the clinical care of patients, because methods of measurement are poorly established. The term tissue perfusion has, in surgery, been used to refer to the functional and circulatory status of a tissue, but no clear definition has been propounded. Some surgeons equate tissue perfusion with blood flow or oxygen delivery, while others regard this as a combined concept to encompass blood flow and nutritional supply including oxygen. If the patient is 'well perfused', tissue function is generally good and undisturbed. During surgery it would

Table 2.1. Main determinants of tissue oxygen perfusion.

I	Oxygen delivery to tissue
	Oxygen in arterial blood
	Delivery to arterial blood to tissues
	Microcirculation
	Oxygen from blood to tissue
II	Oxygen transport in tissue
	Diffusion distance
	Oxygen partial pressure
III	Oxygen consumption of tissue
	Activation status of cells
	Hormones
	Temperature of tissue
	Drugs

therefore be useful to have a parameter that would permit monitoring of both tissue perfusion and tissue oxygenation as a 'mirror' of sufficient nutrition in order to provide optimal cell function. A new concept called tissue oxygen perfusion (TOP) could be useful: a measure of the ability of the central cardiovascular system to deliver an adequate volume of oxygen to the periphery to meet the metabolic demands of tissues. TOP is the net result of the simultaneous changes occurring in the factors shown in Table 2.1.

How can tissue oxygen perfusion be monitored?

Those methods not conducive to repeated monitoring of TOP in surgical practice have been omitted from discussion. Furthermore, routinely measured central haemodynamic monitoring parameters, such as cardiac output, pulmonary pressures, central venous pressure, oxygen delivery, arterial and venous oxygen tension and saturation, are all familiar and will not be specifically described. Methods evaluating peripheral perfusion have not been routinely employed in clinical practice but the following techniques are presently available:

(1) laser Doppler velocimetry (LDV);
(2) post-capillary venous pressure (PCVP) measurements;
(3) skin temperature measurements;
(4) vital capillary microscopy;
(5) pulse oximetry;
(6) intra-mural pH measurements in stomach and colon;
(7) tissue oxygen tension measurements;
(8) other methods (unclear magnetic spectroscopy, infra-red techniques for measuring the functional status of cytochrome a_3).

Methods that may fulfill TOP

Laser Doppler flowmetry (LDV)

The technique of LDV was introduced by Tanaka, Riva, and Ben-Sira (1974) in the early 1970s. Stern (1975) was the first to use the laser Doppler technique for measuring skin blood flow, which is based on the principle that light scattered by moving particles, mainly erythrocytes, undergoes a shift in frequency compared with light reflected by non-moving structures. This frequency shift may be used to evaluate the quantity of blood moving in tissue. The method has been refined with a better signal-to-noise ratio and has become clinically useful (Holloway and Watkins 1977; Nilsson, Tenland, and Öberg 1980).

Results of cutaneous flowmetry have been compared with results of plethysmography, ^{133}Xe clearance and videophotometric capillaroscopy (Engelhart and Kristensen 1983; Johnsson, Taylor, Shepherd, and Park 1984; Winsor, Haumschild, Winsor, Wang, and Luong 1987; Rosen, Östergren, Fagrell, and Stranden 1988). LDV has been applied to measurements of gastric blood flow at gastroscopy (Kvernebo, Lunde, Stranden, and Larsen 1986) to assess intestinal blood flow (Ahn, Lindhagen, and Lundgren 1986*a*; Ahn, Lindhagen, Nitsson, Öberg, and Lundgren 1986*b*) and to assess graft viability in plastic surgery (Bruce-Chwatt 1986; Pietilä, von Smitten, and Sundell 1987). LDV provides information only about relative changes in perfusion rather than absolute values of blood flow. In skin, it has also been difficult to determine which part of the microcirculation produces the signal, and probably only a small fraction of the recorded signal is due to blood flow in nutritional skin capillaries. Marked discrepancies between total circulation, measured by laser Doppler techniques, and nutritional status of the tissue, evaluated by vital capillary microscopy, have been recorded especially in patients with peripheral vascular disorders and/or diabetes (Fagrell 1986*a*). Problems with reproducibility remain unsolved (Sundberg 1984).

The advantage to LDV is that this is a continuous non-invasive measurement which can be used on any of the body surfaces. The major disadvantage is that it does not assess tissue oxygenation and is, therefore, not an assessment of TOP. Other disadvantages are that depth resolution has not been clarified, blood flow may be altered due to tissue compression or mechanical stimulation, and absolute values of blood flow cannot be provided.

Post-capillary venous pressure measurements (PCVP)

The technique of PCVP has been described as in indicator of peripheral perfusion and for providing reliable indices of volume status and perfusion (Sheldon, *et al.* 1983). A specially designed catheter with a small balloon near the tip is inserted into a peripheral vein, placed within a small cutaneous vein in the arm, and an exact position maintained by inflation of the balloon. PCVP is determined by cardiac output and central venous pressure, and has been found to be more sensitive to slowly progressive hypovolaemia than other parameters.

The advantages of this method are that it is a measurement in peripheral tissues; it is a sensitive indicator of cardiac output and blood volume; and it allows the study of capillary perfusion. Disadvantages are that it does not provide an assessment of tissue oxygenation and, therefore, of TOP. Furthermore, it is invasive and sensitive to movement.

Skin temperature measurements

Skin temperature measurements have been used for many years for estimation of tissue circulation and perfusion (Henning, Wiener, Valdes, and Weil 1979; Pietilä, von Smitten, and Sundell 1985). These depend on several factors such as blood flow in adjacent tissues, the activity of nearby muscles, and the rate of evaporation of perspiration. Comparisons between skin temperature and LDV are related in an individual but not between individuals, and digital temperature has been found to respond slowly after vascular occlusion (Bengtsson, Nilsson, and Lofstrom 1983; Ninet and Fronek 1985). Fagrell (1984) noted a crude relationship between skin temperature and capillary circulation, but not close enough to use skin temperature for evaluation of skin microcirculation.

The advantages of this method are that it is a continuous, non-invasive method which is easy to apply. The disadvantage is that it does not assess tissue oxygenation or TOP. Furthermore, it seems a poor indicator of skin capillary flow, which may mainly reflects variations in core temperature, and is dependent on ambient temperature.

Vital capillary microscopy (VCM)

One of the clinically most useful methods for evaluation of nutrition, in an area of skin, is vital capillary microscopy (Fagrell 1986*a*). The papillary capillaries (nutritional vessels) can be studied directly and non-invasively using a light microscopy and a microscopy lamp. The method has been used to study nutritional capillaries during pathological conditions such as arterial and venous insufficiency, to evaluate the risk of developing skin necrosis. Using this system the risk of skin necrosis in an ischaemic area can be assessed accurately, and the effect of therapeutic procedures can be improved.

Dynamic videophotometric capillaroscopy (DVC)

This procedure allows quantitative blood flow parameters to be measured in the nutritional capillaries of the skin (Fagrell 1985). Total microcirculation evaluated by LDV and nutritional blood flow, using DVC, have shown marked discrepancies and, for purposes of evaluating the risk of necrosis, measurements of microcirculation may often be misleading.

The advantages of VCM and DVC are that these are continuous, non-invasive, direct measurements and do not influence the microcirculation of the area studied. They also provide an evaluation of the important nutritional blood flow of the skin. The disadvantages are that these techniques do not assess tissue oxygenation or TOP. They evaluate only a small area of skin and this has primarily been based on the risk of necrosis in patients with diseased vessels. These methods would be difficult to implement in patients for observation in the intensive care unit.

Methods that may fulfill TOP

Pulse oximetry

The combination of an optical method for measuring oxygen and photoplethysmography enables the assessment of oxygen saturation in pulsating arterial blood. Currently, a variety of pulse oximeters are commercially available. More information regarding function and background of this method is provided by Striebel and Kretz (1989).

Pulse oximetry has been widely used in intensive care as well as during anaesthesia. Interpretation of the plethysmographic pulse curve has been related to changes in tissue perfusion and has been suggested as another non-invasive method for assessing circulatory function (Striebel and Kretz 1989). This type of tissue perfusion evaluation has, however, not been proven to be of value in routine clinical use. It cannot indicate the quality of oxygen transport and tissue oxygenation, and during hypoperfusion pulse oximetry reveals only the quality of oxygen uptake providing a value of 93 per cent saturation when tissue oxygen tension is decreased to less than 20 per cent of baseline values (Gottrup, Gellett, Kirkegaard, Hanseen, and Johansen 1989). In view of the 'S'-shaped oxygen dissociation curve, pulse oximetry cannot detect hyperoxaemia. It is not possible to distinguish an oxygen saturation of 100 or 500 mmHg or more in the presence of 98–100 per cent saturation. Furthermore, there may be methodological limitations at low oxygen saturation (Sendak, Harris, and Donham 1988; Severinghaus and Naifeh 1987).

The advantages of this method are that it is a continuous, non-invasive procedure with high accurancy. The disadvantages are that it provides information only on arterial oxygen saturation and this reflects only the quality of oxygen uptake of the lungs. No information regarding oxygen transport, tissue oxygenation, and oxygen supply-and-demand relationships is obtained.

Intramural pH in stomach and colon

Measuring pH in gastrointestinal mucosa in splanchnic ischaemia and multiple organ failure has recently been discribed (Fiddian-Green 1989). The hypothesis is that the splanchnic circulation appears to be consistently affected by endogenous vasoconstrictors when these are released during haemorrhage, cardiac failure, or sepsis. This vasoconstriction may be severe enough to cause visceral ischaemia, primarily in the mucosa. The inadequacy of mucosa oxygenation can be evaluated by measuring the fall of pH which is seen when the decrease of oxygen delivery has reached the point where it cannot continue to meet oxygen demands (Grum, Fiddian-Green, Pittenger, Grant, Rothman, and Dantzer 1984). A further fall in oxygen delivery leads to mucosal ischaemia with acidosis, which is shown by a falling pH of the mucosa. The principle of this method is that saline in a balloon placed in the stomach or sigmoid colon equilibrates rapidly with the carbon dioxide tension of the superficial layers of the mucosa of these organs, enabling intramural (intramucosal) pH (pH_i) to be calculated.

Thus, recording a normal pH_i indicates that oxygenation of the mucosa exceeds the critical values associated with the onset of tissue hypoxia, while low values can be caused by reductions of oxygen delivery and/or utilization in relation to tissue requirements. Transient episodes of mucosal ischaemia, indicative of impaired splanchnic perfusion due to low flow and/or vasospasm, are common in critically ill patients. These episodes are highly predictive of impending complications, sepsis, and death from a low-cardiac output syndrome and from multiple organ failure (Fiddian-Green 1989). The prognostic value of intra-mural (mucosal) pH has been shown to be valid for short-term (within 72 hours of admission) mortality rates of surgical patients, on intensive care, but not for long-term outcome (Gys, Hubens, Neels, Lauwers, and Peeters 1988). Data from patients undergoing cardiovascular surgery have indicated that pH_i may identify patients who have an increased risk of the development of post-operative complications related to mucosal disruption, such as infection from enteric organisms and multiple organ failure (Fiddian-Green and Gantz 1987). However, in elective colorectal surgical patients, pH_i has shown no relationship to postoperative, mainly infective, complications (Gys, van Esbroeck, and Hubens 1990).

The advantages of this method are that it is non-invasive, simple, reliable, and cheap. It is presently the only practical method available for monitoring visceral perfusion in clinical practice and fulfils the requirements of measuring both tissue perfusion and oxygenation. It may be of use in the prediction of outcome in critically ill patients. The disadvantage of the method is that it does not provide continuous assessment and changes in pH_i may take time to develop. This implies that the technique cannot be used for the constant monitoring of rapid changes which may follow haemorrhage, for example.

It is apparently of value in critically ill patients with major changes in haemodynamic status which lead to mucosal ischaemia.

Tissue oxygen tension (P_{tO_2}) Measurements

As described above, the cell has a critical oxygen partial pressure below which level enzymes in the cell fail to function optimally. Thus, the most important criterion on which to judge oxygen supply to organ tissues is the cellular oxygen partial pressure (Grote 1989). Because the cell wall has no diffusion barrier to oxygen, the interstitial fluid close to the cell has the same partial pressure as inside the cell. Measurement of tissue oxygen tension, therefore, becomes the most important parameter to evaluate TOP to the tissue under study. This measurement has not become routine because of methodological problems which do not permit the technique to be used daily at the bedside. Recent developments have, however, made the method so atraumatic, reliable, and constant that measurement of peripheral tissue oxygen tension can now be employed routinely (Gottrup, Niinikoski, and Hunt 1990).

The best evaluation of the adequacy of tissue perfusion in the periphery is measurement of local tissue oxygenation, and both invasive and non-invasive methods are available. In some situations, however, measurement in one tissue may not provide information of what is happening in all tissues of the body. For example, if a leg has an impaired arterial supply, no single measuring site can determine the adequacy of the circulation in the leg. In a surgical patient, however, where information on general tissue perfusion and oxygenation is desired, this may be obtained by measuring tissue oxygen tension in subcutaneous tissue. Subcutaneous tissues are 'non-essential' during hypovolaemia, pain, or fear, are relatively unaffected by heat and cold, and appear to be the best site to measure adequacy of peripheral perfusion and oxygenation. If subcutaneous tissues are well perfused, one would expect a large number of peripheral tissues such as intestine, fascia, bone, and skin also to have an adequate circulation, because innervation by the autonomic nervous system is similar. These considerations are important because we depend on these tissues for healing after injury or surgery. The theory that subcutaneous tissue acts as a 'mirror' of perfusion in other peripheral tissues has been tested by means of microsphere technology (Hunt *et al.* 1991). It has been found that changes in blood flow to bone, skin, spleen, pancreas, and bowel parallel changes in tissue oxygen tension of subcutaneous tissues during haemorrhage. When P_{tO_2} is normal and responding to changes in inspired oxygen tension it can be assumed that perfusion and oxygenation of all other tissues and organs is also normal. After haemorrhage, P_{tO_2} returns to normal only after blood has been re-infused (Gottrup, Firmin, Rabkin, Halliday, and Hunt 1987; Gottrup *et al.* 1989). One can, therefore, assume that if a low P_{tO_2} has returned to normal, perfusion and oxygenation of the tissues may be adequate. Recent work has shown that P_{to_2} measured in subcutaneous tissue is an important parameter for observation of tissue perfusion experimentally as well as in surgical patients (Chang, Goodson, Gottrup, and Hunt 1983; Gottrup *et al.* 1987: Jonsson *et al.* 1987; Kuttila 1989; Hjortdal, Awwad, Gottrup, Kirkegaard, and Gellett 1992). P_{tO_2} in subcutaneous tissue has been shown to be dependent on both cardiac output and tissue perfusion both in normovolaemia and hypovolaemia, and bears a close relationship to oxygen delivery/ oxygen consumption ratios (Gottrup 1992).

During cardiovascular surgery and extra-corporal circulation, P_{tO_2} in subcutaneous tissue was found to fall and stayed low for 3–4 hours after admission to the intensive care unit (Kuttila 1989). During extra-corporal circulation, however, a dissociation between the supply/demand ratio and P_{tO_2} seems to occur (Gellett, Asmussen, and Gottrup 1990). Recent work has also shown that there may be a relationship between P_{tO_2} and postoperative infections (Gys, van Esbroeck, and Hubens 1992) and mortality after colorectal surgery (Göte, Raahave, and Bæch 1989).

Thus, P_{tO_2} in subcutaneous tissue is a measure of TOP in surgical patients. Clinical use of this technique in critically ill patients with multiple organ failure still remains to be investigated.

The advantages of this method are that it is continuous, simple, reliable, rapid, and relatively cheap. It measures the net result of oxygen supply and demand of the tissues, and therefore, it fulfills the criteria of TOP. It may also be a predictor of minor complications after surgery. The disadvantage of the method is that in some versions it is invasive and in certain categories of critically ill patients its use is unsubstantiated.

Other methods

Other techniques provide indications of the cellular energy status. One method is magnetic resonance imaging, which makes it possible to determine the phosphocreatinine: phosphate ratio, adenosine triphosphate: adenosine diphosphate levels, and intracellular pH. Another technique is near infra-red spectroscopy which provides ratios for oxyhaemoglobin and deoxyhaemoglobin as well as reduced and oxidized cytochrome a_3. Despite considerable research activity (Chance 1992; Piantadosi, Parsons, and Griebel 1992) both methods are still not suitable for routine clinical use.

Techniques that measure tissue oxygen perfusion and their use

Intra-mural pH measurements (pH_i)

This method is a non-invasive, indirect measure of pH in gastrointestinal mucosa. The apparatus consists of a catheter with a gas-permeable silicon balloon (Tonomitor®; Tonometrics Incorporated, Bethesda, Maryland,

USA) which is placed in the stomach via the nose (Fig. 2.1) or in the sigmoid colon via the rectum (Fig. 2.2). By substituting the carbon dioxide tension (p_{CO_2}) of saline aspirated from the balloon, and bicarbonate in arterial blood, in the Henderson–Hasselbalch equation it is possible to calculate intra-mural (intra-mucosal) pH.

Tissue oxygen tension measurements (P_{tO_2})

A variety of techniques are available to measure P_{tO_2}, but few are available for clinical use (Hunt, Rabkin, Jensen, Jonsson, and Goodson 1987; Sheffield 1988; Gottrup, Niinikoski, and Hunt 1990). The principal way to measure P_{tO_2} has been by means of polarographic electrodes, but mass spectrometry has also been successfully employed. Newer techniques, especially optical methods, have also shown promise for clinical use. For patient monitoring, direct P_{tO_2} measurement in subcutaneous tissues or the indirect measurements of P_{tO_2} on skin, conjunctiva, or serosal surfaces are the most appropriate techniques.

Directly measured P_{tO_2} *in subcutaneous tissue*

In order to measure P_{tO_2} reproducibly with a sensor, a certain area of tissue, including several capillaries, must be investigated. Such sensors are either placed directly in the tissue (coated in order not to be contaminated; Fig. 2.3) or placed inside a Silastic tissue tonometer (1 mm in outer diameter and 0.8 mm in inner diameter) implanted in the tissue (Fig. 2.4) of the upper arm (Fig. 2.5) (Gottrup, Firmin, Chang, Goodson, and Hunt 1983). Tissue tonometry can also be based on perfusion of anoxic saline through the tonometer with measurement of the equilibrated saline in a Clark gas monitor system (Niinikoski, Heughan, and Hunt 1972; Chang *et al.* 1983) or in a chamber with a membrane-covered transcutaneous oxygen electrode (Larsen, Moesgaard, Gottrup, and Helledie 1989).

Two types of single electrode are currently available. One is a coated polarographic single sensor made of a smooth fibre with a diameter of only 0.55 mm (Biomedical Sensors, UK). This small-sized sensor is stable without calibration for 3–4 days. Another single electrode is based on optical fluorescence and is termed an optode (Innerspace, California, USA). This recently developed optode is the same size as the coated sensor, cost and efficacy are similar, and it may also be used directly in the tissues. The main advantage of the optode compared with the polarographic sensor is that it is not sensitive to changes in temperature, which may be advantageous when no temperature thermistor is included in the sensor. For implantation of the tonometer an 18-gauge spinal needle is used, whereas only a 21-gauge needle is needed for placing the sensor or optode directly into the tissues. This is even less traumatic than inserting an intravenous cannula, and experimental studies evaluating microcirculatory changes after insertion of Silastic tonometers have shown that differences were observed only during

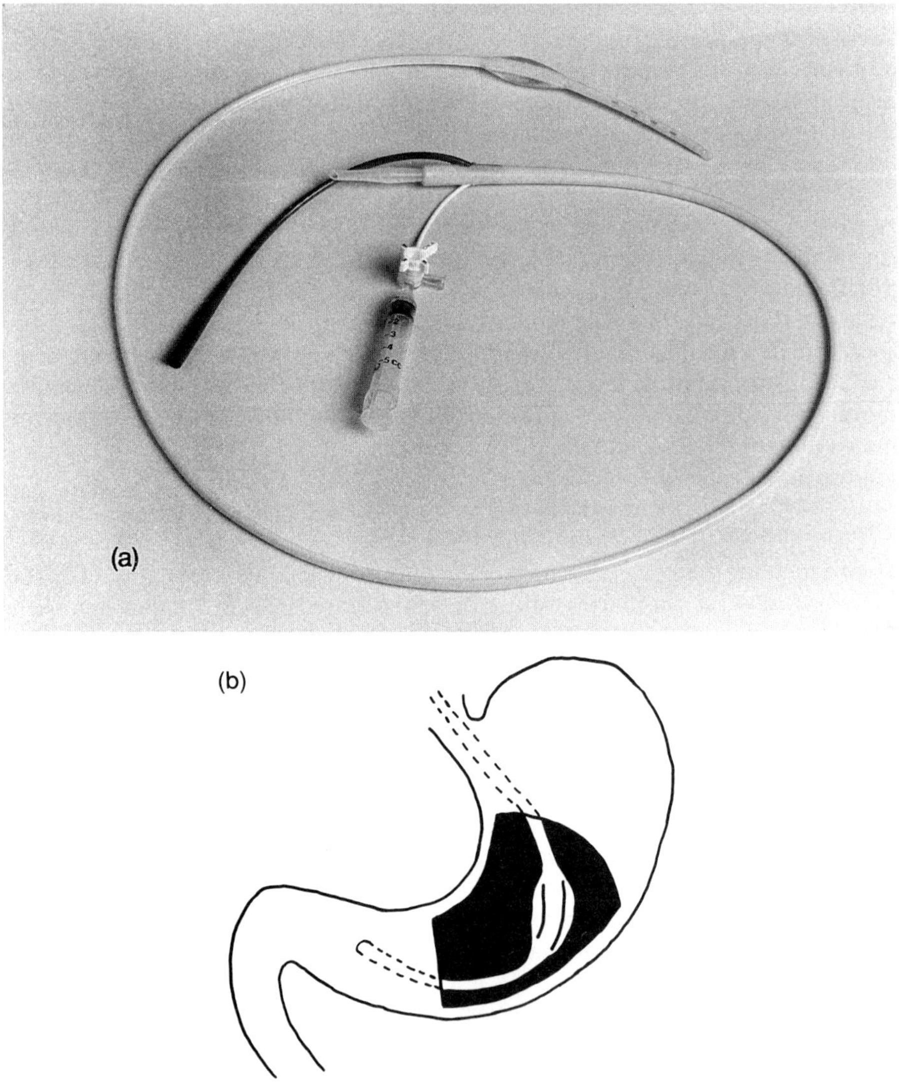

Fig. 2.1. The pH catheter with a gas-permeable Silicon balloon (Tonomitor®). (a) Gastric pH catheter; (b) schematic drawing of the pH catheter placed in the stomach via the nose.

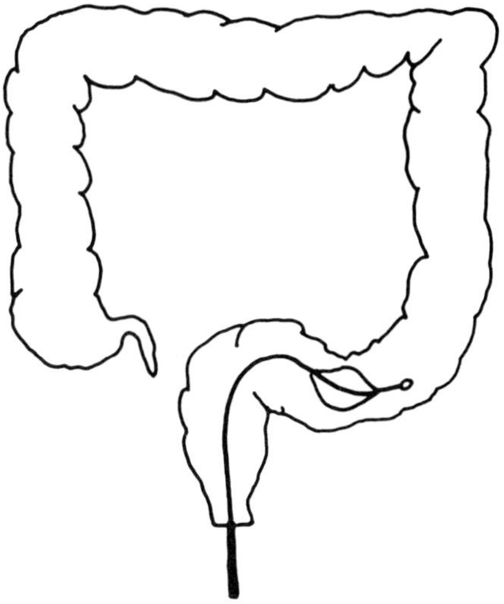

Fig. 2.2. Schematic drawing of the pH catheter placed in the sigmoid colon via the rectum.

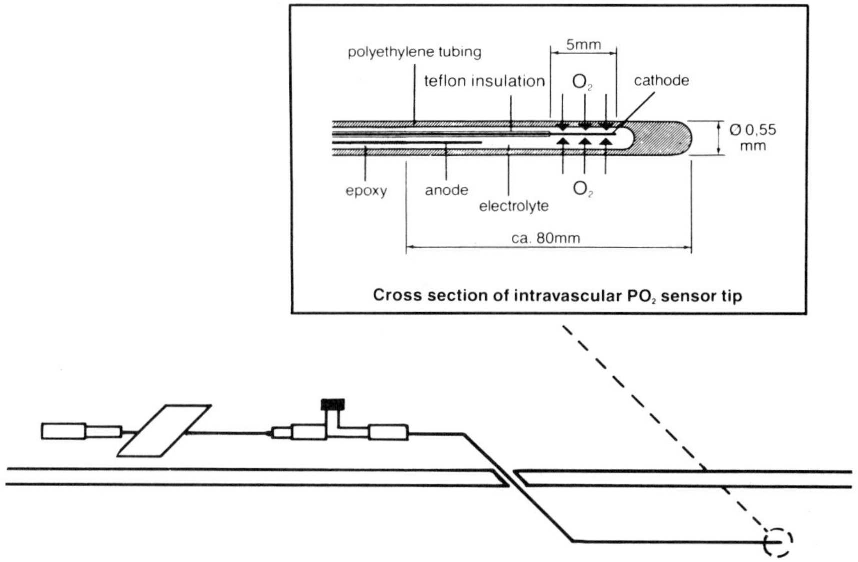

Fig. 2.3. Schematic drawing of coated polarographic oxygen sensor placed in the subcutaneous tissue. The catheter is only 0.55 mm in diameter and measures an area of 5 mm^2.

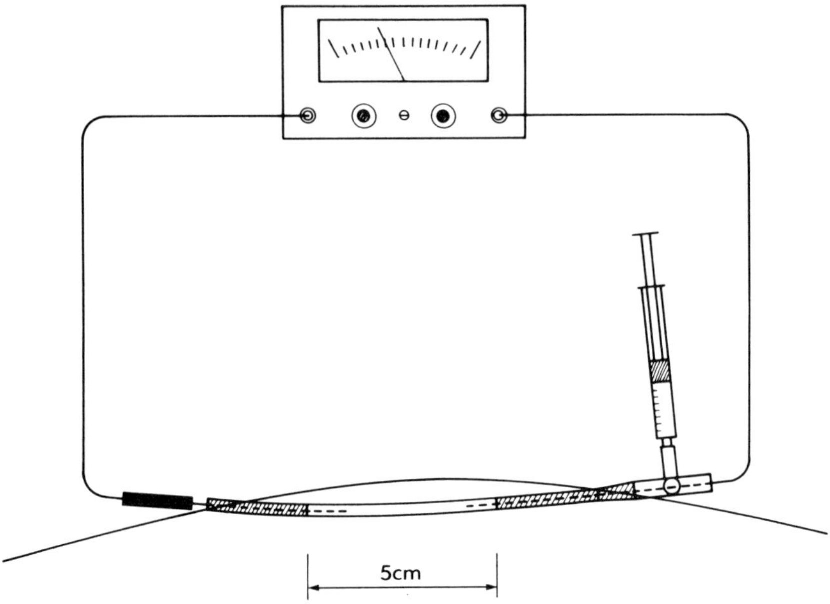

Fig. 2.4. Schematic drawing of one type of Silastic tissue tonometry. The oxygen needle placement and the three-way stopcock assembly containing the reference electrode are shown. A single electrode or optode could also be used inside the tonometer. [Reproduced from Gottrup *et al.* (1988) by kind permission of Williams and Wilkins.]

the first 2.5 hours following insertion (Henriksen, Hjortdal, Kjolseth, Hansen, Djuurhus, and Gottrup 1989).

Indirect P_{tO_2} measurements on skin, conjunctiva, or serosal surfaces

Transcutaneous oxygen tension measurements (P_{tcO_2}) may be made with a Clark polarographic electrode containing a heating element and a thermistor. The electrode must be heated to 43–44°C in order to produce measurable oxygen tension values and these will in most situations approximate to the blood values of the dilated underlying microvessels. This method has primarily been used for evaluation of arterial oxygen tension, but also as a indicator of amputation levels in patients with vascular disease (Katsamouris, Brewster, Megerman, Cina, Darling, and Abott 1984).

Conjunctival oxygen tension measurements assess the only site of the external body surface where oxygen tension can be above zero without heating. The sensor is a membrane-covered Clark electrode and a thermistor. In the conjunctiva the device is placed on a specially designed ophthalmic conformer of a material used in the manufacture of hard contact lenses

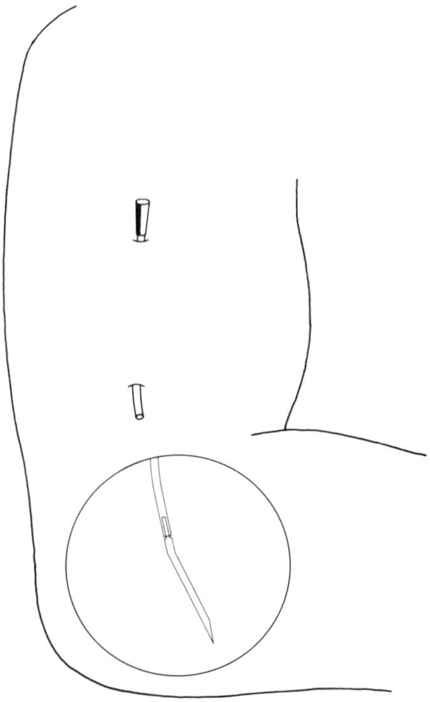

Fig. 2.5. Schematic drawing of a Silastic tonometer placed subcutaneously in an upper arm. The insertion needle is shown in the circle.

(Biomedical Sensors, UK) (Fig. 2.6). The P_{tO_2} can be measured continuously but only for 24 hours for each eye. This method has been used to evaluate arterial oxygen tension, the oxygen delivery to the brain and during unstable haemodynamic conditions, as an indicator of TOP (Abraham, Oye, and Smith 1984; Gottrup *et al.* 1989).

Oxygen tension measurements on serosal surfaces (trans-serosal P_{O_2}*)* typically employ a membrane-covered Clark electrode and a thermistor. This method can be used for intra-operative assessment of perfusion of intra-abdominal organs. Different types for measuring P_{tO_2} on serosal surfaces have been designed. Sheridan, Lowndes, and Young (1987) constructed a special system based on a small sensor, applied directly by hand on the serosal surface (Cardiff tissue oximeter; Fig. 2.7). This system has been used for the prediction of colonic anastomotic healing (Sheridan *et al.* 1987; Sheridan, Lowndes, and Young 1990; Kallehave and Gottrup 1990). Recently, a vacuum-fixed transcutaneous oxygen electrode has been used for P_{tO_2} measurements on serosal surfaces (Larsen, Naver, Helledie, Gottrup,

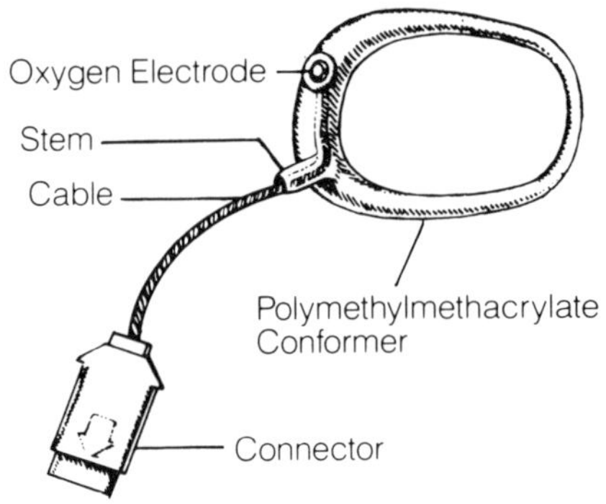

Fig. 2.6. Conjunctival eyelid sensor for indirect measurement of oxygen tension. When the conformer is placed in the eye, tissue oxygen tension can be measured on the palpebral conjunctiva.

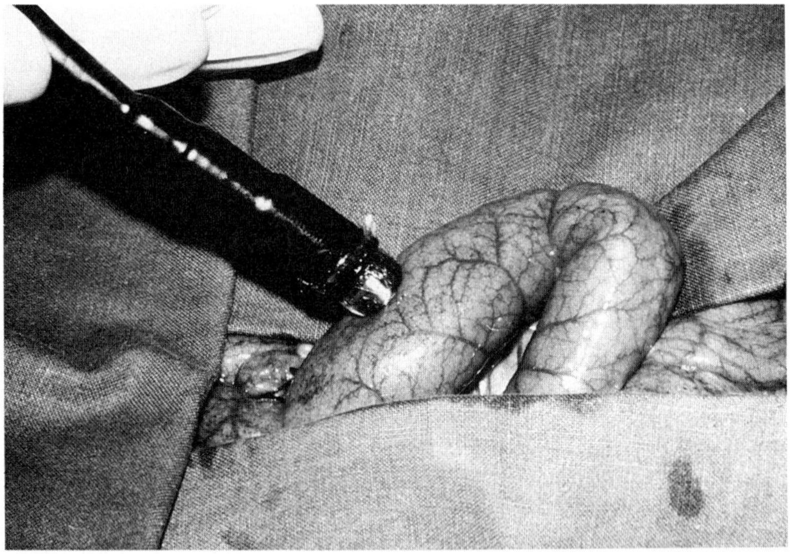

Fig. 2.7. Trans-serosal sensor for indirect measurement of oxygen tension (Cardiff tissue oximeter). The sensor is placed on the surface of the bowel.

Kirkegaard, and Moesgaard 1991). This method has been used for evaluation of perfusion in different intra-abdominal organs and more recently also of the oesophagus (F. Kallehave *et al.*, unpublished data).

Clinical monitoring of tissue oxygen perfusion

In clinical surgical practice TOP can be evaluated systemically or in individual tissues. For these purposes, monitoring of pH_i and P_{tO_2} are available and complementary. Measurement of pH_i is an important method for evaluating visceral perfusion. It is a good predictor of outcome in critically ill patients, whereas the importance of pH_i in elective surgical patients seems more doubtful. Measurements of P_{tO_2} may in these cases be the method of choice. The different methods of P_{tO_2} monitoring can be continuously monitored and react rapidly to changes in haemodynamic status such as hypovolaemia related to bleeding.

During surgery haemodynamic monitoring systems are important to help make TOP optimal for recovery. Presently, monitoring systems evaluate only central perfusion in relation to anaesthesia or haemodynamic stability during surgery. Peripheral perfusion is generally followed only by clinical evaluation and not by more accurate monitoring. The reason for this is that impaired tissue perfusion in peripheral 'non-vital' tissues implies no serious consequences for patients during operation. However, these tissues often develop post-operative complications with impaired wound healing and wound infection, and a decrease of TOP is already established during the surgical procedure. Monitoring of peripheral perfusion should consequently be commenced during surgery.

In intra-abdominal and oesophageal surgery the central haemodynamic monitoring systems used can be supplemented by a trans-serosal P_{tO_2} measurement in the case of a gastrointestinal anastomosis of the oesophagus, gastroduodenal tissues, and colon. Organ assessment of liver, pancreas, and kidney may also be of importance for evaluating organ survival after surgery, but no data are available yet. Assessment of TOP systemically should be performed using subcutaneous or conjunctival oxygen tension techniques.

In other areas of surgery our experience is small, with the exception of cardiac surgery where continuous oxygen tension measurements have been performed in the subcutaneous tissue. Subcutaneous and conjunctival oxygen tension may be employed for assessment of TOP during this type of surgery. Measurement of intramural pH during cardiac surgery may identify patients at risk for the development of serious post-operative complications.

Continuous monitoring of TOP after operation is important in relation to clinical outcome in surgical patients. The goal is to obtain the highest feasible TOP for any given patient. The early post-operative period is important, but observation has to be continued for at least 2 or 3 days.

When patients have left the recovery room, only a clinical evaluation of haemodynamic conditions is maintained and often this results in a peripherally underperfused patient.

In intra-abdominal and oesophageal surgery all patients should be monitored using subcutaneous and conjunctival oxygen tension measurements. Subcutaneous oxygen tension may be undertaken for about 3 days while conjunctival examination is useful only in the first 24 hours, because it then has to be renewed. Intramural pH in the stomach should also be measured in case of complications during surgery or in the recovery period to help predict outcome.

Improvement of TOP measurement

In surgical clinical practice, TOP has been evaluated through subcutaneous measurements of tissue oxygen tension. This has substantial clinical value since the perfusion of subcutaneous tissue is a good indicator of perfusion in other tissues. A relationship between tissue oxygen tension and perfusion is obvious using the Fick principle, and this relationship has also been shown for subcutaneous tissue (Chang *et al.* 1983; Jonsson *et al.* 1987; Gottrup *et al.* 1987; 1989). Subcutaneous oxygen tension can be used for early detection of hypoperfusion in surgical patients. If hypoxia of the subcutaneous tissue is detected, the principle of the investigation has been further to evaluate tissue oxygen tension after oxygen tension is increased in inspired air. If a significant increase in subcutaneous oxygen tension is found, TOP is sufficient for peripheral tissues. If hypoxia is resistant to increased inspired oxygen tension then impaired tissue perfusion of subcutaneous tissue must be expected, and if there is a high arterial oxygen tension it can be assumed that oxygen uptake in the lungs is sufficient. Failure of the subcutaneous oxygen tension to respond to breathing of oxygen must be due to poor perfusion based on decreased oxygen delivery, decreased transport in the tissues, or increased consumption of oxygen in the tissue (Table 2.1). Oxygen consumption in subcutaneous tissues is remarkably constant (Gottrup *et al.* 1987), in which circumstances delivery and transport in such tissues are possible explanations for poor perfusion. This makes measurements of subcutaneous tissues particularly important as predictors of TOP. A tentative diagnosis of hypoperfusion can be tested by a rapid 250–500-ml infusion of normal saline. If tissue oxygen tension rises, the cause of tissue malperfusion is determined and infusion can be continued until no further rise is recorded, or normal P_{tO2} levels have been reached (Chang *et al.* 1983). If a fluid challenge has no effect on tissue oxygen tension, cardiac malfunction is probably the reason for hypoperfusion.

pH_i recordings have been useful for prediction of clinical outcome and in the observation of critically ill patients, but in elective surgical patients pH_i is of only limited value.

Conclusion

Adequate tissue perfusion and oxygenation (TOP) is crucial to successful surgery and can be evaluated with measurements of tissue oxygen tension (P_{tO2}) or intra-mural pH (pH_i) in the gastrointestinal tract. pH_i measurements enable disturbances in splanchnic tissue perfusion to be detected before impairment of core tissue perfusion is evident using conventional means. Transient episodes of mucosal ischaemia are common in the critically ill but are not found in elective surgical patients, and therefore pH_i measurements have not been good predictors of post-operative complications in this latter group of patients. In surgical patients, P_{tO2}, measured directly in tissue or indirectly on tissue surfaces, has been found to provide a continuous, simple, reliable, and rapid assessment of TOP. The level of P_{tO2} in subcutaneous tissues correlates well with wound healing and resistance to infection, as well as epithelialization and angiogenesis in animals. The close relationship to the supply/demand ratio (D_{O2}/V_{O2}) for a wide range of haemodynamic conditions, and the development of atraumatic and stable oxygen sensors, makes subcutaneous oxygen tension measurement an important clinical tool for the evaluation of tissue perfusion and oxygenation in surgical patients. Further clinical studies are necessary to determine the relative merits of the methods in relation to improved healing, decreased infection, and decreased peri-operative mortality rates in surgical patients.

References

Abraham, E., Oye, R.K., and Smith, M. (1984). Detection of blood volume deficits through conjunctival oxygen tension monitoring. *Crit.Care Med.* **12**, 931–4.

Ahn, H., Lindhagen, J., and Lundgren, O. (1986*a*). Measurement of colonic blood flow with laser Doppler flowmetry. *Scand. J. Gastroenterol.* **21**, 871–80.

Ahn, H., Lindhagen, J., Nilsson, G.E., Öberg, P.A., and Lundgren, O. (1986*b*). Assessment of blood flow in the small intestine with laser Doppler flowmetry. *Scand. J. Gastroenterol.* **21**, 63–70.

Ahnefeld, F.W. and Heinrich, H. (1983). Hat sich in der Routine des Anasthesisten die Berucksichtigung von Risikofaktoren bewahrt? *Langenbeck's Arch. Chir.* **361**, 263–7.

Bengtsson, M., Nilsson, G.E., and Lofstrom, J.B. (1983). The effect of spinal analgesia on skin blood flow, evaluated by laser Doppler flowmetry. *Acta Anaesthesiol. Scand.* **27**, 206–10.

Bruce-Chwatt, A.J. (1986). Free flap monitoring using a micro-computer linked to a laser Doppler flowmeter. *Br. J. Plast. Surg.* **39**, 229–38.

Chance, B. (1992). Evaluation of tissue hypoxia by optical methods. In *Update in intensive care and emergency medicine. Vol. 12: Tissue oxygen utilization* (ed. J.L. Vincent). Springer Verlag, Berlin.

Chang, N., Goodson, W.H., Gottrup, F., and Hunt, T.K. (1983). Direct measurement of wound and tissue oxygen tension in postoperative patients. *Ann. Surg.* **197**, 470–8.

Dension, D.M. (1989). Oxygen supply and uses in tissues. In *Clinical aspects of O_2 transport and tissue oxygenation* (ed. K. Reinhart and K. Eyrich) pp. 37–43. Springer, Berlin.
Engelhart, M. and Kristensen, J.K. (1983). Evaluation of cutaneous blood flow responses by ^{133}Xenon washout and laser Doppler flowmeter. *J. Invest. Dermatol.* **80**, 12–15.
Fagrell, B. (1984). Microcirculation in skin. In *The physiology and pharmacology of the microcirculation.* (ed. A.N. Mortillaro) pp. 133–80. Academic Press, New York.
Fagrell, B. (1985). Dynamics of skin microcirculation in humans. *J. Cardiovasc. Pharmacol.* **7** (Supplement 3), 53–8.
Fagrell, B. (1986*a*). The use of capillaroscopy in evaluation of skin viability. *Prog. Appl. Microcirc.* **11**, 40–6.
Fagrell, B. (1986*b*). The relationship between macro- and micro-circulation. Clinical aspects. *Acta Pharmacol. Toxicol.* **58** (Supplement II) 67–72.
Fiddian-Green, R.G. (1989). Studies in splanchnic ischemia and multiple organ failure. In *Splanchnic ischemia and multiple organ failure* (ed. A. Marston, G.B. Bulkley, R.G. Fiddian-Green and U. Haglund) pp. 349–63. Edward Arnold, London.
Fiddian-Green, R.G. and Gantz, N.M. (1987). Transient episodes of sigmoid ischemia and their relation to infection from intestinal organisms after abdominal aortic operations. *Crit. Care Med.* **15**, 835–9.
Fink, M.P. (1989). Clinical care in the ICU: Hemodynamic considerations in the management of the critical ill. In *Splanchnic ischemia and multiple organ failure* (ed. A. Marston, G.B. Bulkley, R.G., Fiddian-Green and U. Haglund) pp. 275–365. Edward Arnold, London.
Gellett, S., Asmussen, J., and Gottrup, F. (1990). Measurement of oxygen in patients during extra-corporal circulation. *J. Intensive Care Med.* **16** (Supplement 1), 98.
Göte, H., Raahave, D., Bæch, J. (1989). Tissue oximetry as a possible predictor of lethal complications after emergency intestinal surgery. *Surg. Res. Commun.* **7**, 243–9.
Gottrup, F. (1992). Tissue oxygen tension monitoring: relation to hemodynamic and oxygen transport variables. In *Update in intensive care in emergency medicine. Vol. 12: Tissue oxygen utilization* (ed. J.L. Vincent). Springer Verlag, Berlin.
Gottrup, F., Niinikoski, J., and Hunt, T.K. (1990). Measurement of tissue oxygen tension in wound repair. In *Wound healing* (ed. H. Janssen) pp. 155–64. Blackwell, Oxford.
Gottrup, F., Firmin, R., Hunt, T.K., and Mathes, S. (1984*a*). The dynamic properties of tissue oxygen in healing flaps. *Surgery* **95**, 527–37.
Gottrup, F., Firmin, R., Chang, N., Goodson, W.H., and Hunt, T.K. (1983). Continuous direct tissue oxygen tension measurement by a new method using an implantable Silastic tonometer and oxygen polarography. *Am. J. Surg.* **146**, 399–403.
Gottrup, F., Firmin, F., Rabkin, J., Halliday, B.J., and Hunt, T.K. (1987). Directly measured tissue oxygen tension and arterial tension assess tissue perfusion. *Crit. Care Med.* **15**, 1030–6.
Gottrup, F., Gellett, S., Kirkegaard, L., Hansen, E.S., and Johansen, G. (1989). Effect of hemorrhage and resuscitation on subcutaneous, conjunctival, and transcutaneous oxygen tension in relation to hemodynamic variables. *Crit. Care Med.* **17**, 904–7.

Gottrup, F., Orredsson, S., Price, D.C., Mathes, S.J., and Hohn, D.C. (1984*b*). A comparative study of skin blood flow in musculocutaneous and random pattern flaps. *J. Surg. Res.* **37**, 443–7.

Gottrup, F., Gellett, S., Kirkegaard, L., Hansen, E.S., and Johansen, G. (1988) Continuous monitoring of tissue oxygen tension during hyperoxia and hypoxia: Relation of subcutaneous, transcutaneous and conjunctival oxygen tension to haemodynamic variables. *Crit. Care Med.* **16**, 1229–34.

Grot, J. (1989). Tissue respiration. In *Human physiology* (ed. R.F. Smidt and G. Thews) pp. 598–612. Springer-Verlag, Berlin.

Grum, C.M., Fiddian-Green, R.G., Pittenger, G.L., Grant, B.J.B., Rothman, E.D., and Dantzer, D.R. (1984). Adequacy of tissue oxygenation in intact dog intestine. *J. Appl. Physiol.* **56**, 1065–9.

Gys, T., van Esbroeck, G., and Hubens, A. (1990). Assessment of the haemodynamics in peripheral tissue beds by subcutaneous oximetry and gastric intramucosal pH measurement in elective colorectal surgery. *Surg. Res. Commun.* **8** (Supplement 1), 67.

Gys, T., van Esbroeck, G., and Hubens, A. (1992). Assessment of the perfusion in peripheral tissue beds by subcutaneous oximetry and gastric intramucosal pH-metry in elective colorectal surgery. *J. Intensive Care Med.*

Gys, T., Hubens, A., Neels, H., Lauwers, L.F., and Peeters, R. (1988). Prognostic value of gastric intramural pH in surgical intensive care patients. *Crit. Care Med.* **16**, 1222–4.

Henning, R.J., Wiener, F., Valdes, S., and Weil, M.H. (1979). Measurement of toe temperature for assessing the severity of acute circulatory failure. *Surg. Gynecol. Obstet.* **149**, 1–7.

Henriksen, T.B., Hjortdal, V.E., Kjolseth, D., Hansen, E.S., Djuurhus, J.C., and Gottrup, F. (1989). The microcirculatory changes in the surroundings of Silastic catheters and the relationship between tissue oxygen tension and microcirculation. An experimental study in pigs. *Eur. Surg. Res.* **21** (Supplement 2), 75–6.

Hjortdal, V.E., Awwad, A., Gottrup, F., Kirkegaard, L., and Gellett, S. (1992). Tissue oxygen tension measurement for monitoring musculocutaneous and cutaneous flaps. *Scand. J. Plast. Reconst. Surg.*

Holloway, G.A. and Watkins, D.W. (1977). Laser Doppler measurements of cutaneous blood flow. *J. Invest. Dermatol.* **69**, 306–9.

Hunt, T.K. (1988). Physiology of wound healing. In *Trauma, sepsis and shock. The physiological basis of therapy*. (ed. G.H.A. Clowes) pp. 443–71. Marcel Dekker, New York.

Hunt, T.K. and Pai, M.P. (1972). Effect of varying ambient oxygen tensions on wound metabolism and collagen synthesis. *Surg. Gynecol. Obstet.* **135**, 561–7.

Hunt, T.K., Rabkin, J, Jensen, J.A., Jonsson, K., and Goodson, W.H. (1987). Tissue oximetry: an interim report. *World J. Surg.* **11**, 126–32.

Hunt, T.K., Halliday, B.J., Hopf, H.W., Gottrup, F., Jonsson, K., and Scheuenstuhl, H. (1991). Measurement and control of tissue oxygen tension in surgical patients. In *Update in intensive care and emergency medicine. Vol 12: Tissue oxygen utilization* (ed. J.L. Vincent). Springer Verlag, Berlin.

Jensen, J.A., Hunt, T.K., Scheuenstuhl, H., and Banda, M.J. (1986). Effect of lactate, pyruvate and pH on secretion of angiogenesis and mitogenesis factors by macrophages. *Lab. Invest.* **54**, 574–8.

Jensen, J.A., Riggs, K., Vasconez, L.O., Goodson, W.H., Rabkin, J., and Hunt,

T.K. (1987). Clinical assessment of postoperative perfusion. *Surg. Forum* **38**, 66–7.

Johnsson, J.M., Taylor, W.F., Shepherd, A.P., and Park, M.K. (1984). Laser-Doppler measurement in skin blood flow: comparison with plethysmography. *J. Appl. Physiol.* **56**, 798–809.

Jonsson, K., Hunt, T.K., and Mathes, S.J. (1988). Oxygen as an isolated variable influences resistance to infection. *Ann. Surg.* **208**, 783–7.

Jonsson, K., Jensen, J.A., Goodson, W.H., West, J.M. and Hunt, T.K. (1987). Assessment of perfusion in postoperative patients using tissue oxygen measurements. *Br. J. Surg.* **74**, 263–7.

Kallehave, F. and Gottrup, F. (1990). Tissue oxygen measurements of the serosal surface in surgical patients. Presented at the Eight Nordic Meeting on Medical and Biological Engineering, Aalborg, Denmark (unpublished data).

Katsamouris, A., Brewster, D.C., Megerman, J., Cina, C., Darling, R.C., and Abott, W.M. (1984). Transcutaneous oxygen tension in selection of amputation level. *Am. J. Surg.* **147**, 510–17.

Knighton, D.R., Silver, I.A., and Hunt, T.K. (1981). Regulation of wound healing angioneogenesis: effect of oxygen gradients and inspired oxygen concentration. *Surgery* **90**, 262–70.

Knighton, D.R., Hunt, T.K., Scheuenstuhl, H., Halliday, B.J., Werb, Z., and Banda, M.J. (1983). Oxygen tension regulates the expression of angiogenesis factor by macrophages. *Science* **221**, 1283–5.

Kuttila, K. (1989). Tissue perfusion and oxygenation in cardiac surgery. *Scand. J. Thorac. Cardiovasc. Surg. Suppl.* **38**.

Kvernebo, K., Lunde, O.C., Stranden, E., and Larsen, S. (1986). Human gastric blood circulation evaluated by endoscopic laser Doppler flowmetry. *Scand. J. Gastroenterol.* **21**, 685–92.

Larsen, P.N., Moesgaard, F., Gottrup, F., and Helledie, N. (1989). Characterization of the Silicone tonometer using a membrane-covered transcutaneous electrode. *Scand. J. Clin. Lab. Invest.* **49**, 513–19.

Larsen, P.N., Naver, L.P.S., Helledie, N., Gottrup, F., Kirkegaard, P., and Moesgaard, F. (1992). Tissue oxygen tension in the gastrointestinal tract measured by a vacuum fixated transcutaneous oxygen electrode. *Scand. J. Gastroenterol.*

Mayr, O. and Hannemann, L. (1989). Preoperative assessment and monitoring of high-risk patients. In *Clinical aspects of O_2 transport and tissue oxygenation* (ed. K. Reinhart and K. Eyrich) pp. 151–61. Springer, Berlin.

Myllyla, R., Tuderman, L., and Kivirikko, K.I. (1977). Mechanism of the prolyl hydroxylase reaction. 2. Kinetic analyses of the reaction sequence. *Eur. J. Biochem.* **80**, 349–57.

Niinikoski, J. (1977). Oxygen and wound healing. *Clin. Plast. Surg.* **4**, 361–74.

Niinikoski, J., Heughan, C., and Hunt, T.K. (1972). Oxygen tension in human wounds. *J. Surg. Res.* **12**, 77–82.

Nilsson, G.E., Tenland, T., and Öberg, P.A. (1980). A new instrument for continuous measurement of tissue blood flow by light beating spectroscopy. *IEEE Trans. Biomed. Eng.* **27**, 12–19.

Ninet, J. and Fronek, A. (1985). Cutaneous postocclusive reactive hyperemia monitored by laser Doppler flux metering and skin temperature. *Microvasc. Res.* **30**, 125–32.

Piantadosi, C.A., Parsons, W.J., and Griebel, J.A. (1992). Application of NIR spectroscopy to problems of tissue oxygenation. In *Update in intensive care and*

emergency medicine. Vol. 12: Tissue oxygen utilization (ed. J.L. Vincent). Springer Verlag, Berlin.
Pietilä, von Smitten, K., and Sundell, B. (1985). The effect of perfusion on post-operative viability in the reimplanted rabbit ear: measured by laser Doppler flowmetry and skin temperature. *Scand. J. Plast. Reconst. Surg.* **19**, 251–4.
Pietilä, J.P., von Smitten, K., and Sundell, B. (1987). The rabbit ear pedicle flap. A new model for evaluating factors affecting the circulation in flaps. *Scand. J. Plast. Reconstr. Surg.* **21**, 145–7.
Prockop, D.J., Kivirikko, K.I., Tuderman, L., and Guzman, N.A. (1979). The biosynthesis of collagen and its disorders, part I. *N. Engl. J. Med.* **301**, 13–23.
Rosen, L., Östergren, J., Fagrell, B., and Stranden, E. (1988). Skin microvascular circulation in the sympathetic dystrophies evaluated by videophotometric capillaroscopy and laser Doppler fluxmetry. *Eur. J. Clin. Invest.* **18**, 305–8.
Sendak, M.J., Harris, A.P., and Donham, R.T. (1988). Accuracy of pulse oximetry during arterial oxyhemoglobin desaturation in dogs. *Anesthesiology* **68**, 111–14.
Severinghaus, J.W. and Naifeh, K.H. (1987) Accuracy of response of six pulse oximeters to profound hypoxia. *Anesthesiology* **67**, 551–8.
Sheffield, P.J. (1988). Tissue oxygen measurements. In *Problem wounds. The role of oxygen* (ed. J.C. Davis and T.K. Hunt) pp. 17–51. Elsevier, New York.
Sheldon, C.A., Cerra, F.P., Bonhoff, N., Belani, K., Frieswyk, D., and Dhanalal, K. (1983). Peripheral postcapillary venous pressure: a new more sensitive monitor of effective blood volume during hemorrhagic shock and resuscitation. *Surgery* **94**, 399–406.
Sheridan, W.G., Lowndes, R.H., and Young, H.L. (1987). Tissue oxygen tension as a predictor of colonic anastomotic healing. *Dis. Colon Rectum* **30**, 867–71.
Sheridan, W.G., Lowndes, R.H., and Young, H.L. (1990). Intra-operative tissue oximetry in the human gastrointestinal tract. *Am. J. Surg.* **159**, 314–19.
Sorensen, M.B. (1986). Haemodynamisk monitorering. In *Kirurgisk patofysiologi* (ed. H.C., Engell, A. Enquist, and M. Blichert-Toft) pp. 145–59. Munksgaard, Copenhagen.
Stern, M.D. (1975). *In vivo* evaluation of microcirculation by coherent light scattering. *Nature* **254**, 56–8.
Striebel, H.W. and Kretz, F.J. (1989). Advantages and limitations of pulse oximetry. In *Clinical aspects of O_2 transport and tissue oxygenation* (ed. K. Reinhart and K. Eyrich) pp. 212–29. Springer, Berlin.
Sundberg, S. (1984). Acute effectss and long-term variations in skin blood flow measured with laser Doppler flowmetry. *Scand. J. Clin. Lab. Invest.* **44**, 341–5.
Tanaka, T., Riva, C., and Ben-Sira, I. (1974). Blood velocity measurements in human retinal vessels. *Science* **186**, 830–1.
Viidik, A. and Gottrup, F. (1986). Mechanics of healing soft tissue wounds. In *Frontiers in biomechanics* (ed. G.W. Schmid-Schonbein, S.L.Y. Woo, and B.W. Zweifach) pp. 263–79. Springer, New York.
Winsor, T., Haumschild, D.J., Winsor, D.W., Wang, Y., and Luong, T.N. (1987). Clinical application of laser Doppler flowmetry for measurement of cutaneous circulation in health and disease. *Angiology* **38**, 727–36.
Winter, G.D. (1972). Epidermal regeneration studied in the dogmestic pig. In *Epidermal wound healing* (ed. H.I. Maibach and D.T. Rovee) pp. 71–112. Year Book Medical Publishers, Chicago.

3. Preventing surgical infection

Eric W. Taylor

Infection is the most common form of morbidity and a common cause of mortality following surgical procedures. The influence of the bacterium on surgical practice has been aptly expressed by Lord Moynihan (1920) when he stated: 'every operation in surgery is an experiment in bacteriology'. Humans live in symbiosis with bacteria and it has been estimated that each of us plays host to some 1×10^{14} bacteria from more than 500 different species (Williams 1973; Moore and Holdeman 1974). Indeed, there may be more bacteria in and on our bodies than cells forming our body. This symbiotic balance may be disturbed by modern antibiotic therapy which allows colonization by new, or more pathogenic, species. It may be disturbed by an operation, which breaks down the barriers between the body and bacteria, and allows the bacteria access to areas where they can behave in a different, pathogenic role. The world of surgery is changing rapidly and, in particular, an increasing number of implant procedures are being performed, which has given new opportunities of pathogenesis to bacteria previously considered harmless.

In this chapter the classification of operations, the incidence of infection, and methods to prevent infection are reviewed, together with the indications for antibiotic prophylaxis.

Classification of operations

The incidence of post-operative infection is proportional to the contamination of the operative field and to the ability of the body to resist that contamination. Different operations carry different risks, determined by the degree of contamination which has already occurred, or which occurs at the time of operation. A classification system has been developed which differentiates degrees of contamination.

All surgeons see some patients undergoing surgery who develop infection after operation, and inevitably they feel a sense of failure. Some comfort is available from the fact that their colleagues also observe infection after similar operations, and audit enables comparison of results. Nevertheless, if audit is to provide an accurate comparison then 'like must be compared with like', and a system of classification of operations has been in use for some years which allows appropriate comparison (Table 3.1). When infectious

Table 3.1. Classification of operations.

Type of operation	Description
Clean	No infection encountered No break in aseptic technique No bacterially colonized viscus opened
Clean–contaminated	Bacterially colonized viscus opened but minimal contamination Minor break in aseptic technique
Contaminated	Greater contamination from bacterially colonized viscus Acute inflammation without suppuration Traumatic wounds within 4 hours of injury
Dirty	Frank pus encountered Perforated viscus or traumatic wound more than 4 hours after injury

complications of surgical procedures are audited, it is important to review the patient after discharge from hospital, because many operation-related infections become apparent only when the patient has returned home. In one recent series 49 (59 per cent) of the 83 infections which occurred after operation in 1242 patients presented after the patient had left hospital (Law, Mishriki, and Jeffrey 1990).

The classification does not allow for variation in host resistance, and any change in the ability of the patient to resist contamination must be considered separately.

The classification of operations is useful, if not essential, when conducting audit, but it is also important to recognize that all operations impart some risk to the patient and to ensure that the patient is prepared appropriately and that antibiotic prophylaxis and, if appropriate, therapy, is instituted. As might be expected there are differing incidences of infection, dependent upon the category or class of operation, and several major reviews have been published which have demonstrated this difference. The largest series is that published by Cruse and Foord (1980), the results of which are summarized in Table 3.2. It is against a background of data such as these that the results of any individual or of a group conducting audit or assessing the results of prospective trials must be compared.

Clean operations

Clean operations are those in which the operative field is not contaminated by bacteria from within the patient, and there is minimal contamination from the environment. There should be no break in strict, aseptic technique

Table 3.2. Infection according to classification of operation.

Class of operation	No.	No. infected
Clean	47 054	732 (1.6)
Clean–contaminated	9 370	720 (7.7)
Contaminated	4 442	676 (15.2)
Dirty	2 093	832 (39.8)

Values in parentheses are percentages. [From Cruse and Foord (1980).]

in the operating theatre. This category of operation usually includes neurosurgical procedures, peripheral vascular surgery including varicose veins, herniorrhaphy, and operations on the salivary glands and breasts. Whilst salivary gland and breast tissue is potentially contaminated, in that the ducts are open to the environment and have been shown to be colonized, such operations have traditionally been considered clean with a low incidence of infection.

Clean–contaminated operations

Clean–contaminated operations are those that open the bacterially contaminated tracts within the body. These include the gastrointestinal, genitourinary, and pancreatico-biliary tracts, the bronchial tree, and the paranasal sinuses. All are open to the exterior of the body and to a greater or lesser extent are colonized by bacteria. In clean–contaminated operations there should be minimal spillage of the luminal contents of the tract, which ought to have been prepared before operation, and a minor break in sterile technique at the operating table would move a clean operation into this category.

Contaminated operations

Operations are considered contaminated if there is a break in aseptic technique, or if there is a degree of spillage of the luminal contents of one of the bacterially colonized tracts within the body, at the time of operation. Both situations lead to a greater degree of contamination. Patients in whom there has been a compound injury to bones or soft tissues, or perforation of a bacterially contaminated viscus, are classified as contaminated, provided they are operated on within 4 hours of the incident. Within this time bacterial contamination will have initiated the inflammatory process associated with infection but suppuration will not yet have occurred.

Dirty operations

An operation should be considered as being dirty when more than 4 hours has elapsed from the time of injury in the case of an open wound, or from the time of perforation of a viscus. This allows sufficient time for suppuration to commence. An operation where frank pus is encountered during the course of the operation, such as when a diverticular abscess is opened or where the patient is found to have a pyosalpinx, is classified as dirty.

Factors influencing contamination

Bacterial contamination of the operative field can come either from within the patient (endogenous) or from the external environment (exogenous). The challenge posed by the bacterial flora from endogenous contamination is frequently quite different from that posed by exogenous contamination, and the steps taken to eliminate or to minimize both must be considered separately.

There is little doubt that the most important factor in reducing contamination, be it endogenous or exogenous, is surgical expertise at the time of operation. Clumsy, careless surgery will increase bacterial contamination of the wound and lead to a higher incidence of wound infection despite all the precautions taken to reduce infection.

Endogenous contamination

The surface and internal environment of each patient pose a potential hazard at the time of operation (Raahave, Friis-Moller, Bjerre-Jepsen, Thiis-Knudsen, and Rasmussen 1986). We live in a symbiotic relationship with the bacterial flora of the gastrointestinal tract, and many of the other systems within the body are colonized even if we gain no obvious advantage from that colonization. Whenever these tracts are opened at operation there will be some degree of contamination of the operative field. The factors influencing endogenous bacterial contamination of the operative field are listed in Table 3.3. It may be possible to lower the risk to the patient by pre-operative preparation which should reduce the bacterial load. Skin cleansing, emptying the stomach of the patient with pyloric stenosis, and bowel preparation before colonic surgery are obvious examples of this.

Skin preparation

Attempts should be made to reduce the bacterial colonization of the skin prior to operation to prevent organisms being carried into the wound from the skin surface. Large amounts of antibiotics are used in most hospitals and organisms, resistant to many antibiotics, rapidly colonize patients after admission to hospital. Therefore it is important to try to minimize the interval between admission to hospital and operation.

Reduction of the bacterial count on the skin by pre-operative whole body washing with chlorhexidine has given mixed results. Brandburg, Holm, Hammersten, and Scherston (1980) reported a reduction in groin wound infections from 17.5 to 8.0 per cent after pre-operative chlorhexidine

Table 3.3. Factors influencing endogenous bacterial contamination of the operative field.

Skin cleanliness
Skin preparation
Pre-operataive shaving
Pre-operative bowel preparation
Duration of pre-operative hospitalisation
Duration of operation
Surgical expertise

showering, and in a study of 2015 patients Hayek and Emerson (1988) also showed a fall in the incidence of infection, but no such benefit was seen by Ayliffe, Noy, Babb, Davies, and Jackson (1983) when they compared pre-operative bathing with chlorhexidine detergent with non-medicated soap in the prevention of wound infection. However, chlorhexidine does apparently have a more persistent effect, and emergence of resistant strains of *Staphylococcus* appears to be unlikely (Newsom and Rowland 1988). In healthy volunteers two showers with chlorhexidine have been shown to produce maximal decrease in skin flora but three showers or baths before operation have been advocated in patients who may be able to shower or wash less thoroughly (Byrne, Napier, and Cushieri 1990).

It has been traditional to shave the hair from the skin in the region of the incision before operation, and in many hospitals this is done on the day before operation. Nevertheless, in the largest study of its kind, Cruse and Foord (1980) found a significantly lower incidence of wound infection in patients who were not shaved, shaved immediately before operation, or had the hair removed with depilatory cream than in those who were shaved on the day before operation. Microscopic examination of the skin surface after shaving shows multiple small lacerations. If these occur immediately before operation they pose a risk no different from the main operative incision. However, if shaving with microscopic lacerations occurs the day before operation these become contaminated and infected before the operation commences.

In the operating room the skin at the site of the incision is cleaned with antiseptic solution. Alcoholic solutions of chlorhexidine or iodine are usually employed for this purpose, but attempts to reduce the contamination further by the use of plastic adhesive drapes have not proved beneficial (Lilly, Loudon, Lowbury, and Porter, 1970; Jackson, Pollock, and Tindal 1971). The skin organism most commonly associated with post-operative wound contamination and infection is *Staphylococcus aureus* but there is increasing awareness of the importance of *S. epidermidis*, or coagulase-negative staphylococci, which are particularly associated with breast (Freedman and

Jackson 1989), orthopaedic (Fitzgerald, Nolan, Ilstrup, van Scoy, Washington, and Coventry 1977; Hope, Kristinsson, Norman, and Elson 1989), prosthetic implant and vascular graft infection (Strachan 1988). These organisms caused 60 per cent of graft infections in one series (Bandyke, Berni, Thiele, and Towne 1984) and are resistant to many antibiotics probably because they are slime producers (Edmiston, Schmitt, and Seabrook 1989). Many patients enter the ward before operation with resistant coagulase-negative staphylococcal colonies in both groin and perineum, and attempts have been made to clear these organisms by bathing in chlorhexidine before operation, with some success (Mannion, Thom, Reynolds, and Strachan 1989).

Bowel preparation

Bacteria exist throughout the gastrointestinal tract, although the acidity of the stomach is thought to be effective in reducing the progress of organisms lower into the tract (Howden and Hunt 1987). However, the stomach cannot be regarded as being sterile, and in patients who have undergone vagotomy or an operation diverting bile and pancreatic fluid into the stomach, in patients with pyloric stenosis, and in those with gastric ulcer or gastric cancer, significant colonization occurs (Nichols and Condon 1975). This is also true of those patients who are receiving histamine receptor antagonist therapy, and recent evidence suggests that even parenteral hyperalimentation may be a source of nosocomial infection in patients receiving intensive care (Thurn, Crossley, Gordts, Maki, and Johnson 1990).

If gastric surgery is to be performed for peptic ulceration which has led to pyloric stenosis, it is logical to remove as much food debris as possible from the stomach by pre-operative gastric lavage. Similarly, in patients with small bowel obstruction there is rapid bacterial multiplication in the luminal contents which can be removed at operation by retrograde 'stripping' into the stomach or by aspiration via a Foley catheter passed into the lumen.

Bowel preparation is usually considered to refer to colonic preparation, and clearly evacuation of faeces reduces the total load of organisms present in the bowel, but even an apparently empty colon is still heavily contaminated (Nichols, Gorbach, and Condon 1971). Traditionally patients were admitted to hospital several days before colorectal surgery and given a fluid diet only, together with repeated doses of a cathartic agent such as magnesium sulphate, in order to evacuate their bowel. Not only was this expensive in terms of bed utilization, but it ensured that the patient came to operation hungry, frequently demoralized, and colonized with antibiotic-resistant, hospital-acquired organisms.

In order to shorten this process, whole bowel irrigation was introduced (Crapp, Powis, Tillotson, Cooke, and Alexander-Williams 1975), at which large volumes of normal saline were administered via a nasogastric tube. Over a period of 6–8 hours the colon was irrigated and evacuated. Whilst

Table 3.4. Factors influencing exogenous bacterial contamination of the operative field.

Theatre ventilation
Sterility of instruments
Gloves (?)
Masks (?)
Caps (?)
Gowns (?)
Wound dressings (?)
Surgical expertise

this was effective, there was considerable fluid absorption from the colon and cardiac failure developed in some elderly patients. Attempts were made to overcome this problem by the use of osmotically balanced solutions such as 10 per cent mannitol, which would not be absorbed. However, the incidence of post-operative infection was higher when mannitol bowel preparation was used (Hares, Greca, Youngs, Burdon, and Keighley 1981*a*) and it was shown that, whilst solid faecal material was removed from the colon, the mucus remaining on the colonic mucosa was more heavily contaminated after mannitol bowel preparation than after whole gut lavage. The high molecular weight sugar is broken down by bacteria and forms a nutrient for their growth (Keighley, *et al.* 1981). This also leads to increased methane production and an increased risk of explosion at polypectomy (Taylor, Bently, Youngs, and Keighley 1981). The use of polyethylene glycol seems to have overcome this problem (Fleites, Marshall, Eckhauser, Mausour, Imbembo, and McCullough 1985).

Whilst some surgeons maintain that bowel preparation is unnecessary (Irving and Scrimgeour 1987), most surgeons administer some form of preoperative bowel preparation before conducting elective colorectal surgery, or undertake irrigation of the colon with saline at the time of operation (Dudley, Radcliffe, and McGeehan 1980).

The use of oral antimicrobial agents further to reduce microbial contamination at the time of operation is discussed below in the section dealing with antimicrobial prophylaxis in colorectal surgery.

Exogenous contamination

The operating room is an area beset by customs and traditions, with little proven justification. Some of the factors thought to be involved in reducing exogenous contamination are listed in Table 3.4. Filtration of the air entering the operating theatre via the ventilation system has been shown to reduce the incidence of infection (Lidwell, Lowbury, Whyte, Blowers, Stanley, and Lowe 1982), but this is probably of any significant importance only when prosthetic implant surgery is being performed and when every other precaution relating to surgical technique has been taken. Similarly swabs and instruments, including the hands of the operating team, that come into contact with the body tissues should be sterile. Sterilization of instruments and swabs is now routine and it has become traditional for surgeons to scrub their hands before donning sterile gloves. Fortunately, the days of prolonged (5–10 minutes) scrubbing before each operation is now recognized to be quite unnecessary, and an initial 2-minute wash with chlorhexidine, followed by the application of 70 per cent alcoholic chlorhexidine, is sufficient. Between operations the further application of alcoholic chlorhexidine is probably all that is required (Lilly, Lowbury, and Wilkins 1979).

Hand washing reduces the spread of infection both in theatre and in wards where the more difficult problem is to persuade staff, most particularly the senior medical staff, that their hands are just as capable of transmitting infection as those of the nurses and their juniors. In a recent report the incidence of nosocomial infection fell from 33 to 10 per cent when the staff of an intensive therapy unit were reminded to wash their hands. The infection rate crept up to pre-trial levels when habits returned to normal, and fell again on a further reminder (Conley, Hill, Ross, Lertzman, and Louie 1989).

It has become traditional for all attending the operating table to wear sterile surgical gloves, but the incidence of puncture of gloves during operation is high (Berg, Kirk, and Bain 1987; Dodds, Guy, Peacock, Duffy, Barker, and Thomas 1988). The significance of glove puncture on the incidence of post-operative infection is unclear and it may well be that gloves, like masks (Orr 1981), are not essential and do not reduce the incidence of infection. Close woven cotton gowns or the more recently introduced non-woven disposal theatre gowns prevent transfer of bacteria from the surgeon and assistants to the patient (Nagai, Katoda, Takechi, Kumamoto, Nakano, and Jitsukawa 1986; Jalovaara and Puranen 1989).

Again, it has been traditional to dress the wound on completion of the operation, but provided there has been adequate haemostasis the wound seals within a few hours, and recent evidence has confirmed that dressing the wound beyond this time does not influence the incidence of infection (Chrintz, Vibits, Corditz, Harreby, Waaddegaard, and Larsen 1989).

Whilst many of these traditions may be of little inherent value they do set aside the operating room as an area where particular care must be taken, and they are a constant reminder to all that strict precautions in aseptic technique should be taken at all times. Furthermore, there is increasing concern about the spread of the hepatitis and the human immunodeficiency virus (HIV) from patient to surgeon. Even if the patient does not benefit

Table 3.5. Factors reducing host resistance.

Patient-dependent factors	Surgeon-dependent factors
Extreme old age	Tissue oxygenation
Obesity	Foreign body implantation
Diabetes	Haemostasis
Cirrhosis	Prolonged pre-operative hospitalization
Uraemia	Prolonged operation time
Malignancy	Blood transfusion
Malnutrition	
Leukopenia	
Steroid therapy	
Antimitotic therapy	

from the use of caps, gowns, masks, etc., it is possible that the surgeon does because these may offer protection from exposure to the body fluids of the patient.

Factors influencing host resistance

The ability of the body to resist a bacterial challenge is the other major determinant of the incidence of infection, after contamination has occurred during an operation. Despite the preparation of the patient before operation, and the precautions taken in the operating theatre, some bacteria will gain access to the tissues either from the external environment or from within the patient. A bacterial challenge that would be resisted by most fit healthy patients may be sufficient to lead to infection or sepsis in a patient with reduced resistance. Factors that reduce the body's ability to resist bacterial challenge are listed in Table 3.5. Many of the factors are patient dependent and cannot be obviated at the time of operation, but there are a number of factors over which the surgeon does have control.

Hypoxia and poor tissue perfusion increase the risk of infection. Whilst modern anaesthesia and cardiac support render most operations very safe, local hypoxia and reduced tissue perfusion frequently occur when self-retaining retractors are used for prolonged periods, when skin or other sutures encompassing large volumes of tissue are inserted too tightly, and when large volumes of tissue are rendered necrotic by excessive use of diathermy.

Foreign body implantation, which may be anything from a total hip replacement to a ligature, forms a nidus around which infection can occur. In an elegantly simple experiment, Elek (1956) showed that injection of 1×10^6 staphylococcal organisms in the forearm produced no reaction, whereas

1×10^3 of the same organism together with a silk suture produced an abscess (Elek and Conen 1957).

Haemostasis is important. A residual haematoma, or one that forms in the wound after closure of the skin, is an ideal culture medium for bacteria and may lead to the formation of a wound abscess.

As has been mentioned above, prolonged pre-operative hospitalization leads to colonization of the body by organisms from within the hospital environment which are resistant to many antibiotics, and prolonged operation times are associated with a higher incidence of infection. This may be because the operation is more difficult, or the surgeon encounters more complications, but the longer the wound is open the longer it is at risk of contamination.

Blood transfusion

Blood transfusion is expensive and the risks of transfusion reactions, as well as the transfer of hepatitis and HIV virus, are well known. Intra-operative blood transfusion may reduce the resistance of the body to tumour growth, and may increase the incidence of tumour recurrence, after surgery for malignant disease (Burrows and Tartter 1982; Blumberg, Agarwhal, and Chuang 1985; Crowson, Hallissay, Kiff, Kingston, and Fielding 1989). Blood transfusion has been used before renal transplantation to reduce the incidence of rejection (Opelz, Senger, Mickey, and Terasaki 1981), and evidence is growing that blood transfusion reduces the body's resistance to infection and leads to a higher post-operative infection rate (Maetani, Nishikawa, Hirakawa, and Tobe 1986; Jensen, *et al.* 1990). However meticulous the surgical technique, there will be operations where blood loss will be such that the patient needs to be transfused, but an awareness of the short-term effect on the body's resistance should impose some caution and blood should be transfused only when absolutely necessary.

Immunomodulation

Various bacterial products including BCG, muramyl dipeptide, *Corynebacterium parvum* and zymosan are known to cause non-specific stimulation of the immune system. Some synthetic products such as levamisole hydrochloride and lithium carbonate improve neutrophil response and the delayed-type hypersensitivity reaction (Polk 1987). This is an area of increasing interest but the clinical role of these products has yet to be defined and none is yet available commercially.

Prophylactic antibiotics

In order to reduce the incidence of endogenous contamination, before the surgeon undertakes any operation it is important to ensure that the patient is adequately prepared and that the operative environment has adequate elimination or reduction of exogenous contamination. Nevertheless, all surgeons are aware that whatever preparation and precautions are taken, in some patients a degree of contamination is likely, or may be inevitable, and it is the surgeon's responsibility to try to prevent progress to infection, and ensure that the patient does not pass down the slippery slope of suppuration, sepsis, multiple organ failure, and death.

The role of prophylactic antibiotics is to aid and support the body's ability to resist the contamination that occurs at the time of operation. Thus, if the antibiotic is to be effective as a prophylactic agent to prevent infection, it must be administered before (optimally) or immediately after bacterial inoculation of the tissues. Where a surgeon believes it likely that an operation will be contaminated to such an extent that infection may ensue, then the antibiotic should be given before the operation commences, and when contamination occurs unexpectedly during the course of an operation the antibiotic should be administered immediately.

Prophylactic antibiotics are not a substitute for, and will not compensate for, inappropriate patient preparation, nor are they a substitute for good surgical technique. Prophylactic antibiotics will not compensate for bad technique and if the bacterial challenge is sufficiently high, for whatever reason, or the patient's resistance is abnormally low, prophylactic antibiotics will not prevent the development of infection.

It is important to differentiate 'prophylaxis' and 'therapy'. Prophylactic antibiotics are administered to assist the body's host resistance during the period of bacterial contamination. This usually extends for the duration of the operation, or possibly for a few hours thereafter until bacteria remaining in the wound have been removed by phagocytosis. However, if infection or suppuration has already occurred as, for example, in the patient with acute appendicitis, it is inappropriate to regard the use of antibiotics as prophylactic. Host resistance has already been breached, infection has occurred, and therapy is indicated.

Choice of prophylactic antibiotic therapy

Factors that will influence the choice of antibiotics to be used for chemoprophylaxis are listed in Table 3.6. Clearly the antibiotic chosen should have a spectrum sufficiently wide to be effective against organisms most likely to contaminate the wound. The antibiotic must be capable of being administered in such a way as to ensure a high circulating blood level at the time of maximal contamination; in practice this usually implies intramuscular or intravenous injection. Administering the antibiotic after the operation confers no benefit (Stone, Hooper, Kolb, Geheber, and Dawkins 1976) but an antibiotic given during the course of the operation would appear to be as effective as if it had been given before operation (Bates, *et al.* 1989). Intra-

Table 3.6. Factors influencing the choice of antibiotic for chemoprophylaxis.

Antibacterial spectrum
Route of administration
Frequency of administration
Monitoring of toxicity
Complications
Cost

incisional injection also seems to be as effective as the intravenous or intramuscular route and gives high wound and blood levels (Taylor, Walker Mason, Richmond, and Lee 1982; Dixon, Armstrong, Duffy, Chetty, and Davies 1984; Taylor, Dawson, de Silva, Shaw, Durans, and Makin 1985).

The half-life of the antibiotic affects the frequency of administration, and the long half-life of the third-generation cephalosporin, ceftriaxone, is particularly useful from this point of view. The aminoglycosides cause nephrotoxicity and ototoxicity, and if these agents are to be used then blood levels should be monitored to ensure that toxic levels are not approached.

In addition some other drugs have specific complications: chloramphenicol may cause blood dyscrasias, and the penicillins and cephalosporins may give rise to allergic reactions. Almost all antibiotics have now been shown to be potential causes of pseudomembranous colitis, and *Clostridium difficile* may appear in stool cultures even after one dose of many of the cephalosporins (Ambrose, Johnson, Burdon, and Keighley 1985).

However, one of the most important factors regarding the choice of a chemoprophylactic agent is the cost. It has been estimated that in the UK, approximately 50 per cent of the annual budget for injectable antibiotics is for agents used for prophylaxis. There is an inevitable temptation to use the latest, most expensive, and most heavily marketed antibiotic, when a cheaper agent would be perfectly adequate.

Duration of administration

In some surgical specialties it has become traditional to administer 'prophylactic' antibiotic for prolonged periods (up to 2 weeks), and even amongst general surgeons 3 or 4-day courses of prophylaxis are not uncommon (Scher, Bernstein, Arenstein, and Sorensen 1990). Few studies have been conducted to investigate specifically the results of prolonged or shortened courses of prophylaxis. Strachan, *et al.* (1977) showed no benefit from one pre-operative dose plus a 5-day post-operative course of cephazolin when compared with one pre-operative dose alone in biliary tract operations, the infection rates being 5.5 and 3.2 per cent respectively. A review of published antibiotic trials shows an increasing trend towards single-dose prophylaxis and even in colorectal operations, where the risk of post-operative infection is highest, no benefit has been demonstrated by continuing the duration of antibiotic cover for more than one dose (Giercksky, *et al.* 1982; Bergman and Solhaug 1987; Jagelman, Fabian, Nichols, Stone, Wilson, and Zellner 1988). However, if the operation is prolonged for more than 2 hours, or if there is blood loss in excess of 2 litres, a second dose of antibiotic is indicated to ensure that the circulating blood concentration remains high throughout the period of exposure to contamination.

Nevertheless, many surgeons favour a 'belt and braces' approach and choose to continue to administer antibiotics after operation, believing that the additional cost, and presumably the additional risks of bacterial resistance, superinfection, and pseudomembranous colitis, for example, are outweighed by the benefit to the patient. In the era of increasing financial stringency it is of interest that in one study an enforced policy, restricting prophylactic antibiotics to 24 hours, not only produced considerable cost saving, but actually lowered the infection rate from 3.8 to 2.1 per cent in clean contaminated operations (Scher *et al.* 1990). Furthermore, there is evidence that prolonging the duration of antibiotic prophylaxis is of no benefit even in those patients with impaired host defences (Moesgaard and Lukkegaard-Neilsen 1989).

It is the author's practice to give a single dose of antibiotic to all patients who require prophylaxis when undergoing elective surgery. If excessive intra-abdominal contamination occurs then the peritoneal cavity is lavaged with 1 litre of 0.1 per cent tetracycline in saline (Krukowski, Stewart, Alsayer, and Matheson 1984).

Indications for antibiotic prophylaxis

It has been traditional teaching that antibiotic prophylaxis should be given only if there is likely to be contamination of the operative field, or if the patient is at particular risk of infection because of reduced resistance. Where infection and suppuration have already occurred, therapy is appropriate for a longer period. Therefore, antibiotic prophylaxis should be considered mandatory for patients with reduced resistance undergoing clean operations, for all patients undergoing clean–contaminated operations, and for contaminated operations, where a therapeutic extension of the course of treatment may be appropriate.

Prosthetic implant procedures

The number of prostheses implanted into patients is rapidly increasing and now involve most, if not all, surgical specialties. These implants are usually inserted during clean operations but there may be particular problems when orthopaedic implants are inserted into compound fractures. The risk of infection around the implant should be small (0–2 per cent), but when it does occur the results may be disastrous. An infected total hip replacement leading to a Girdlestone revision is a considerable morbidity, and an infected aorto-femoral bifurcation graft may frequently lead to the death of the patient (Gordon-Smith, Taylor, Nicolaides, Goldman, Kenyon, and Eastcott 1978).

To prove that antibiotic prophylaxis benefits the patient undergoing an implant procedure is difficult, because a trial of adequate statistical power would require the recruitment of many thousands of patients, and would involve a placebo or no treatment group which would no longer be considered ethical. Infection in some implants presents late, and the follow-up of such a trial would need to be continued for many years. It is now considered normal surgical practice to administer antibiotic prophylaxis at least for the peri-operative period.

The spectrum of the antibiotic administered depends upon the implant and the site into which it is to be inserted. In most sites, *Staphylococcus epidermidis* is the most serious contaminant carried into the wound from the skin. In some areas, such as the lumen of an abdominal aortic aneurysm, many other organisms may be present and an anti-staphylococcal agent is no longer considered sufficient (Earnshaw, Slack, Hopkinson, and Makin 1988). A single dose of antibiotic will suffice unless the operation lasts for more than 2 hours, or if there is excessive blood loss.

Prosthetic implants are now being inserted into patients at a younger age and it is no longer uncommon for operations to be performed subsequently on patients who have already received a prosthetic implant. For many years it has been recognized that dental procedures cause a bacteraemia and it has been traditional to protect patients with rheumatic heart disease with antibiotics when undergoing dental or other operative procedures. There is an increasing suspicion that 'late' infections of prosthetic implants, which may present many years after the original operation, are not simply reactivation of infection which has lain dormant since the primary procedure, but that these are in fact secondary, haematogenous, infections resulting from subsequent procedures. These suspicions are difficult to prove, but evidence is accumulating (Sullivan, Johnston, and Kelley 1990), and it would seem prudent to accord the same respect to an indwelling prosthesis as to a rheumatically damaged heart valve. Urinary manipulation, such as catheterization, is the procedure most associated with bacteraemia and would seem particularly dangerous to these patients.

Clean operations

All operations carry some risk of bacterial contamination and if host resistance is diminished then the patient should receive prophylactic antibiotics. However, there is now evidence to suggest that prophylactic antibiotics may confer some benefit even in patients with normal resistance. Platt, *et al.* (1990), in a well-constructed trial of 1218 patients undergoing groin hernia

Table 3.7. Prophylactic antibiotics in clean surgery.

	Placebo ($n = 614$)	Cefonicid ($n = 604$)
Hernia (n)	311	301
Wound infection	6	4
Urinary tract infection	2	1
Total	8	5
Breast (n)	303	303
Wound infection	26	17
Urinary tract infection	8	3
Total	34	20
Total (all infections)	50	27*

* $p < 0.01$ (cefonicid *versus* placebo). [From Platt *et al.* (1989).]

repairs and breast operations, have demonstrated a significant reduction in the incidence of infection using cefonicid, a second-generation cephalosporin (Table 3.7). This paper has major medico-legal implications and if the results are confirmed by other, equally well-constructed, studies of sufficient statistical power there will need to be a review of surgical practice.

Clean–contaminated operations

Most gastrointestinal operations are classified as clean–contaminated. Staphylococci, streptococci, *Haemophilus*, *Neisseria*, and micrococci are the common aerobic bacteria, and bifidabacteria, lactobacilli, fusobacteria, *Bacteroides* species, and *Veillonella* are the common anaerobic organisms colonizing the oesophagus and stomach. Colonization by the Enterobacteriaceae may occur in health but is more commonly seen when gastric pH is raised in conditions such as gastric carcinoma and gastric ulcer, and in patients who have had acid-lowering operations or who have been receiving histamine receptor antagonists. The fastidious organism *Helicobacter pylori* has been associated with ulceration but not with post-operative wound infection. Most gastric operations are performed for pathology which is associated with gastric bacterial colonization of the stomach and there is a significant risk of post-operative infection (Lewis 1977; Gatehouse, Dimock, Burdon, Alexander-Williams, and Keighley 1978). Whilst some have advocated antibiotic prophylaxis only for patients undergoing gastric operation when the pathology is associated with hypochlorhydria and retention (Hares, *et al.* 1981*b*; Nichols, Webb, Jones, Smith, and LoCicero 1982),

Sjostedy, Levin, Malmbourg, Bergman, and Kager (1989) reported an overall rate of primary infection of 23 per cent after 750 gastric operations in 674 patients, and advocated antibiotic prophylaxis in all patients undergoing gastric surgery. In the author's view this applies to all surgery of the oesophagus, stomach, and small bowel.

Biliary tract surgery

Chetlin and Elliott (1971) showed that the biliary tract is increasingly colonized with advancing age and that 63 per cent of patients have bactobilia by the age of 70–80 years. These authors also showed that patients with bactobilia had a 40-fold incidence of post-operative infectious complications, compared with those in whom the bile was sterile at the time of surgery. Subsequently, surgeons became aware that certain conditions — acute cholecystitis, stones in the common bile duct, and jaundice (whether caused by benign or malignant pathology) — in patients with common bile duct strictures and those over the age of 70 years had a high incidence of bactobilia. This has led some to advise prophylactic antibiotics in so-called 'high-risk' patients only and not for routine uncomplicated elective cholecystectomy in patients under 70 years of age (Cahill and Pain 1988). Nevertheless, doubt remains as to whether bacteria in the bile are responsible for subsequent infections. Van Leeuwen, Keeman, Butzelar, and van den Bogaard (1985), when reviewing the data of 840 patients, showed that the most common pathogen was *Staphylococcus aureus*, and not organisms cultured from the bile at the time of operation.

If the bile is not colonized, then operations on the biliary tract are clean operations and it is justifiable to withhold prophylactic antibiotics. This raises the question of whether bactobilia can be predicted accurately before operation, and whether the 'high-risk factors' are a reliable guide. In a study of 644 patients, all of whom received pre-operative antibiotic prophylaxis with ampicillin and the beta-lactamase inhibitor sulbactam, the bile was found to be colonized in 121 (19 per cent) patients (Wells, Taylor, Lindsay, Morton, and the West of Scotland Surgical Infection Study Group 1989). Whilst the frequency of bile colonization was higher in those patients with a recognizable high-risk factor, more than half of the patients who had colonized bile (65 of 121) had no high-risk factor to suggest this (Table 3.8). Table 3.8 also demonstrates the high rate of infection (22 per cent) which occurs when the bile is colonized compared with a rate of 2 per cent when the bile is sterile. Further examination of the data derived from this study (Edwards, Lindsay, Taylor, and the West of Scotland Surgical Infection Study Group 1990) showed that where a single organism was isolated from the bile (86 patients) the rate of infection was 17.4 per cent but when the bile culture was polybacterial 12 (34 per cent) of 35 patients developed

Table 3.8. Bile colonisation, 'high-risk' factors and post-operative infection.

	Colonized bile		Sterile bile	
Risk	No. of patients	Post-operative infection	No. of patients	Post-operative infection
High ($n = 177$)	56	12 (21)	121	5(4)
Low ($n = 467$)	65	15 (23)	402	8(2)
Total	121	27 (22)*	523	13 (2)*

Values in parentheses are percentages. * $\chi^2 = 66.3$; $p < 0.0001$. [From Wells *et al.* (1989).]

post-operative infection despite prophylactic antibiotic therapy. From these data it would appear that prophylactic antibiotics should be given to all patients undergoing biliary tract operations until it is possible to predict bactobilia before operation with greater accuracy.

An alternative approach is to delay surgery until action has been taken to sterilize the bile before operation. It may well be that 24 or 48 hours of antibiotic therapy will sterilize the bile in all patients before operation, and thus reduce the incidence of infection to a very low rate. The administration of antibiotics on this basis would reduce bacterial contamination rather than enhance host resistance, but the longer course of therapy which would be needed, either parenteral or oral, may affect bowel flora and increase the likelihood of bacterial resistance and pseudomembranous colitis. This remains to be investigated.

Appendicectomy

Many papers have been published advocating the use of antibiotics as 'prophylaxis' in appendicectomy. It has been argued that the antibiotics are therapeutic as far as the peritoneal infection is concerned, and prophylactic in preventing infection in the wound through which the appendix is removed. In the author's view, appendicitis is an inflammatory condition requiring antibiotic therapy, usually for 2–5 days. Metronidazole has been the antibiotic of choice in the management of appendicitis (Tanner, Alis, Collins, Fahy, Lane, and McCormack 1980; Kortelainen, Huttunen, Kairaluoma, Mokka, Laitinen, and Larmi 1982), and variable results have been obtained by the addition of an antibiotic active against aerobic organisms (Flannigan, Clifford, Carver, Yule, and Madden 1983; Lau, Fan, Yiu, and Wong 1983). In the author's experience a single dose of such an antibiotic confers benefit (Wilson, Taylor, Lindsay, Dreghorn, and Thompson 1987) and it may well be that early elimination of the aerobic Gram-negative organisms disrupts the synergy between aerobes and anaerobes which leads to abscess formation.

Even when the appendix is not infected transection of its lumen leads to bacterial contamination and to an increased incidence of infection. In an unpublished review of papers reporting the benefit of antibiotic treatment compared with placebo, the author found a 10 per cent infection rate when the normal appendix was removed without antibiotic cover, compared with a 3 per cent frequency of infection when metronidazole with or without an antibiotic active against aerobic organisms was administered.

Colorectal surgery

The colon and rectum contain the greatest bacterial load and this is maximal in the sigmoid colon and rectum. Therefore, it is not surprising that operations on both descending and sigmoid colon and on the rectum are associated with the highest rates of post-operative infection. The infection rate after colorectal operations is high, not only because the frequency of bacterial contamination may be high (although with careful surgical techniques this need be no higher than in any other operation) but because the high concentration of anaerobic organisms present creates the right environment for the synergy known to exist between aerobic and anaerobic organisms in the aetiology of infection (Onderdonk, Bartlett, Laine, Sullivan-Seigler, and Gorbach 1976; Kelly 1980). In Onderdonk *et al.*'s study in rats, a low rate of abscess formation was seen after intra-abdominal injection of aerobic organisms alone, or of anaerobic organisms alone. However, any combination or aerobic and anaerobic organisms led to a very high rate of abscess formation.

The concentration of anaerobic organisms in the colon is high and oral pre-operative antibiotics do not reduce this concentration sufficiently to disturb the synergistic action with aerobes. The numbers of aerobic organisms can be reduced by cathartics and oral antibiotics sufficiently to disturb this synergy (Taylor, Lindsay, and Hellyar 1989) and it is possible that this is the mechanism of action of the oral antibiotics given as pre-operative antibiotic prophylaxis. Whether or not it is necessary to administer parenteral antibiotics, which are active against anaerobic organisms at the time of operation, remains an open question but it is usual practice for these to be administered. The use of antibiotics to reduce the considerable morbidity and mortality rates associated with colonic surgery have progressed along two lines: oral or parenteral administration. A combination of both routes needs also to be considered.

Oral antibiotics In 1972, Nichols, Condon, Gorbach, and Nyhus showed that oral antibiotics given before operation reduced the incidence of post-operative infectious complications after colorectal operations. Their regimen has become standard throughout the US, and the administration of the non-absorbable antibiotics neomycin and erythromycin base, 1 g of each given orally at 13.00, 14.00 and 23.00 hours on the day before surgery, remains the recommended antibiotic prophylaxis for colonic surgery (Kaiser 1986). When emergency colonic surgery is undertaken, or in situations which preclude pre-operative oral antibiotic prophylaxis, systemic antibiotics are administered. The rationale for the use of oral antibiotics is to reduce the bacterial load in the colon, and hence reduce the contamination at the time of operation. This regimen is claimed to reduce the overall septic complication rate to 7.8 per cent (Condon, *et al.* 1983). Other oral antibiotic regimens have been advocated but few series have reported such a low incidence of infection with oral antibiotics alone (Weaver, Burdon, Youngs, and Keighley 1986; Lau, Chu, Poon, and Ho 1988).

Parenteral antibiotics It has long been recognized that mechanical bowel preparation does not alter the bacterial concentration in the fluid which remains in the colonic lumen (Nichols *et al.* 1971; Arabi, Dimock, Burdon, Alexander-Williams, and Keighley 1978) and, therefore, contamination is inevitable at the time of operation. Antibiotics are required to complement host resistance but the choice of an oral or parenteral route for the administration of antibiotics remains controversial (Keighley, Arabi, Alexander-Williams, Youngs, and Burdon 1979; Figueras-Felip, *et al.* 1984). There seem to be no reason to believe that a combination of both routes may give the best results of all.

Combined oral and parenteral antibiotics Lazorthes, *et al.* (1981) reported infectious complications in 9 of 30 patients given oral kanamycin and metronidazole, in 7 of 30 patients given systemic cephradine and metronidazole, but in only 1 of 30 patients given both the pre-operative oral regimen together with systemic peri-operative antibiotics. Whilst the infection rates reported after combined oral and systemic antibiotic prophylaxis have not always approached the low figures reported by Condon and colleagues (1983), the incidence is most frequently lower than that reported after both the oral or systemic route alone (Coppa, Eng, Gouge, Rauson, and Localio 1983; Kaiser, Harrington, Jacobs, Mulherin, Roach, and Sawyer 1983).

It is the author's practice to purge the bowel with two doses of sodium picasulphate (Picolax®) and to give two doses of a quinolone antibiotic (500 mg ciprofloxacin) by mouth on the day before operation. These antibiotics have been shown to eliminate aerobic organisms from the colon in volunteers (Shah, Enzensberger, Glogau, and Knothe 1987), and this combination of cathartic and antibiotic therapy has been shown significantly to reduce Gram-negative aerobic bacteria in the colonic lumen within 24 hours

(Taylor *et al.* 1989). A single dose of a broad-spectrum third-generation cephalosporin together with metronidazole is given intravenously on induction of anaesthesia.

Summary

Infection rates following surgery are dependent upon contamination occurring at the time of the operation and the body's ability to resist this. Preparation of the patient before operation and careful operative technique will reduce the level of contamination, and appropriate systemic antibiotics given to cover the operative period will assist the body to resist any accidental or inevitable contamination.

Prophylactic antibiotics should be administered whenever a prosthesis is to be implanted, or has already been implanted into the patient; when the patient is recognized as having reduced resistance; or when a clean–contaminated or contaminated operation is being performed. The role of prophylactic antibiotics in healthy patients undergoing non-implant, clean operations remains open to question.

References

Ambrose, N.S., Johnson, M., Burdon, D.W., and Keighley, M.R.B. (1985). The influence of single dose intravenous antibiotics on faecal flora and emergence of Clostridium difficile. *J. Antimicrob. Chemother.* **15**, 319–26.

Arabi, Y., Dimock, F., Burdon, D.W., Alexander-Williams, J., and Keighley, M.R.B. (1978). Influence of bowel preparation and antimicrobials on colonic microflora. *Br. J. Surg.* **65**, 555–9.

Ayliffe, G.A.J., Noy, M.F., Babb, J.R., Davies, J.E., and Jackson, J. (1983). A comparison of pre-operative bathing with chlorhexidine detergent and non medicated soap in the prevention of wound infection. *J. Hosp. Infect.* **4**, 237–44.

Bandyke, D.F., Berni, G.A., Thiele, B.L., and Towne, J.B. (1984). Aortofemoral graft infection due to *Staphylococcus epidermidis*. *Arch. Surg.* **119**, 102–8.

Bates, T., Siller, G., Crathern, B.C., Bradley, S.P., Zlotnik, R.D., Couch, C., *et al.* (1989). Timing of prophylactic antibiotics in abdominal surgery: trial of pre-operative *versus* an intra-operative first dose. *Br. J. Surg.* **76**, 52–6.

Berg, G.A., Kirk, A.S., and Bain, W.H. (1987). Punctured surgical gloves and bacterial recolonisation of hands during open heart surgery: implications for prosthetic valve replacement. *Br. J. Clin. Pract.* **41**, 903–6.

Bergman, L. and Solhaug, J.H. (1987). Single dose chemoprophylaxis in elective colorectal surgery. *Ann. Surg.* **205**, 77–81.

Blumberg, N., Agarwhal, M.M., and Chuang, C. (1985). Relation between recurrence of cancer of the colon and blood transfusion. *Br. Med. J.* **290**, 1037–9.

Brandberg, A., Holm, J., Hammersten, J., and Scherston, J. (1980). Post-operative wound infection in vascular surgery — effect of pre-operative whole body bathing by showering with chlorhexidine soap. In *Problems in the control of hospital infection* (ed. S.W.B. Newson and A.D.S. Caldwell) pp. 72–6. Royal Society of Medicine, London.

Burrows, L. and Tartter, P. (1982). Effect of blood transfusion on colonic malignancy recurrence rates. *Lancet* **ii**, 662.
Byrne, D.J., Napier, A., and Cushieri, A. (1990). Rationalising whole body disinfection. *J. Hosp. Infect.* **15**, 183–7.
Cahill, C.J. and Pain, J.A. (1988). Current practice in biliary surgery. *Br. J. Surg.* **75**, 1169–72.
Chetlin, S.H. and Elliott, D.W. (1971). Biliary bacteraemia. *Arch. Surg.* **102**, 303–7.
Chrintz, H., Vibits, H., Corditz, T.O., Harreby, J.S., Waaddegaard, P., and Larsen, S.O. (1989). Need for surgical wound dressing. *Br. J. Surg.* **76**, 204–5.
Condon, R.E., Bartlett, J.G., Greenlea, H., Schulte, W.J., Ochi, S., Abbe, R., *et al.* (1983). Efficacy of oral and systemic antibiotic prophylaxis in colorectal operations. *Arch. Surg.* **118**, 496–501.
Conley, J.M., Hill, S., Ross, J., Lertzman, J., and Louie, T.J. (1989). Hand washing practices in an intensive care unit: the effects of an educational programme and its relationship to infection rates. *Am. J. Infect. Control* **17**, 330–9.
Coppa, G.F., Eng, K., Gouge, T.H., Ranson, J.H.C., and Localio, S.A. (1983). Parenteral and oral antibiotics in elective colon and rectal surgery. *Am. J. Surg.* **145**, 62–5.
Crapp, A.R., Powis, S.J.A., Tillotson, P., Cooke, W.T., and Alexander-Williams, J. (1975). Preparation of the bowel by whole-gut irrigation. *Lancet* **ii**, 1239–40.
Crowson, M.C., Hallissay, M.T., Kiff, R.S., Kingston, R.D., and Fielding, J.W.L. (1989). Blood transfusion in colorectal cancer. *Br. J. Surg.* **76**, 522–3.
Cruse, P.J.E. and Foord, R. (1980). The epidemiology of wound infection. A 10 year prospective study of 62939 wounds. *Surg. Clin. North Am.* **60**, 27–40.
Dixon, J.M., Armstrong, C.P., Duffy, S.W., Chetty, U., and Davies, G.C. (1984). A randomised prospective trial comparing the value of intravenous and preincisional cefamandol in reducing post-operative sepsis after operations upon the gastrointestinal tract. *Surg. Gynecol. Obstet.* **158**, 303–7.
Dodds, R.D.A., Guy, P.J., Peacock, A.M., Duffy, S.R., Barker, S.G.E., and Thomas, M.H. (1988). Surgical glove perforation. *Br. J. Surg.* **75**, 966–8.
Dudley, H.A.F., Radcliffe, A.G., and McGeehan, D. (1980). Intra-operative irrigation of the colon to permit primary anastomosis. *Br. J. Surg.* **67**, 80–1.
Earnshaw, J.J., Slack, R.C., Hopkinson, B.R., and Makin, G.S. (1988). Risk factors in vascular surgical sepsis. *Ann. R. Coll. Surg. Engl.* **70**, 139–43.
Edmiston, C.E., Schmitt, D.D., and Seabrook, G.R. (1989). Coagulase-negative staphylococcal infections in vascular surgery. Epidemiology and Pathogenesis. *Infect. Control Hosp. Epidemiol.* **10**, 111–17.
Edwards, G.S.F., Lindsay, G., Taylor, E.W., and the West of Scotland Surgical Infection Study Group (1990). A bacteriological assessment of ampicillin with sulbactam as antibiotic prophylaxis in patients undergoing biliary tract operations. *J. Hosp. Infect.* (In press, 1992).
Elek, S.D. (1956). Experimental staphylococcal infections in the skin of man. *Ann. N. Y. Acad. Sci.* **65**, 85.
Elek, S.D. and Conen, P.E. (1957). The virulence of *Staphylococcus pyogenes* for man. A study of the problems of wound infection. *Br. J. Exp. Pathol.* **38**, 573–86.
Figueras-Felip, J., Basilio-Bonet, E., Lara-Eisman, F., Caride-Garcia, P., Isamat-Baro, E., Fara-Bargallo, P., *et al.* (1984). Oral is superior to systemic antibiotic prophylaxis in operations upon the colon and rectum. *Surg. Gynecol. Obstet.* **155**, 359–62.
Fitzgerald, R.H., Nolan, D.R., Ilstrup, D.M., van Scoy, R.E., Washington, J.A.,

and Coventry, M.B. (1977). Deep wound sepsis following total hip arthroplasty. *J. Bone Joint Surg.* **59A**, 847–55.

Flannigan, G.M., Clifford, R.P., Carver, R.A., Yule, A.G., and Madden, N.P. (1983). Antibiotic prophylaxis in acute appendicitis. *Surg. Gynecol. Obstet.* **150**, 209–11.

Freedman, A.M. and Jackson, I.T. (1989). Infection in breast implants. *Infect. Dis. Clin. North Am.* **3**, 275–87.

Fleites, R.A., Marshall, J.B., Eckhauser, M.L., Mansour, E.G., Imbembo, A.L., and McCullough, A.J. (1985). The efficacy of polythylene glycol-electrolyte lavage solution *versus* traditional mechanical bowel preparation for elective colonic surgery: a randomised, prospective, blinded clinical trial. *Surgery* **98**, 708–16.

Gatehouse, D., Dimock, F., Burdon, D.W., Alexander-Williams, J., and Keighley, M.R.B. (1978). Prediction of wound sepsis following gastric operations. *Br. J. Surg.* **65**, 551–4.

Giercksky, K.E., Danielsen, S., Garberg, O., Gruner, B.P.N., Holter, O., Johnson, J.A., *et al.* (1982). A single dose of tinidazole and doxycycline prophylaxis in elective surgery of the colon and rectum. *Ann. Surg.* **195**, 227–31.

Gordon-Smith, I.C., Taylor, E.W., Nicolaides, A.N., Goldman, L., Kenyon, J., and Eastcott, H.H.G. (1978). Management of abdominal aortic aneurysm. *Br. J. Surg.* **65**, 834–8.

Hares, M.M., Greca, F., Youngs, D., Burdon, D.W., Keighley, M.R.B. (1981*a*). Failure of antimicrobial prophylaxis with cefoxitin, or metronidazole and gentamicin in colorectal surgery. Is mannitol to blame? *J. Hosp. Infect.* **2**, 127–33.

Hares, M.M., Hegarty, M.A., Warlow, J., Malins, D., Youngs, D., Bently, S., *et al.* (1981*b*). A controlled trial to compare systemic and intra-incisional cefuroxime prophylaxis in high risk gastric surgery. *Br. J. Surg.* **68**, 276–80.

Hayek, L.J. and Emerson, J.M. (1988). Pre-operative whole body disinfection — a controlled clinical study. *J. Hosp. Infect.* **11** (Supplement B), 15–19.

Hope, P.G., Kristinsson, K.G., Norman, P., and Elson, R.A. (1989). Deep infection of cemented total hip arthroplasties caused by coagulase negative staphylococci. *J. Bone Joint Surg.* **71**, 851–5.

Howden, C.W. and Hunt, R.H. (1987). Relationship between gastric secretion and infection. *Gut* **28**, 96–9.

Irving, A.D. and Scrimgeour, D. (1987). Mechanical bowel preparation for colonic resection and anastomosis. *Br. J. Surg.* **74**, 580–1.

Jackson, D.W., Pollock, A.V., and Tindal, D.S. (1971). The use of a plastic adhesive drape in the prevention of wound infection. *Br. J. Surg.* **58**, 340–2.

Jagelman, D.G., Fabian, T.C., Nichols, R.L., Stone, H.H., Wilson, S.E., and Zellner, S.R. (1988). Single dose cefotetan *versus* multiple dose cefoxitin as prophylaxis in elective colorectal surgery. *Am. J. Surg.* **155**, 71–6.

Jalovaara, P. and Puranen, J. (1989). Air bacterial and particle counts in total hip replacement operations using non-woven and cotton gowns and drapes. *J. Hosp. Infect.* **14**, 333–8.

Jensen, L.S., Anderson, A., Fristrup, S.L., Holme, J.B., Hvid, H.M., Kraglund, K., *et al.* (1990). Comparison of one dose *versus* three doses of prophylactic antibiotics, and the influence of blood transfusion, on infectious complications in acute and elective colorectal surgery. *Br. J. Surg.* **77**, 513–18.

Kaiser, A.B. (1986). Antimicrobial prophylaxis in surgery. *N. Engl. J. Med.* **315**, 1129–38.

Kaiser, A.B., Harrington, J.L., Jacobs, K.J., Mulherin, J.L., Roach, A.C., and

Sawyer, J.L. (1983). Cefoxitin *versus* erythromycin, neomycin and cefazolin in colorectal operations. *Ann. Surg.* **198**, 525–30.

Keighley, M.R.B., Arabi, Y., Alexander-Williams, J., Youngs, D., and Burdon, D.W. (1979). Comparison between systemic and oral antimicrobial prophylaxis in colorectal surgery. *Lancet* **i**, 894–7.

Keighley, M.R.B., Taylor, E.W., Hares, M.M., Arabi, Y., Youngs, D., Bently, S., *et al.* (1981). Influence of oral mannitol bowel preparation on colonic microflora and the risk of explosion during endoscopic diathermy. *Br. J. Surg.* **68**, 554–6.

Kelly, M.J. (1980). Wound infection: a controlled clinical and experimental demonstration of synergy between aerobic (*Escherichia coli*) and anaerobic (*Bacteroides fragilis*) bacteria. *Ann. R. Coll. Surg. Engl.* **62**, 52–9.

Kortelainen, P., Huttunen, R., Kairaluoma, M.I., Mokka, R.E., Laitinen, S., and Larmi, T.K.I. (1982). Single dose intra-rectal metronidazole prophylaxis against wound infection after appendicectomy. *Am. J. Surg.* **143**, 244–5.

Krukowski, Z.H., Stewart, M.P.M., Alsayer, H.M., and Matheson, N.A. (1984). Infection after abdominal surgery: a five year prospective study. *Br. Med. J.* **288**, 278–80.

Lau, W.Y., Chu, K.W., Poon, G.P., and Ho, K.K. (1988). Prophylactic antibiotics in elective colorectal surgery. *Br. J. Surg.* **75**, 782–5.

Lau, W., Fan, S.T., Yiu, T.F., and Wong, S.H. (1983). Prophylaxis of post appendicectomy sepsis by metronidazole and ampicillin: a randomised prospective double blind trial. *Br. J. Surg.* **70**, 155–7.

Law, D.J.W., Mishriki, S.F., and Jeffrey, P.J. (1990). The importance of surveillance after discharge from hospital in the diagnosis of post-operative wound infection. *Ann. R. Coll. Surg. Engl.* **72**, 207–9.

Lazorthes, F., Legrand, G., Monrozies, X., Fretigny, E., Pugnet, G., Cordova, J.A., *et al.* (1982). Comparison between oral and systemic antibiotics and their combined use for the prevention of complications in colorectal surgery. *Dis. Colon Rectum* **25**, 309–11.

Lewis, R.T. (1977). Wound infection after gastroduodenal operations: a 10 year review. *Can. J. Surg.* **29**, 435–40.

Lidwell, O.M., Lowbury, E.J.L., Whyte, W., Blowers, R., Stanley, S.J., and Lowe, D. (1982). Effect of ultraclean air in operating rooms on deep sepsis in the joint after total hip or knee replacement: a randomised study. *Br. Med. J.* **285**, 10–14.

Lilly, H.A., Lowbury, E.J.L., and Wilkins, M.D. (1979). Limits to the progressive reduction of resident skin bacteria by disinfection. *J. Clin. Pathol.* **32**, 382–5.

Lilly, H.A., Loudon, P.S., Lowbury, E.J.L., and Porter, M.F. (1970). Effects of adhesive drapes on contamination of operative wounds. *Lancet* **ii**, 431–2.

Maetani, S., Nishikawa, T., Hirakawa, A., and Tobe, T. (1986). Role of blood transfusion in organ system failure following major abdominal surgery. *Ann. Surg.* **203**, 275–81.

Mannion, P.T., Thom, B.T., Reynolds, C.S., and Strachan, C.J.L. (1989). The acquisition of antibiotic resistant coagulase negative staphylococci by aortic graft recipients. *J. Hosp. Infect.* **14**, 313–23.

Moesgaard, F. and Lukkegaard-Neilsen, M. (1989). Pre-operative cell mediated immunity and duration of antibiotic prophylaxis in relation to postoperative infective complications. A controlled trial in biliary, gastroduodenal and colorectal surgery. *Acta Chir. Scand.* **155**, 281–6.

Moore, W.E.C. and Holdeman, L.V. (1974). Human fecal flora: the normal flora of 20 Japanese-Hawaiians. *Appl. Microbiol.* **27**, 961–79.

Moynihan, B.G.A. (1920). The ritual of a surgical operation. *Br. J. Surg.* **8**, 27–35.
Nagai, I., Katoda, M., Takechi, M., Kumamoto, R., Nakano, S., and Jitsukawa, S. (1986). Studies on the bacterial permeability of non-woven fabrics and cotton fabrics. *J. Hosp. Infect.* **7**, 261–8.
Newsom, S.W. and Rowland, C. (1988). Studies on perioperative skin flora. *J. Hosp. Infect.* **11** (Supplement B), 21–6.
Nichols, R.L. and Condon, R.E. (1975). Role of the endogenous gastrointestinal microflora in postoperative wound sepsis. In *Surgery Annual* (ed. L.M. Nyhus), pp. 279–93. Appleton Century Crofts, New York.
Nichols, R.L., Gorbach, S.L., and Condon, R.E. (1971). Alterations of intestinal microflora following pre-operative mechanical preparation of the colon. *Dis. Colon Rectum*, **14**, 123–7.
Nichols, R.L., Condon, R.E., Gorbach, S.L., and Nyhus, L.M. (1972). Efficacy of pre-operative antimicrobial preparation of the bowel. *Ann. Surg.* **176**, 227–32.
Nichols, R.L., Webb, W.R., Jones, J.W., Smith, J.W., and LoCicero, J. (1982). Efficacy of antibiotic prophylaxis in high risk gastroduodenal operations. *Am. J. Surg.* **143**, 94–8.
Onderdonk, A.B., Bartlett, J.G., Laine, T., Sullivan-Seigler, N., and Gorbach, S.L. (1976). Microbial synergy in experimental intra-abdominal abscess. *Infect. Immun.* **13**, 22–6.
Opelz, G., Senger, D.P.S., Mickey, M.R., and Terasaki, P.I. (1981). Effect of blood transfusion on subsequent kidney transplants. *Transplant Proc.* **ii**, 253–9.
Orr, N.W.M. (1981). Is a mask necessary in the operating theatre? *Ann. R. Coll. Surg. Engl.* **63**, 390–2.
Platt, R., Zaleznik, D.F., Hopkins, C.C., Dellinger, E.P., Karchmer, A.W., Bryan, C.S., *et al.* (1989). Perioperative antibiotic prophylaxis for herniorrhaphy and breast surgery. *N. Engl. J. Med.* **322**, 153–60.
Polk, H.C. (1987). Non-specific host defence stimulation in the reduction of surgical infection in man. *Br. J. Surg.* **74**, 969–70.
Raahave, D., Friis-Moller, A., Bjerre-Jepsen, K., Thiis-Knudsen, J., and Rasmussen, L.B. (1986). The infective dose of aerobic and anaerobic bacteria in post-operative wound sepsis. *Arch. Surg.* **121**, 924–9.
Scher, K.S., Bernstein, J.M., Arenstein, G.L., and Sorensen, C. (1990). Reducing the cost of surgical prophylaxis. *Am. Surg.* **56**, 32–5.
Shah, P.M., Enzensberger, R., Glogau, O., and Knothe, H. (1987). Influence of oral ciprofloxacin and ofloxacin on the faecal flora of healthy volunteers. *Am. J. Med.* **82**, 332–5.
Sjostedt, S., Levin, P., Malmbourg, A.S., Bergman, U., and Kager, L. (1989). Septic complications in relation to factors influencing the gastric microflora in patients undergoing gastric surgery. *J. Hosp. Infect.* **13**, 191–6.
Stone, H.H., Hooper, C.A., Kolb, L.D., Geheber, C., and Dawkins, E.J. (1976). Antibiotic prophylaxis in gastric, biliary and colonic surgery. *Ann. Surg.* **184**, 443–52.
Strachan, C.J.L. (1988). Current thoughts on *Staphylococcus epidermidis* in vascular surgery. *J. Hosp. Infect.* **11** (Supplement B), 33–41.
Strachan, C.J.L., Black, J., Powis, S.J.A., Waterworth, T.A., Wise, R., Wilkinson, A.R., *et al.* (1977). Prophylactic use of cephazolin against wound sepsis after cholecystectomy. *Br. Med. J.* **i**, 1254–6.
Sullivan, P.M., Johnston, R.C., and Kelley, S.S. (1990). Late infection after total

hip replacement, caused by an oral organism after dental manipulation. A case report. *J. Bone Joint Surg.* **72**, 121–3.

Tanner, W.A., Ali, A.E., Collins, P.G., Fahy, A.M., Lane, B.E., and McCormack, T. (1980). Single dose intra-rectal metronidazole as prophylaxis against wound infection following emergency appendicectomy. *Br. J. Surg.* **67**, 809–10.

Taylor, E.W., Lindsay, G., and Hellyar, A.G. (1989). Preoperative selective decontamination of the colon by ciprofloxacin and mechanical catharsis in patients undergoing elective colorectal operations. *Surg. Res. Commun.* **7**, 351–5.

Taylor, E.W., Bently, S., Youngs, D., and Keighley, M.R.B. (1981) Bowel preparation and the safety of colonoscopic polypectomy. *Gastroenterology* **81**, 1–4.

Taylor, T.V., Walker, W.S., Mason, R.C., Richmond, J., and Lee, D. (1982). Pre-operative intra-parietal (intra-incisional) cefoxatin in abdominal surgery. *Br. J. Surg.* **69**, 461–2.

Taylor, T.V., Dawson, D.L., de Silva, M., Shaw, S.J., Durans, D., Makin, D. (1985). Pre-operative intra-incisional cefamandole reduces wound infection and post-operative in patient stay in upper abdominal surgery. *Ann. R. Coll. Surg. Engl.* **67**, 235–7.

Thurn, J., Crossley, K., Gordts, A., Maki, M., and Johnson, J. (1990). Enteral hyperalimentation as a source of nosocomial infection. *J. Hosp. Infect.* **15**, 203–17.

van Leeuwen, P.A.M., Keeman, J.N., Butzelar, R.J.M., and van den Bogaard, A.E.J.M. (1985). Correlation between a positive gallbladder culture and subsequent wound infection after biliary surgery. A retrospective study of 840 patients. *Neth. J. Surg.* **37**, 179–82.

Weaver, M., Burdon, D.W., Youngs, D.J., and Keighley, M.R.B. (1986). Oral neomycin and erythromycin compared with single-dose systemic metronidazole and ceftriaxone prophylaxis in elective colorectal surgery. *Am. J. Surg.* **151**, 437–42.

Wells, G.R., Taylor, E.W., Lindsay, G., Morton, L., and the West of Scotland Surgical Infection Study Group (1989). The relationship of bile colonization, high risk factors and post-operative sepsis in patients undergoing biliary tract operations whilst receiving a prophylactic antibiotic. *Br. J. Surg.* **76**, 374–7.

Williams, R.E.O. (1973). Benefit and mischief from commensal bacteria. *J. Clin. Pathol.* **26**, 811–18.

Wilson, R.G., Taylor, E.W., Lindsay, G., Dreghorn, C., Thompson, G., McGavigan, J., *et al.* (1987). A comparative study of cefotetan and metronidazole against metronidazole alone to prevent infection after appendicectomy. *Surg. Gynecol. Obstet.* **164**, 447–51.

4. Surgery for HIV-infected patients

Anne C. Bayley, John E. Jellis, and David K. Watters

HIV and the surgeon

It is still less than a decade since publication of the first descriptions of disease caused by the human immunodeficiency virus (HIV). The evolution of a global pandemic since 1981 has resulted in an explosion of research effort and accomplishment, recorded in many papers and in conferences attended by thousands of people, including men and women living with acquired immune deficiency syndrome (AIDS), economists, sociologists, politicians, and theologians, as well as scientists. Despite all this activity, surgical aspects are under-represented: for example, at the Sixth International Conference on AIDS in June, 1990, surgery merited two posters (plus two unpresented items included in the abstract volume), compared with 75 abstracts on 'surveillance' and 72 concerned with 'public policy'.

Only some aspects of the pandemic have had close attention from surgeons: notably how to protect the surgical team from occupational infection (particularly in the operating theatre), and how to ensure the safety of blood for transfusion. Other consequences, such as changing surgical pathology in cities with high seroprevalence rates, changing demands for surgical services (with implications for the allocation of resources), and effects on the personal and professional lives of surgeons have had little or no public discussion.

We begin this chapter with an overview of how the pandemic is affecting surgical practice. Next we describe how we recognize HIV-infected patients in Zambia, and survey changing pathologies in general and orthopaedic surgery, before considering effects on intensive care and blood transfusion practice. Finally, we shall mention some social, economic, and political implications of HIV infection in surgical patients. In 1990 our knowledge remains provisional and qualitative, as we are learning from day to day. Although quantitative studies have begun, few have been completed.

Overview

The World Health Organization (WHO) recognizes three patterns of HIV infection in countries and continents (Fig. 4.1), by reference to major mode(s) of transmission and numbers of persons infected (Chin and Mann 1988).

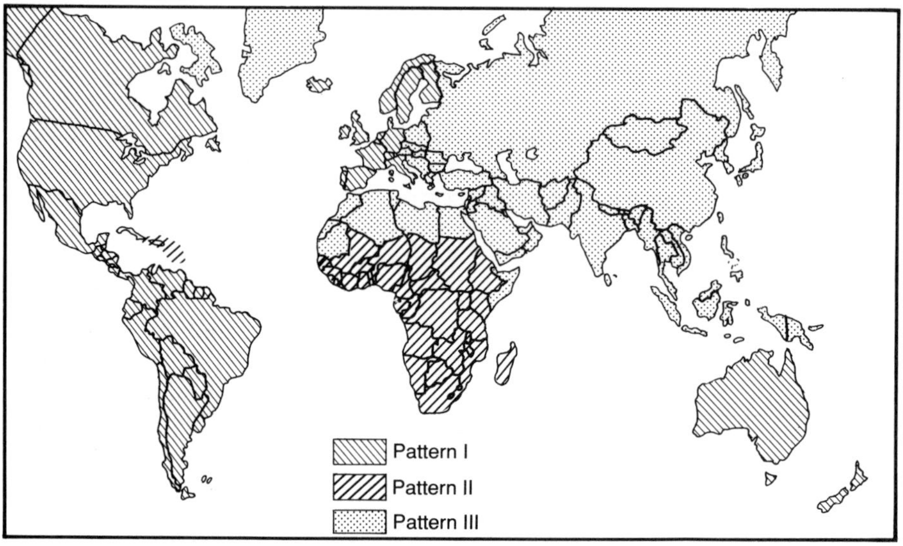

Fig. 4.1. Global patterns of HIV infection and AIDS. [Reproduced from Chin and Mann (1988) by kind permission.]

- Pattern I: countries where transmission occurs mostly during homosexual activity or by needle-sharing (intravenous drug users);
- Pattern II: countries where transmission is through heterosexual coitus and vertically from mother to fetus, with a few infections from blood or unsterilized skin-piercing instruments;
- Pattern III: areas where infection is absent or infrequent at present.

In the western World, pattern I encourages surgeons to regard HIV-infected patients as a local problem in large cities. However, spread of HIV into the general population is occurring insidiously and if preventive messages are unheard or unheeded a pattern II situation will result, perhaps within a decade. Studies of stored sera from some African cities showed no antibodies to HIV 10 years ago in places where seropositivity rates amongst adults were 15 per cent or more in 1990.

In parts of Africa and of South America a pattern II epidemic already exists and is spreading. Here the key concepts are that all sexually active adults are in a 'risk group', and that HIV destroys families by killing first one parent, then the other, and often the youngest child, leaving orphans with an uncertain future. These orphans grow up in societies stressed by loss of many adults during their most productive years and by the social, economic, and political consequences of this.

In pattern II countries, seroprevalence rates are not uniform. Children between the ages of 4 and 15 years are rarely affected, and infection is uncommon over the age of 60 years. Seroprevalence is low in rural areas, except in proximity to trunk roads or in towns where illicit trading takes place across borders. Seroprevalence is higher in provincial centres and highest in major cities, where more than 15 per cent of adults between the ages of 16 and 55 years may be infected, with higher rates in subgroups such as young single women (who may be forced to sell sex in order to eat) or patients attending clinics for the treatment of sexually transmitted diseases (Melbye, *et al.* 1986). Seroprevalence rates amongst hospitalized patients are generally higher than rates for the same age group in the local community.

Most curves showing the development of the pandemic are exponential in shape, although in some pattern I cities (notably San Francisco) the curve is flattening as risk behaviours change. Several predictions of future numbers of infected persons or patients with AIDS have been published, but these are difficult for non-mathematicians to understand, and ignore factors which may not seem relevant at a distance, but which seem all too relevant to clinicians seeing patients (or funeral processions) every day.

In the cities of pattern II countries, surgeons have already found that HIV dominates pathology in their clinics, is responsible for half of all surgical infections, and disturbs the efficient use of beds, because many patients cannot be discharged quickly. The increasing prevalence of surgical sepsis and surgical tuberculosis will have implications for the use of antibiotics, and for infection control policies, which need to be investigated urgently.

The advent of HIV introduces not a new disease amongst many, but a new dimension to first contacts with all patients. It becomes necessary to ask in respect of each one: is this person likely or not to be HIV infected? If the answer is 'infected', then alterations in the presentation of progress of familiar pathologies must be expected and a watch kept for new and unfamiliar disease. It will be the rule rather than the exception for multiple pathologies to coexist. Management decisions will have to take into account patients' unpredictable and possibly abnormal responses to surgery, as well as measures to minimize the risk of transmitting HIV to the surgical team and the wise deployment of resources.

A broad division of all patients, to guide physical aspects of care, has metaphysical implications: HIV-infected people are not (at least not at present) likely to reach middle age, so that the quality of life for the intense living of a few years has great importance to them and their children. At the same time uninfected people who can survive to old age must do so: they are the base from which communities will be stabilized and replenished, and they must not be excluded from surgical services by overcrowding or failure of morale in staff.

Recognizing HIV-infected persons

With experience it becomes painfully easy to recognize many HIV-infected persons in the street but, in the clinic or ward, diagnosis is based on symptoms and signs, and on the known association of HIV with certain pathologies.

Soon after infection some patients experience seroconversion as an acute febrile illness. In Africa this is attributed, usually to 'malaria', but it may be followed by a period of chronic ill-health with mild weight loss, sore throat, malaise, and enlarged lymph nodes which the patient is likely to notice in the occipital area. After a few weeks or months, health improves and the patient feels and looks well for some years, although numerous small nodes are easily felt if sought for.

As health begins to decline patients develop many symptoms, often in several organ systems simultaneously. A conviction that 'I am ill' is usual, night sweats occur, with intermittent fever with skin rashes, mild weight loss, lack of energy, difficult-to-treat sexually transmitted diseases, headache, and cough. Later attacks of diarrhoea, more severe wasting, oral thrush, dysphagia, herpes zoster, herpes simplex, or Kaposi's lesions declare the diagnosis.

No clothes and a good light

Many persons who look fit, sitting up in bed with a newspaper awaiting a hernia repair, look very different when undressed and examined in good daylight. Estimate the patient's age before asking for it: an estimate 10 or more years older than the stated age is a warning sign. Study hair texture and colour: early greying is common, and in Africans it takes the form of scattered white hairs over the whole scalp (Fig. 4.2) instead of following the normal path backwards from temples and frontal scalp, leaving occipital hair dark for months or years. Hair thins, lacks lustre, and may be lost from the occipital pressure area.

Recognition of early effects of HIV on the brain depends on experience, and to some extent on knowledge of the patient's previous personality, but slow (though accurate) answers to questions, and a performance at variance with that expected for the patient's occupation are signs to watch for. Tremor or an unchanging and haunted expression are easier to recognize (Fig. 4.3), but confusion is a late and uncommon sign.

The skin is rarely unblemished: in a dermatology clinic in Lusaka, Hira, *et al.* (1988) found that 99 per cent of 113 patients with AIDS and 54 per cent of 1009 with the AIDS-related complex (ARC) had one or more cutaneous lesions. HIV-infected patients are predisposed to suffer severe drug reactions, particularly to antituberculous therapy. In some group II countries the incidence of herpes zoster has increased 20-fold in young adults, of whom more than 90 per cent are positive for antibodies to HIV. They

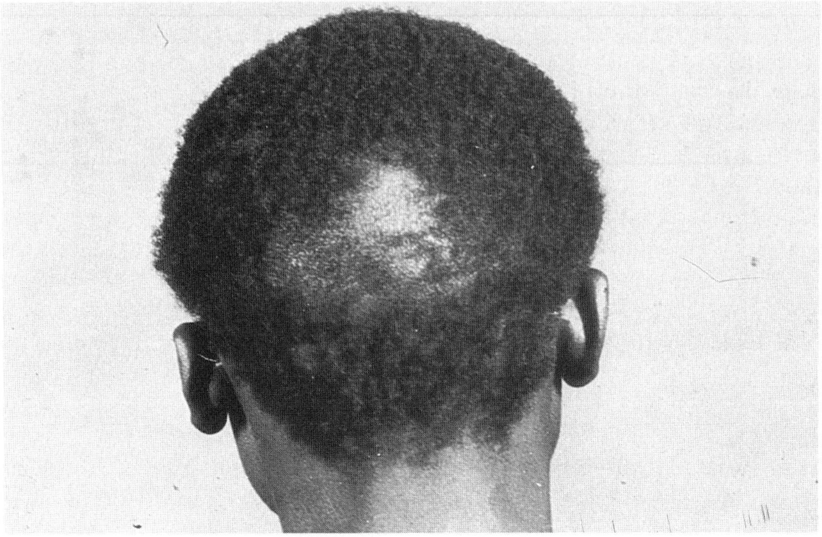

Fig. 4.2. Sparse hair with occipital baldness in HIV-infected patient.

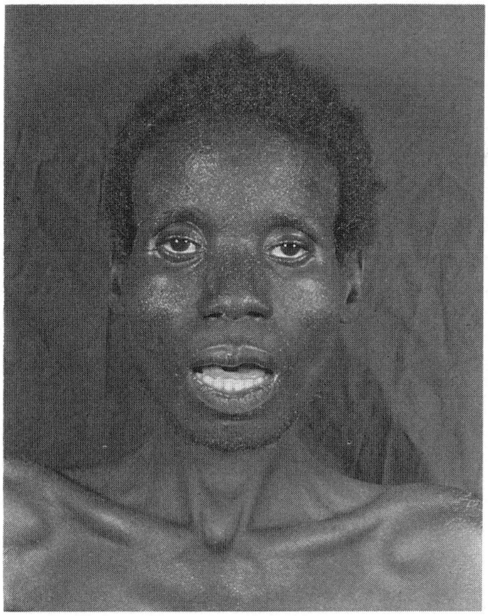

Fig. 4.3. Haunted stare of man with AIDS-related encephalopathy.

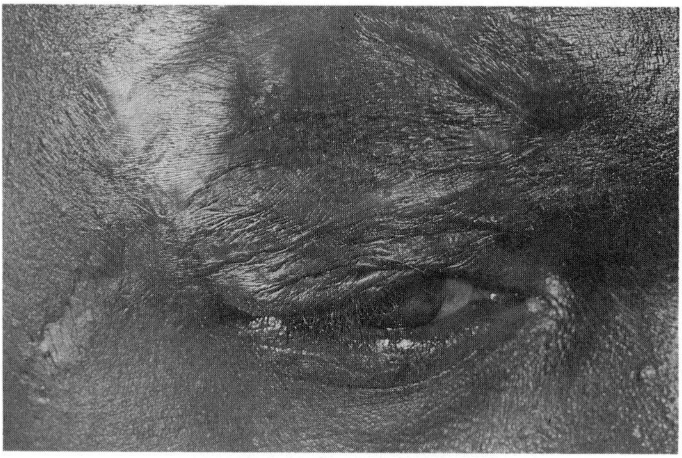

Fig. 4.4. Scarring caused by herpes zoster ophthalmicus.

develop severe multi-dermatomal or recurrent disease leading to marked scarring, which should be carefully looked for. The ophthalmic division of the fifth nerve is often affected, and corneal scarring, performation, iritis, or secondary glaucoma may lead to blindness (Fig. 4.4).

Alterations in pigmentation are common, and dryness with scaling, darkening of the facial skin, folliculitis, seborrhoeic dermatitis, extensive tinea versicolor, and molluscum contagiosum in an adult are all non-specific but suggestive signs of HIV infection. Characteristic scars are left by an HIV-related intracutaneous lymphoplasmacytic angiitis (Hira *et al.* 1988), which causes an itchy rash and often occurs for the first time soon after infection. In the acute stage tiny macules or papules develop (often on the upper chest, both back and front), which ooze fluid when scratched. Minute ulcers heal to leave characteristic 'target' scars with a centre lighter than normal skin, outlined by a fine line of deeper pigmentation. More than three or four such scars are pathognomonic for HIV infection. Many patients suffer recurrent bouts of this maculopapular dermatosis and develop widespread scarring as a result (Fig. 4.5).

Lymphadenopathy is not usually detectable in seropositive patients until a late stage of disease, when other signs make the diagnosis obvious. In the asymptomatic it is symmetrical in relation to the sagittal plane, the nodes are usually 2 cm or less in average diameter (except in the axilla), firm, numerous, mobile, and separate from each other. Simultaneous and symmetrical enlargement of both epitrochlear and iliac nodes is common and almost pathognomonic for HIV infection. However, patients who have

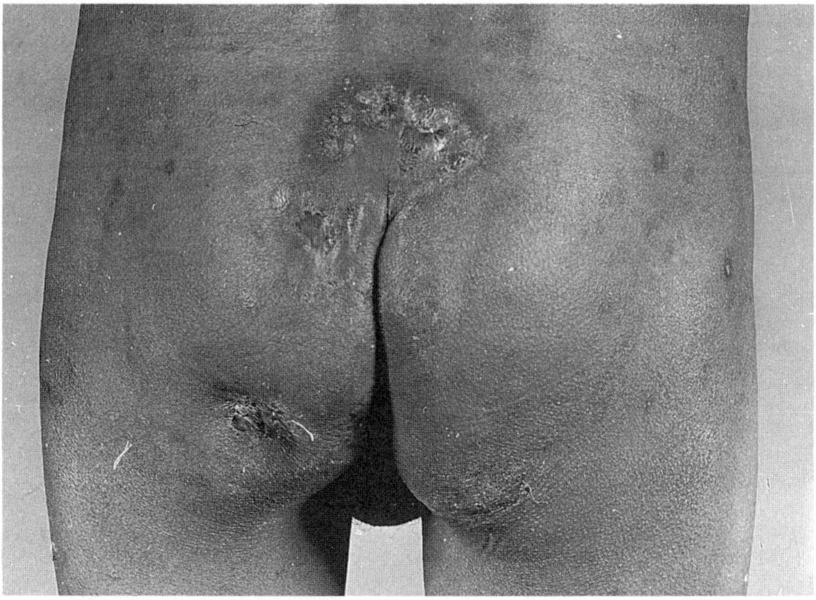

Fig. 4.5. Target scars of maculopapular dermatosis.

marked asymmetry in the size or distribution of nodes may have opportunist lymphoma or tuberculosis, and node biopsy is indicated.

Finally, the mouth is examined thoroughly with the aid of a spatula and torch, looking for early candidiasis (erythematous patches on the palate or flakes of white in the gingivobuccal sulcus or retro-molar fossa); oral hairy leukoplakia (Fig. 4.6), which is symptomless but seen as groups of fine white parallel lines at right angles to the lateral border of the tongue; early purple stains of Kaposi's disease on the hard palate; marked tonsillar enlargement without acute soreness (Fig. 4.7) and a non-specific but common appearance of general erythema and wetness.

Endoscopic procedures

Endoscopy is not required for the diagnosis of HIV infection but may be needed to distinguish between treatable consequences of immunosuppression. Hanson, *et al.* (1989) found that 7 of 20 unwashed endoscopes used on HIV-infected patients were indeed contaminated with HIV, but washing removed this and other organisms. The British Society of Gastroenterology (1988) recommended thorough washing of endoscopes followed by a 20-minute soak in 2 per cent glutaraldehyde; the endoscopist should wear gloves and goggles or spectacles.

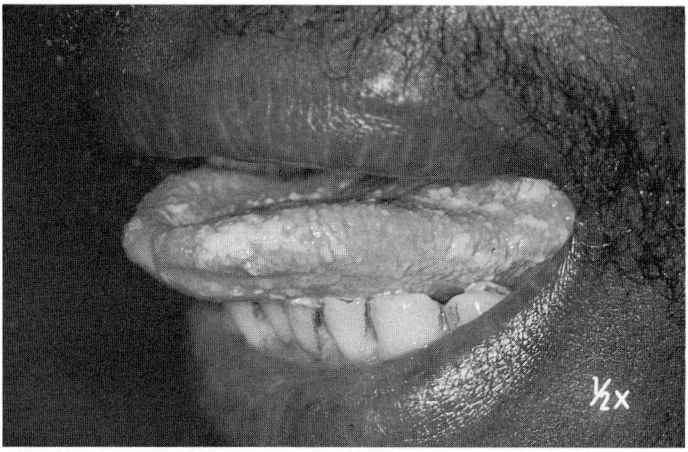

Fig. 4.6. Oral hairy leukoplakia with candidiasis.

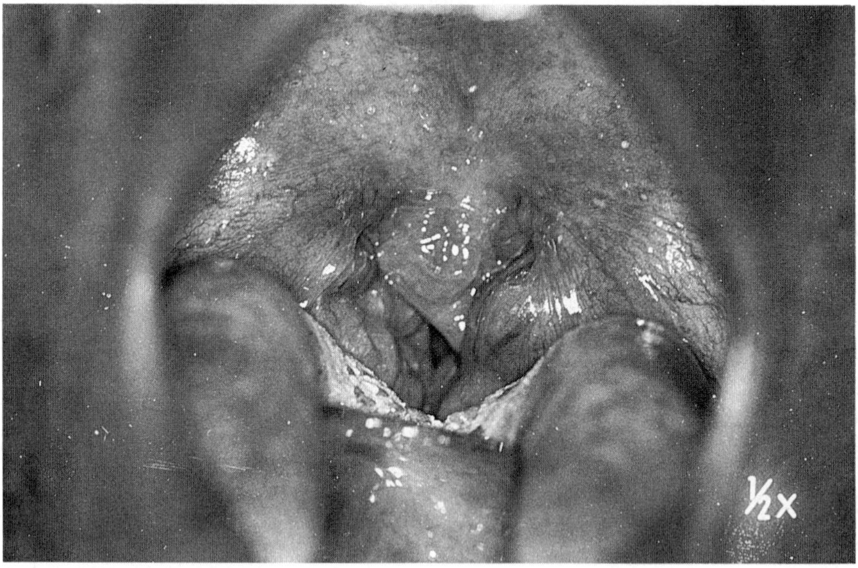

Fig. 4.7. Gross tonsillar enlargement.

Table 4.1. Survey: Results of serological tests.

	Male	Female	Total (n = 363)
Refused			3
Negative	170	67	237
Equivocal	2	3	5
Positive	62	31	93
?False negative	11	4	15
Lost or mislabelled			10

Survey of HIV-related pathology in Zambia

A prospective survey of the surgical pathology of uninfected and HIV-infected patients in Zambia showed a statistically significant association between some diagnoses and HIV infection (Bayley and Tembo 1990). We examined, and tested for antibodies to HIV, consecutive adult patients admitted to emergency surgical beds at the University Teaching Hospital in Lusaka during four 24-hour periods, and all adults found in designated surgical beds during unannounced visits to selected provincial and district hospitals.

We saw 363 persons with a sex ratio of 2.4:1 (M:F). Only three declined HIV testing, and Table 4.1 shows the results obtained in the others. Fifteen patients were seronegative on testing but had signs (Kaposi's disease, hairy leukoplakia, herpes zoster scars, or candidiasis) which strongly suggested HIV infection. The mean age for seropositive males was 28 years, and for females, 25 years. Table 4.2 shows the proportions of patients who were seropositive at rural, provincial, and city hospitals; there is a significant difference ($P < 0.001$) between rural and provincial hospitals, but the difference between 1989 and 1990 admissions in Lusaka did not reach statistical significance. Table 4.3 shows common diagnoses in HIV-negative and HIV-positive patients, emphasizing the importance of sepsis at any site as a warning sign, and the need to give special attention to accident and emergency departments when planning measures to protect staff.

In summary, the following diagnoses were significantly associated with HIV infection: sepsis of soft tissues (including the anorectal area and genital tracts in both sexes) and infection of bones and joints; tuberculosis of lymph nodes, non-infective anorectal disease and Kaposi's 'sarcoma'. In this survey 57 per cent of all patients presenting with sepsis were HIV infected, but few had diabetes. Seropositivity for patients admitted with trauma reflected the seropositivity of the general community.

Unusual pathology should be viewed with suspicion, but subjected to critical testing: an hypothesis that a recent increase in the incidence of

Table 4.2. Survey: Seropositivity at individual hospitals.

	Total	Seropositive
Rural		
Katete	58	8 (13.8)
Chikankata	17	2 (11.8)
Chilonga	23	4 (17.4)
Provincial		
Mongu	33	8 (24.2)
Kasama	32	8 (25.0)
Livingstone	32	8 (25.0)
Main Road (Monze)	48	22 (45.8)
City (Lusaka)		
March 1989	57	19 (33.3)
March 1990	64	27 (42.2)

Values in parentheses are percentages.

Table 4.3. Survey: common diagnostic groups.

Diagnosis	HIV negative	HIV positive	p
Trauma	95 (40)	17 (16)	< 0.001
Sepsis, all sites	29 (12)	38 (35)	< 0.001
Non-septic anorectal	5 (2)	8 (7)	< 0.04
Tuberculosis of nodes	1 (0.24)	8 (7)	< 0.001
Genital ulcers	5 (2)	9 (8)	< 0.02
Kaposi's disease (old)	1 (0.24)	0	
Kaposi's disease (new)	0	3 (2.8)	< 0.05
All other diagnoses	106 (45)	25 (24)	

Values in parentheses are percentages.
Fifty-seven per cent of all patients presenting with sepsis at any site were seropositive for HIV antibodies.

typhoid performations of the ileum in Lusaka might be HIV related was examined — and found wanting (C. Bem, personal communication, 1990).

Surgical sepsis

The commonest sites for HIV-related sepsis are the female genital tract, the pleural space, large joints, and the anal canal, but a few patients have multiple abscesses or abscesses in unusual sites such as the thyroid gland, or lesions which extend repeatedly. Severe necrotizing fasciitis is becoming more common (Fig. 4.8). Soft tissue sepsis forms part of a sequence of illnesses, individually apparently unimportant, which yield a thick in-patient

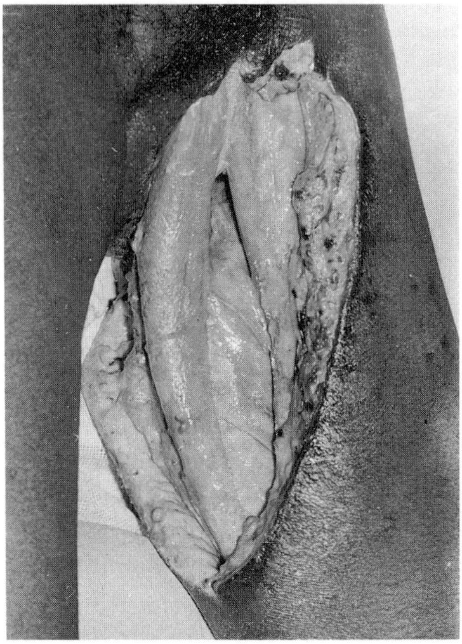

Fig. 4.8. Necrotizing fasciitis of thigh after excision.

file over a period of a year or two. Gynaecological and orthopaedic sepsis are described below.

Empyema thoracis occurs more frequently than in the past, so a prospective study was initiated in Lusaka in 1989; to date most patients are male and most are seropositive for HIV. Usually a pleural effusion rather than an empyema is suspected because symptoms are subacute, but there are signs of AIDS, such as severe wasting. After intercostal drainage the lungs may re-expand with unusual rapidity (suggesting an absence of the fibrinous exudate which normally organizes quickly to form a limiting membrane) or fail to re-expand at all. Broncho-pleural fistulae are common, but the prognosis is poor and most patients die quickly.

Anorectal sepsis is common wherever HIV infection is seen, but in Africa anal intercourse is exceedingly rare, so that local trauma cannot be a determining factor. We have seen relatively painless peri-anal ulcers of spontaneous onset, which are not purple (as in Crohn's disease) but have a pale base with little or no granulation tissue. In one general ward four of five recent patients with high fistula-*in-ano* (Fig. 4.9) were seropositive for HIV, but on the same unit only one HIV-infected patient has presented with anorectal tuberculosis (D.A.K. Watters, unpublished data). A postgraduate researcher in Lusaka found that 16 of 25 patients with anorectal sepsis were HIV positive (D.A., Echun personal communication).

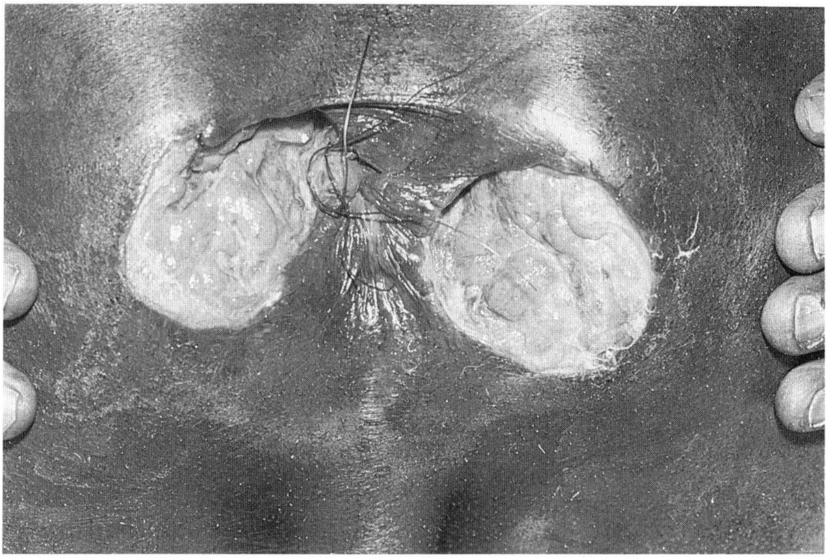

Fig. 4.9. High fistula-*in-ano* treated with a seton.

In our opinion both fistula-*in-ano* and haemorrhoids should be managed conservatively because anal wounds heal poorly and either anal dilatation or sphincterotomy may impair continence for fluid diarrhoea; indeed the focus of treatment should be control of the diarrhoea responsible for anal pathology. Ulcerative colitis is rare in Africans, but salazopyrin-responsive proctitis has been seen in a few HIV-positive men in Lusaka.

In one general unit, with wide experience of abdominal surgery, no specific changes have occurred, either in diagnoses made or in the behaviour of peritonitis, and necessary major surgery has not resulted in accelerated progression to ARC or AIDS. However, the surgical pathology survey found four seropositive patients who had chronic abdominal pain of undetermined cause following laparotomies for various reasons, whereas no seronegative persons had similar sequelae.

In Lusaka, 84 per cent of patients with tuberculosis of lymph nodes are HIV positive (Bem, Patil, Elliot, and Mulenga, in press), and tuberculosis is the commonest reason for asymmetric node enlargement, which occurs at classical sites but also in the abdomen, where signs may suggest a retroperitoneal tumour. Multiple sinuses develop (sometimes at more than one site), which was common 50 years ago. Aspiration rarely yields a diagnosis, so a biopsy is needed, as drug treatment is rewarding.

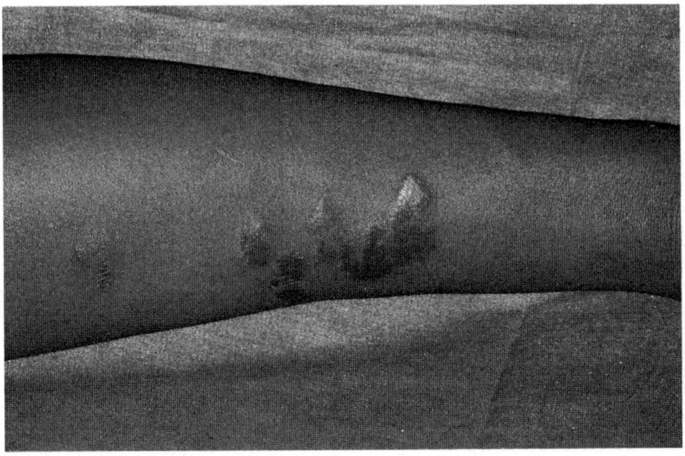

Fig. 4.10. Kaposi's sarcoma: skin plaques.

HIV-related Kaposi's disease

Kaposi's disease was part of the original case definition for AIDS, and in Africa about 95 per cent of patients with generalized signs of antibodies to HIV in their blood (Bayley, Cheingsong-Popov, Dalgleish, Downing, Tedder, and Weiss 1985). There is still uncertainty about the malignant nature of Kaposi's disease (Bayley and Lucas 1990), and because lesions often develop at an early stage of immunosuppression, it may not be correct to equate Kaposi's disease with AIDS. In most patients the diagnosis is obvious from inspection of typical oral or cutaneous plaques, so that biopsy is rarely necessary.

The commonest sign of HIV-related Kaposi's disease is symmetrical node enlargement (71 per cent), followed in frequency by dark red or purple patches or plaques on the hard palate, gums, or tongue (58 per cent), and irregular hyperpigmented plaques on the skin (40 per cent) (Fig. 4.10; Bayley 1988). Unlike endemic African Kaposi's sarcoma, skin lesions occur (often symmetrically) on the face, trunk, or proximal parts of limbs rather than on hands and feet, and may show the influence of physical factors (Langer's lines or pressure). This behaviour is difficult to explain if Kaposi's disease is indeed sarcomatous (Bayley 1991). There is never an identifiable primary and at first presentation there are always multiple lesions at many sites and in several different tissues. In Lusaka two adults developed acute obstructive intussusception due to multiple Kaposi's disease nodules in the ileum, but endoscopic evidence suggests that more than half of all patients with African Kaposi's disease have multiple gut nodules, so this complication is surprisingly rare (Khorshid, Erzingatzian, Watters, and Bayley 1987).

HIV-associated tumours

In the West there is a well-established association between malignant lymphomas of B-cell origin and HIV infection, but this association, although present, is less frequent in Africa. Anecdotal evidence suggests that other tumours, notably carcinoma of the cervix, adult Burkitt's lymphoma, and possibly nasopharyngeal carcinoma, are becoming more common, occurring in younger patients and taking an unusually aggressive course in HIV-infected persons. In pattern II countries, case-controlled prospective studies of these and other common tumours are needed, to confirm or refute suspected associations, and to identify HIV-related changes in tumour behaviour. However, there were fewer malignancies than expected in the Zambian survey of surgical pathology, giving support to the opinion of one surgeon who said that HIV-infected and tumour patients form 'two separate populations'.

Defects of healing and skin ulcers

There is debate amongst surgeons about the quality and speed of wound healing, and the aetiology of spontaneous skin ulcers in HIV-infected patients. Clearly standard wound care and maintenance of a normal haemoglobin level facilitate healing, even in persons with advanced immunosuppression, and skin grafting is often surprisingly successful. However, many wounds are observed to heal slowly, or to heal and then break down again, sometimes after several weeks (Fig. 4.11). Closed fractures heal normally, but in one man with Kaposi's disease a fracture of the tibia healed unusually quickly, probably because of the enhanced limb blood supply evoked by Kaposi's disease. Problems in the management of open fractures are considered below.

Wound breakdown after repair of obstetric fistulae is becoming more common, and a urologist in Tanzania has begun a prospective study of such fistulae. In Lusaka, urologists see an increase in the incidence of perineal fistulae in association with urethral strictures. Urinary diversion results in healing of the fistulae only after some delay, but, once achieved, underlying strictures can be managed by endoscopic urethrotomy in the usual way.

Specific genital ulcers, especially those due to *Haemophilus ducreyi*, are large, aggressive, difficult to treat, and quick to recur in HIV-infected patients (Ansary, Hira, Bayley, Chintu, and Nyawa 1988). Likewise, genital warts recur often and may defy treatment to spread over large areas of the perineum; both problems cause much misery and take up a good deal of clinicians' time.

New pathology

So far, we have described florid examples of familiar diseases and unexpected complications of surgery but, in addition, we see some pathological

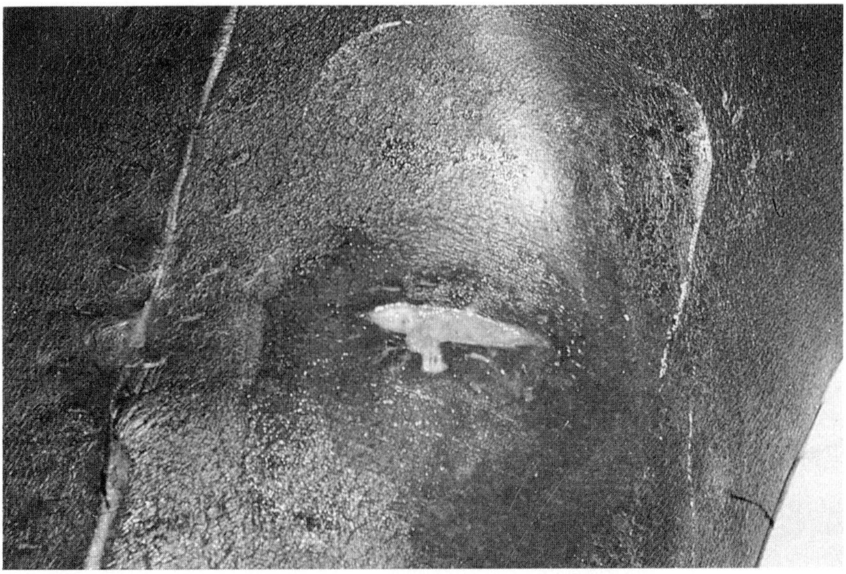

Fig. 4.11. Breakdown of colostomy closure.

processes which appear to be new. For example, a urologist in Lusaka has seen inflammation of the urinary bladder causing microscopic haematuria in HIV-positive men which is not associated with recognized bladder pathogens (B. Elem, personal communication). In Zambia cytomegalovirus-associated enlargement of Peyer's patches is seen in the ileum, which led to perforation and fatal peritonitis in two HIV-infected infants. A new subacute symmetrical osteitis has also been recognized (see orthopaedic section of this chapter).

Does HIV infection predispose to arterial disease?

We suspect that some arterial disease may be related to AIDS as we have seen severe vascular insufficiency of unknown aetiology and multiple aneurysms occurring in young HIV-infected adults, even though arterial pathology is rare in Zambia. For example, we have seen five HIV-infected patients with aneurysms; three had external iliac aneurysms, one had a mycotic aneurysm of the carotid, and one man with Kaposi's disease had multiple aneurysms of the aortic arch and branches. One young woman presented with painful swelling of one leg, but both legs were found to be cool and swollen, with normal sensation but absent pulses. On one leg several patches of full-thickness skin loss followed (Fig. 4.12), but the limb

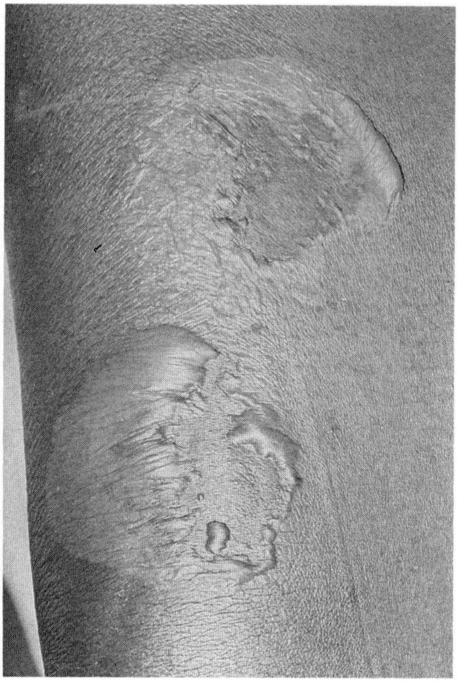

Fig. 4.12. Necrotic skin resulting from arterial insufficiency.

remained viable though pulseless; distal pulses returned in the other leg. Other young people were less fortunate: we have seen unexplained gangrene progress proximally and require high amputations (Bayley 1990).

Conclusions

Some consequences of HIV-infection for surgery which we think need urgent attention, both in debate and in the planning of operational and clinical research, can be summarized:

1. In pattern II countries, all sexually active adults are at risk; this situation could spread within a decade to the West.
2. Where heterosexual transmission is dominant, AIDS destroys families and creates a population of orphans needing long-term care.
3. Economic and social factors have facilitated the rapid spread of HIV in pattern II countries since 1981, and no prevention campaigns which ignore these primary factors will succeed in 'stopping' the pandemic.
4. Once seropositivity reaches 10 per cent in a young adult population (1985 in Zambia) surgeons will notice a change in surgical pathology; when

seropositivity in adults reaches 20 per cent, they must expect HIV-related problems to begin to dominate their professional practice.

5. The response to surgery is modified by HIV infection, and established treatments need re-evaluation: some can be continued with success, others (e.g. use of internal fixation for some fractures) will have to be abandoned.
6. Multiple pathology, sepsis, slow healing, surgical tuberculosis, new disease processes, and increased bed-occupancy are the main issues in central Africa. However, consequences of HIV infection are locally determined by the absence or presence of pathogens (we do not have either *Toxoplasma* or *Pneumocystis carinii* in Zambia) and by social or political factors, such as the health budget and the physical distribution of resources.
7. We need, urgently, several (operational research) studies:
   (a) to predict effects of the pandemic on demand for surgical services;
   (b) to design and evaluate alternative methods for the provision of surgical care in town and country;
   (c) to re-evaluate the goals of individual treatments and of community services;
   (d) to re-consider resources available to meet chosen goals and how already available or new resources could be used more effectively.
8. We should write a 'Surgical pathology of the HIV-infected patient' to be used in parallel with established texts describing the pathology of persons with normal immune defences. This text is needed soon and a draft edition should be written within the next 2 years.

The operational research and re-writing of surgical pathology which we demand are large tasks requiring time, energy, analytical skills, and a capacity to stand back from daily experience. The men and women working in high incidence areas for HIV infection do not lack these resources but find their personal quotas exhausted by large clinics, battles for basic materials (which would be taken for granted in other environments), and by their sadness at seeing too many young people die. If early answers are to be given to urgent questions, then the experience of local surgeons needs to be milked, and their day-to-day observations supplemented by formal prospective studies.

This could be achieved quite quickly, for example by small groups of surgeons (supported by appropriate laboratory staff) who are willing to go to work in large hospitals in high-incidence cities for at least 1 year, preferably 2 years. Such teams would ask questions, record their own and others' observations, provide for accurate microbiology and biochemistry, and share the clinical and emotional burden with local colleagues.

Effects of HIV disease on orthopaedic practice

The rising incidence of HIV infection has profoundly affected orthopaedic practice. The incidence of bone and joint tuberculosis has increased, both in HIV-positive and HIV-negative patients. Osteomyelitis and septic arthritis, until recently diseases of children, are regularly seen in adults, and metal implants are becoming infected years after insertion. Chronic bone and joint sepsis is proving impossible to eradicate and many such patients occupy a hospital bed until they die.

The countries most seriously affected by HIV disease are not those best able to investigate these problems. Cultures of infecting organisms are difficult to obtain. HIV-positive patients are not a homogeneous group as far as their immune status is concerned, and patients may show fluctuations in immune competence. Our inability to investigate their immune status other than by clinical examination has been a major constraint. White cell counts are difficult to obtain while T-cell subsets or skin tests for anergy are not available. Response to surgery is therefore difficult to predict.

Traumatology

In Zambia, a very conservative attitude has been developed to the treatment of fractures because implants are expensive and there are very few skilled orthopaedic surgeons. However, approximately 10 per cent of fractures can be treated effectively only by internal fixation.

Careful examination will often indicate that a patient has HIV disease, but in the early stages the presence of the virus is not detectable clinically. So far, our experience seems to indicate that HIV has no effect upon primary wound or bone healing as long as infection does not occur. A careful atraumatic and aseptic technique, intra-operative wound irrigation, and the use of prophylactic antibiotics will produce a successful result initially. There is increasing evidence, however, that implanted materials are at great risk of haematogenous infection from the frequent bacteraemias that such patients experience (Gold 1985).

Open fractures frequently become infected despite vigorous debridement, lavage, and high-dose antibiotic therapy, and internal fixation should certainly be avoided in affected patients. There is a strong tendency for external fixator screws to become infected, even when all the usual precautions have been taken and the screws have been placed far from the fracture site. Once infection has occurred, it has usually proved impossible to eradicate, despite repeated surgical drainage and aggressive antibiotic therapy. It would seem wise to remove all implants at the earliest possible time as the risks of further surgery are probably less than those of infection of the implant.

The fate of orthopaedic implants

It is well known that a few orthopaedic implants become infected years after insertion from bacteraemia, which may arise from dental manipulations (Sullivan, Johnston, and Kelly 1990) or from other sites of sepsis. The risk of such infection is greatly increased in HIV-positive patients and it may well be in these patients that all implanted materials will become infected in time.

In Lusaka during the past year, late infection has necessitated removal of two hip prostheses, a Smith-Petersen pin, a Kuntscher nail, and three plates and screws which have become infected with a variety of organisms at between 1 and 13 years after insertion. The infecting organisms have included *Proteus*, *Pseudomonas* and non-typhoid *Salmonella* species, as well as *Staphylococcus aureus*. Characteristically, there has been bone resorption with a remarkable lack of periosteal new bone formation. The sepsis has proved difficult to eradicate and continued until death in several patients, and followed a relapsing course in others.

Haematogenous osteomyelitis and septic arthritis

Before the HIV epidemic, we saw occasional cases of haematogenous osteomyelitis in adults, but invariably the pelvis and vertebrae were the affected bones. Adult haematogenous septic arthritis was usually confined to the knees and due to gonococcal infection.

Over the past 3 years, haematogenous osteomyelitis of the long bones has become quite common in HIV-positive adults. The upper metaphysis of the tibia and the lower metaphysis of the femur, with early diaphyseal spread, have been the areas most frequently involved. The knee is often infected by direct extension. The onset is subacute and there is a strong tendency for the condition to become bilateral and symmetrical. There is very little periosteal reaction or new bone formation, but lysis of cancellous and cortical bone occurs from within the medullary cavity with little tendency to form sequestra. Those cases presenting soon after onset have produced cultures of non-typhoid *Salmonella* species from the pus, while others have produced mixed cultures of staphylococcal and coliform organisms. Despite surgical drainage and high doses of appropriate antibiotics, the illness runs a chronic and relapsing course, and so far we have been unable to eradicate these infections.

Bone and joint tuberculosis

There has been a significant increase in all forms of tuberculosis since the HIV epidemic began. More than 60 per cent of tuberculous patients are HIV positive (Elliott, Luo, Tembo, Steenbergen, Machiels, Probee, Nunn, Hayes, and McAdam, 1991).

Five years ago, our orthopaedic wards usually contained one or two patients with spinal tuberculosis (one of whom would be a child) and one patient with tuberculosis of another major joint. Currently, the number of such patients has more than doubled, related to an increase of HIV-infected adults.

Some HIV-positive patients were seen with recurrence of spinal tuberculosis which had been effectively treated and had been quiescent for up to 30 years. One such patient presented with complete paraplegia, showed no response to conventional antituberculous chemotherapy and developed huge pressure sores before she could be operated on.

In HIV-positive patients, bone and joint tuberculosis tends to progress rapidly. The patients have very high sedimentation rates and are Mantoux negative with a poor lymphocyte response. Those with spinal or large-joint tuberculosis generally show a poor response to antituberculous drug therapy. Some show an initial improvement and then relapse.

We have not attempted radical surgery for spinal tuberculosis in HIV-positive patients because of the theoretical possibilities of dissemination of the tuberculosis or of worsening the course of the HIV disease by the stress of thoracotomy or other major surgery (Okong 1988).

There is a distinct tendency for all spinal bone infections to be labelled as tuberculous and treated as such. It is increasingly apparent that, especially in the immune-compromised patient, an accurate bacteriological diagnosis is essential. *Salmonella* and other types of bone infection cannot be differentiated from tuberculosis on clinical or radiological grounds (Govender and Chotai 1990), so open or needle biopsy is mandatory.

Polyarthropathy

Typical rheumatoid arthritis is rare in Zambia, but polyarthropathy (usually affecting the knees, ankles, elbows, and wrists) is regularly seen. The onset is insidious, and the disease runs a chronic and relapsing course. The patients are only mildly unwell, but they have a raised sedimentation rate and negative rheumatoid serology. We have been unable to culture any organisms from the joint effusions and the synovial biopsies have shown only chronic, non-specific inflammation. We have assumed that this is a variation of rheumatoid arthritis or Reiter's disease. Over the past 3 years, we have seen far more patients with this syndrome and most of them are HIV positive. Although it is possible that these cases of polyarthropathy are due to infection with an organism which we have not yet detected, our impression is that they are a rheumatoid-like disease, and it seems that this has become a common orthopaedic presentation of HIV-positive patients.

Neurological problems in HIV disease

A considerable variety of neurological problems have now been documented in HIV disease. Spinal disease may mimic a prolapsed disc (Crawfurd,

Baird, and Clark 1987), and a sudden onset of complete paraplegia is not uncommon (Byarumanga, 1987; Dhaffala-Adupa, Kiryabwire, Carswell, Kahsw, and Yuri 1987). The latter patients show no evidence of a spinal block; they have normal myelograms and no evidence of infection in the cerebrospinal fluid. HIV-positive patients with paraplegia frequently develop huge decubitus ulcers and rapidly die from a combination of blood and protein loss and septicaemia.

Herpes zoster infection is very common in HIV-positive patients. The rash is usually severe and may cover several adjacent dermatomes. The limb dermatomes are frequently affected and the limb is often weakened with marked muscle wasting. Occasionally, there may be severe joint pains and tenderness with marked osteoporosis reminiscent of Sudeck's atrophy, which continues long after the rash has healed. Whether this response is due to disuse atrophy of a painful limb, or whether there is direct viral involvement of the motor nerves, is uncertain.

Conclusion

In areas where a significant proportion of the adult population now carries the human immunodeficiency virus, orthopaedic practice must change radically. Apart from risks to medical staff, the possibility that a patient is infected with HIV will profoundly affect the methods of treatment available. If HIV infection becomes common in developed countries, the training of orthopaedic surgeons in prosthetic implant surgery and early internal fixation of fractures will become wholly inappropriate. Effective methods of conservative treatment will have to be re-evaluated and re-learnt.

HIV infection in the critically ill

Who should be admitted?

Intensive care does not benefit patients with chronic terminal disease, whatever the cause, so as a general rule patients with full blown AIDS should not be admitted to an intensive care unit. We have found that patients with AIDS-related pneumonia causing respiratory failure (Fig. 4.13) or altered consciousness due to AIDS encephalopathy usually die. Similar findings have been reported from the UK (Deam, Kimberley, Anderson, and Soni 1988) and the US (Schein, Fischl, Pitchenik, and Sprung 1986). In one study a better understanding of the prognosis of critically ill AIDS patients led to reduced admissions to intensive care (Wachter, Cooke, Hopewell, and Luce 1988).

However, a distinction needs to be made between patients dying from AIDS and HIV-positive patients who are critically ill because of associated or coincidental diseases. The latter are likely to benefit from aggressive treatment and should not be denied intensive care (Watters and Wilson 1988).

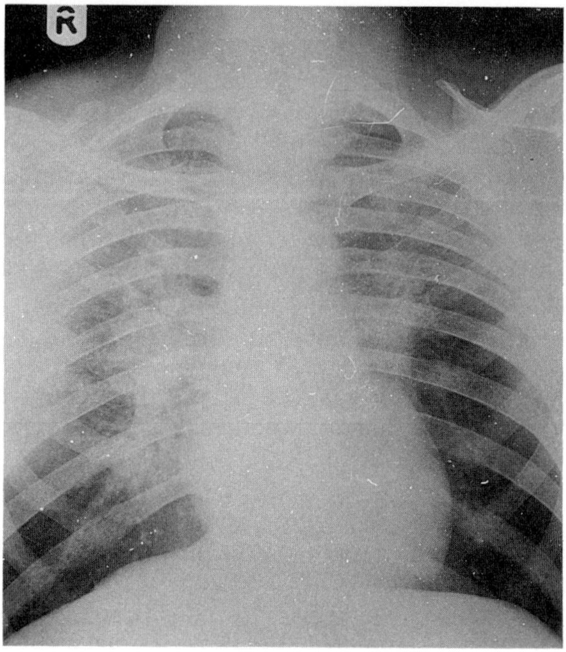

Fig. 4.13. Chest radiograph showing bilateral bronchopneumonia in HIV-positive make aged 36 years. No microbiological or histological diagnosis was obtained but this appearance would also be consistent with Kaposi's sarcoma.

Incidence of HIV infection in critically ill patients

In pattern II countries, the incidence of HIV infection in critically ill patients is likely to be significant. In 1986, in Lusaka, 396 patients were tested on admission to intensive care for HIV antibodies (Watters, Sinclair, Luo, and Verma 1988). Only one patient was known to have AIDS and two others with upper airway obstruction due to tonsillar enlargement had Kaposi's sarcoma proven by biopsy. Forty-three of 240 males were seropositive (17.9 per cent) and 38 of 156 females (24.4 per cent). The highest seropositivity rates were in the 21–30 (28 per cent) and 31–40 (25 per cent) age groups; 26.7 per cent of surgical and 18.2 per cent of trauma admissions were seropositive. Even in pattern I countries the incidence of HIV infection in patients in intensive care is rising (Kelen, *et al.* 1989).

Does HIV infection influence outcome from critical illness?

When all diagnoses were grouped together we found no statistically significant difference in hospital mortality rates between seropositive and seronegative patients. Forty-one of 81 seropositive patients (50.6 per cent) died in hospital compared with 138 of 315 seronegatives (43.8 per cent). However, there is little doubt that some patients with HIV infection fail to respond, or succumb to secondary infection. Since T-cell studies are generally not available in sub-Saharan Africa, a clinical staging system is needed to predict which patients have a good prognosis.

Follow-up of the patients over a 2–3-year period would provide information to determine whether acute illness adversely affects the balance between the patient's immune system and the retrovirus infection. Deterioration in immune status may occur in pregnancy (Pinching and Jeffries 1985) and is possible after major illness.

Anaemia

HIV infection may cause anaemia, granulocytopenia, and thrombocytopenia (Perkocha and Rodgers, 1986; Mehta, Gascon, Tannir, Lambardo, and Robboy 1989). In Lusaka, HIV-positive patients are more likely to require blood transfusion during the management of their critical illness. Twenty-eight of 69 seropositive patients (40.6 per cent) required transfusion as opposed to 45 of 208 seronegatives (21.6 per cent). Where blood for transfusion is in short supply it is all the more important to select carefully who should be admitted to intensive care.

Sepsis

Patients with impaired immune systems respond poorly to sepsis and may not exhibit the normal clinical signs of infection. Close monitoring for bacteraemia, pneumonia, urinary tract infection, and recurrent intra-abdominal sepsis is important. Intravascular and other catheters should be kept in place for the minimum possible time. When sepsis is detected, antibiotic therapy needs to be aggressive and appropriate.

Severe peritonitis arising from female genital tract sepsis

The commonest source of generalized peritonitis in tropical Africa is the female genital tract (Watters 1988). Patients often present late and the mortality rate can be high, particularly when aggressive treatment of severe infection is delayed.

Women with pelvic infection are a high-risk group for HIV infection. This may be because HIV-positive individuals have a reduced resistance to infection and also to increased opportunity of contracting infection due to their own or their partner's sexual habits. Other coexistent sexually transmitted diseases, especially genital ulcers, may enhance the likelihood of becoming infected (Pinching 1986). If female patients with HIV infection have residual salpingeal infection this may become invasive when immune surveillance is impaired.

During 1986 and 1987 we admitted 83 patients with a mean age of 24 years to the intensive care unit with severe female genital tract sepsis (Table

Table 4.4. Causes, outcome, and HIV serology of cases with peritonitis of female genital tract origin.

	HIV positive		HIV negative		HIV unknown			
Aetiology	Lived	Died	Lived	Died	Lived	Died	Total	(died)
Tubo-ovarian	5	3	7	3	4	1	23	(7)
Pueperal sepsis	0	2	4	3	1	3	13	(8)
Post-LSCS	0	2	4	1	2	1	10	(4)
Abortion	3	10	2	6	2	1	24	(17)
Miscellaneous	1	2	2	2	1	2	10	(6)

LSCS – lower segment caesarean section.

4.4), either before or after laparotomy, depending upon their pre-operative condition. They usually presented late to hospital and were severely ill. Sixty-five patients had HIV serology performed and 29 (44.6 per cent) were positive. Of 70 obstetric patients admitted to the unit without sepsis during the same period, only nine (12.9 per cent) were HIV seropositive (χ^2 = 15.27, $p < 0.001$). The seropositive patients had a higher mortality rate, although this was not statistically significant. Nineteen of 29 seropositive patients died in hospital (65.5 per cent) as opposed to 15 of the 36 seronegative patients (41.7 per cent).

Those patients admitted during 1986 were treated without a strict protocol by whichever unit was on duty. Laparotomy was often delayed or inadequate, the incision and exploration being confined to the lower abdomen, and the skin was sutured. The indications for hysterectomy were not clearly understood by some registrars performing laparotomy. Only 9 of 35 patients survived (mortality rate 74.3 per cent). In 1987 a more aggressive surgical approach was promoted and 34 of 48 patients survived (mortality rate 29 per cent). This remarkable reduction in the hospital mortality rate demonstrates the benefit of a more radical and aggressive approach to severe female genital tract sepsis, even when there is an associated HIV infection. However, a trial of antibiotic therapy and repeated re-examination of the patient for 24 or 48 hours is certainly justified for patients with pelvic peritonitis in whom criminal abortion is not suspected and whose general condition is satisfactory. The treatment of pelvic inflammatory disease has been well reviewed by Brown (1982) and de Muylder (1987, 1988), and we have no reason to believe that HIV infection should influence treatment, although it may affect outcome.

The susceptibility of HIV-positive female patients to genital tract sepsis has implications for obstetric management (Pinching and Jeffries 1985). There is need for a study of HIV status and outcome from caesarean section. If it is found that emergency caesarean section tends to be complicated by a septic, gangrenous, and non-healing uterus, then either greater efforts will have to be made to avoid caesarean section, or to perform the operation electively before the membranes have ruptured and with appropriate antibiotic cover. Whether antibiotic cover should be given for uncomplicated, spontaneous vaginal delivery in all HIV-seropositive patients is yet to be determined.

Necrotizing fasciitis and Fournier's gangrene

Fournier's gangrene due to neglected peri-urethral or peri-anal infection was common in the tropics long before the advent of HIV. Although infection may be limited to the perineum and scrotum it may also spread into the abdominal wall or thigh. Necrotizing fasciitis in the female usually arises from the vulva. Patients with peri-urethral or vulval infections are a high-risk group for HIV infection, and many of the cases we see now are HIV positive. Figures 4.14(a) and (b) show Fournier's gangrene in an HIV-positive male after excision which, once healthy granulations were obtained, was later grafted. Figure 4.15 shows an extensive abdominal wall excision for necrotizing fasciitis in a 24-year-old HIV-positive female, successfully grafted 2 months later.

At presentation, the patient is usually critically ill with septicaemic shock. Aggressive resuscitation is required but surgery should not be delayed for long. Penicillin and broad-spectrum antibiotics with good anaerobic cover should be given. Definitive treatment entails wide excision of all necrotic tissue, which includes the overlying skin, subcutaneous fat, and fascia beyond the visible extent of the infection. The edges of the excision (which can sometimes extend from above the costal margin to the upper thigh) must be vertical or sloping, but not undermined since this would enable further growth of anaerobic organisms beneath the margin of the wound. Post-operatively the wound should be irrigated and dressed three to four times daily. The surgeon should expect to perform further excisions within the first few days before the spread of infection is halted.

Autologous blood transfusion

Eshelman, working as a urologist in Tanzania, investigated the safety and scope of autologous transfusion in his practice, where previously 51 per cent of patients undergoing prostatectomy had received homologous blood (Eshelman, Young, and Eshelman, in press). By using autologous blood he reduced the use of homologous blood to 4 per cent in 179 consecutive patients having a prostatectomy. He found that healthy Tanzanians, living around his hospital at an altitude of 3000–6000 feet (900–1800 metres), had haematocrits 5 per cent lower than American Blacks of corresponding age. In spite of this, it was shown that the accepted haematocrit level for an autologous donation of 34 per cent could be lowered safely to 28 per cent.

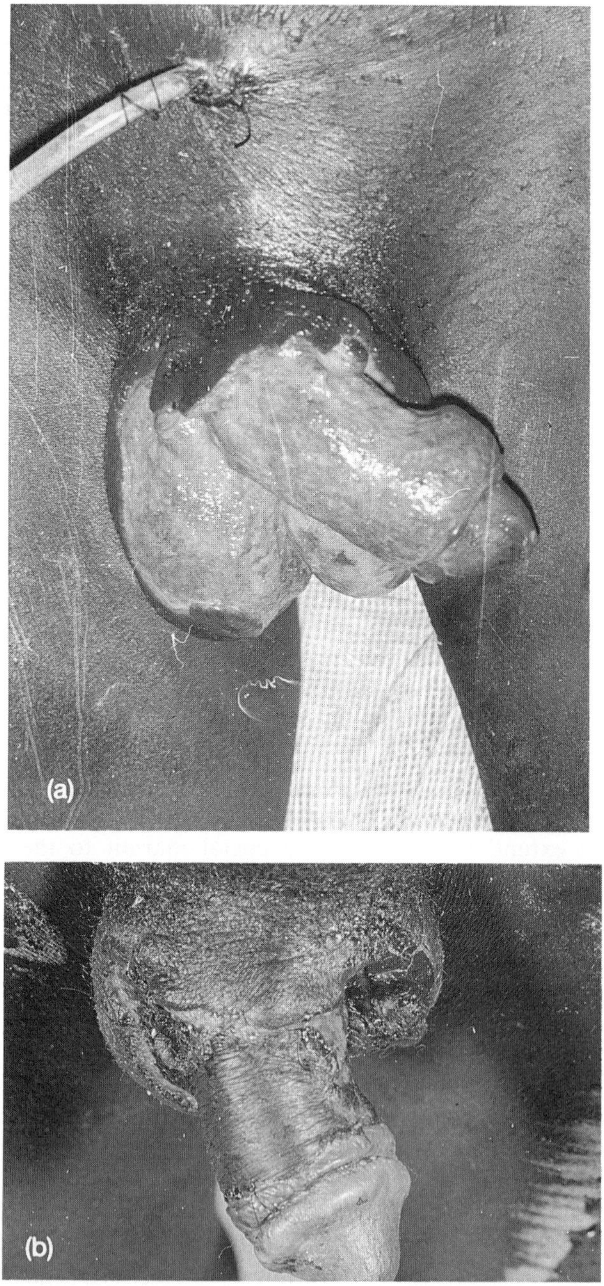

Fig. 4.14. (a) The wound after excision of Fournier's gangrene arising from peri-urethral infection in a HIV-positive male. Suprapubic cystotomy was required to provide urinary drainage. (b) Successful skin grafting in the same patient after 3 weeks.

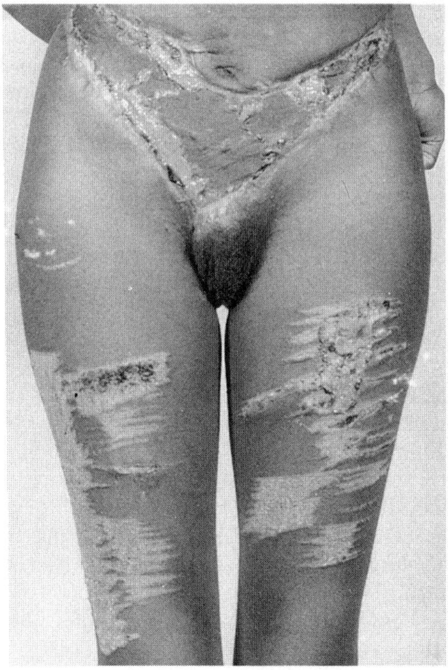

Fig. 4.15. Necrotizing fasciitis of the anterior abdominal wall arising from vulval ulceration and infection in a 24-year-old HIV-positive woman. This required three excisions and 10 days of intensive care before the infection was controlled. This picture was taken after successful skin grafting at 2 months.

In patients with haemoglobin levels in the range of 9.3–11.0 g/100 ml he recommended taking blood at least 2 days before surgery and giving oral ferrous sulphate, but patients who had a haematocrit greater than 33 per cent could safely undergo surgery within 2 days from donation. Patients with unacceptably low haematocrits were given a trial of iron dextran (no allergic reactions were observed) before deciding whether or not to give homologous blood.

Acknowledgements

We are very grateful to colleagues who have shared their experience with us and allowed us to mention the early findings of studies which are not yet complete. In particular, we are in debt to members of the Council of the Association of Surgeons of East Africa whose questions and critical comments have helped us to see new signs and meanings in those signs.

References

Ansary, A., Hira, S.K., Bayley, A.C., Chintu, C., and Nyawa, S. (1988). *A colour atlas of AIDS in the tropics*. Wolffe, London.

Bayley, A.C., Cheingsong-Popov, R., Dalgleish, A.G., Downing, R.G., Tedder, R.S., and Weiss, R.A. (1985). HTLV III serology distinguishes atypical and endemic Kaposi's sarcoma in Africa. *Lancet* **i**, 359–61.

Bayley, A.C. (1988). Atypical African Kaposi's sarcoma. In *AIDS and associated cancers in Africa* (ed. G. Giraldo, E. Beth-Giraldo, N. Clumeck, Md.-R. Gharbi, S.K. Kyalwazi, and G. de The) pp. 152–64. Karger, Basel.

Bayley, A.C. (1990). Surgical pathology of HIV infection: lessons from Africa. *Br. J. Surg.* **77**, 863–8.

Bayley, A.C. (1991). Occurrence, clinical behaviour and management of Kaposi's sarcoma in Zambia. In *Cancer, HIV and AIDS* (ed. V. Beral, W. Bodmer, H. Calvert, C. Dickson, P. Goodfellow, D. Lane, B. Ponder, G. Stark, and J. Wyke) *Cancer Surveys* (ed. L.M. Franks) (in press).

Bayley, A.C. and Tembo, G. (1990). Abstract. Sixth International Conference on AIDS, San Francisco, June 1990.

Bayley, A.C. and Lucas, S.B. (1990). Kaposi's sarcoma or Kaposi's disease? A revaluation. In *Pathobiology of soft tissue tumours* (ed. C. Fletcher) Churchill Livingston, Edinburgh.

Bem, C., Patil, P.S., Elliot, A.M., and Mulenga, R.C. One hundred lymph node biopsies. *Proc. Assoc. Surg. East Africa* (in press).

British Society of Gastroenterology (1988). Cleaning and disinfection of equipment for gastrointestinal flexible endoscopy: interim recommendations of a working party. *Gut* **29**, 1134–51.

Brown, I. (1982). The management of pelvic sepsis. *Prog. Obstet. Gynaecol.* **2**, 274–83.

Byarumanga, R.B. (1987). Three AIDS patients with neurological signs. *Proc. Assoc. Surg. East Africa* **10**, 50–1.

Chin, J. and Mann, J.M. (1988). The global patterns and prevalence of AIDS and HIV infection. *AIDS* **2** (Supplement 1); S247–S252.

Crawfurd, E.J.P., Baird, P.R.E., and Clark, A.L. (1987). Cauda equina and lumbar nerve root compression in patients with AIDS. *J. Bone Joint Surg.* **69**, 36–7.

De Muylder, X. (1987). Management of pelvic sepsis. *Proc. Assoc. Surg. East Africa* **10**, 24–6.

De Muylder, X. (1988). Pelvic inflammatory disease in Zimbabwe. *Trop. Doct.* **18**, 84–8.

Deam, R., Kimberley, A.P.S., Anderson, M., and Soni, N. (1988). Aids in ICU: outcome. *Anaesthesia* **43**, 150–1.

Dhaffala-Adupa, P., Kiryabwire, J.W.M., Carswell, J.W., Kahsw, M., and Yuri, C. (1987). Neurological manifestations of AIDS in Uganda. *Proc. Assoc. Surg. East Africa* **10**, 47–9.

Elliott, A.E., Luo, N., Tembo, G., Halwindi, B., Steenbergen, G., Machiels, L., Probee, J., Nunn, P., Hayes, R.J., and McAdam, K.P.W.J. (1990). Impact of human immunodeficiency virus on tuberculosis in Zambia: a cross-sectional study. *Br. Med. J.*, **301**: 412–15

Eshelman, J.L., Young, E.R., and Eshelman, L.L. Blood transfusion and the use of autologous blood in urologic surgery. *Proc. Assoc. Surg. East Africa* (in press).

Gold, J.W.M. (1985). Clinical spectrum of infection in patients with HTLV III associated diseases. *Cancer Res* (supplement): 4652.

Govender, S. and Chotai, P.R. (1990). Salmonella osteitis and septic arthritis. *J. Bone Joint Surg.* **72**, 504–6.

Hanson, P.J.V., Clarke, J.R., Nicholson, G., *et al.* (1989). Contamination of endoscopes used in AIDS patients. *Lancet* **ii**, 86–8.

Hira, S.K., Wadhavan, D., Kamanga, J., *et al.* (1988). Cutaneous manifestations of the human immunodeficiency virus in Zambia. *J. Am. Acad. Dermatol.* **19**, 451–7.

Kelen, G.D., Fritz, S., Qaquish, D., *et al.* (1989). Substantial increase in human immunodeficiency virus (HIV-1) infection in critically ill emergency patients: 1986 and 1987 compared. *Ann. Emerg. Med.* **18**, 378–82.

Khorshid, K.A., Erzingatzian, K., Watters, D.A.K., and Bayley, A.C. (1987). Intussusception due to Kaposi's sarcoma. *J. R. Coll., Surg. Edinb.* **32**, 339–41.

Mehta, K.U., Gascon, P., Tannir, N., Lambardo, J., and Robboy, S. (1989). Impaired bone marrow in AIDS. *N. Engl. J. Med.* **86**, 623–7.

Melbye, M., Njelesani, K., Bayley, A.C., *et al.* (1986). Evidence for heterosexual transmission and clinical manifestations of human immunodeficiency virus infection and related conditions in Lusaka, Zambia. *Lancet* **ii**, 1113–15.

Okong, P. (1988). Response of HIV-positive patients to surgery. *Proc. Assoc. Surg. East Africa* **11**, 41–2.

Perkocha, L.A. and Rodgers, G.M. (1986). Haematological aspects of human immunodeficiency virus infection: laboratory and clinical considerations. *Am. J. Hematol.* **29**, 94–105.

Pinching, A.J. (1986). The spectrum of human immunodeficiency virus (HIV) infection: routes of infection, natural history, prevention and treatment. *Clinics in Immunology and Allergy* W.B. Saunders, London.

Pinching, A.J. and Jeffries, D.J. (1985). AIDS and HTLV-III/LAV infection: consequences for obstetrics and perinatal medicine. *Br. J. Obstet. Gynaecol.* **92**, 1211–17.

Schein, R.M.H., Fischl, M.A., Pitchenik, A.E., and Sprung, C.L. (1986). ICU survival of patients with the acquired immune deficiency syndrome. *Crit. Care Med.* **14**, 1026–7.

Sullivan, P.M., Johnston, R.C., and Kelly, S.S. (1990). Late infection after total hip replacement caused by an oral organism after dental manipulation. *J. Bone Joint Surg.* **72**, 121–3.

Wachter, R.M., Cooke, M. Hopewell, P.C., and Luce, J.M. (1988). Attitudes of medical residents regarding intensive care for patients with the acquired immunodeficiency syndrome. *Arch. Intern. Med.* **148**, 149–52.

Watters, D.A.K. (1988). Severe peritoneal sepsis. *Clin. Trop. Med. Comm. Dis.* **3**, 275–300.

Watters, D.A.K., Sinclair, J.R., Luo, N., and Verma, R. (1988). HIV seroprevalence in critically ill patients in Zambia. *AIDS* **2**, 142–3.

Watters, D.A.K. and Wilson, I.H. (1988). HIV infection, AIDS and ICU in central Africa. *Anaesthesia* **43**, 980–95.

5. Surgery in patients with bleeding disorders

Sven-Erik Bergentz and Ulla Hedner

Bleeding is one of the most feared post-operative complications. It may result in a prolonged hospital stay and may give rise to a number of secondary surgical complications, and even death (Bergqvist and Källerö 1985). The necessary blood transfusions may cause transmission of disease (Bergentz 1987) and, furthermore, multiple blood transfusions have been found to have an immunosuppressive effect which may increase the risk for tumour spread in surgery for malignant disease (Salo 1988).

Surgeons have a tendency to blame bleeding disorders, rather than deficient surgical technique, when their patients suffer from post-operative bleeding complications. It is important to appreciate that bleeding disorders do occur, to recognize these early and, if possible, before surgery, and to treat disorders correctly. It is however, also salutary to recall that the vast majority of post-operative bleeding complications are caused by errors in surgical technique. In a review of 527 post-operative haemorrhagic complications requiring reoperations, Bergqvist and Källerö (1985) found that only 55 occurred in patients with bleeding disorders or diseases known to be associated with an increased bleeding tendency. Thirteen of these had thrombocytopenia (platelet count below 100 000/ml), six had uraemia, four had haemophilia, two had Ehlers–Danlos syndrome, and one had von Willebrand's disease. In addition, eight patients were on treatment with oral anticoagulants and 21 were receiving platelet-inhibiting drugs. In all the other cases, no other factor than errors in the surgical technique could be held responsible, or the cause was unknown.

This chapter reviews the most common types of bleeding disorders of surgical interest, particularly with regard to diagnosis and to management in connection with surgery.

Normal haemostasis

Haemostasis is initiated at the site of injury of a vessel wall and has been fully reviewed by Nilsson (1979). As an immediate response to injury, platelets adhere to the vessel wall, change their shape, and aggregate to each other to form a white haemostatic plug which may momentarily stop bleeding. The platelets secrete serotonin, causing vasoconstriction and substances which aggregate the platelets (adenosine diphosphate, thromboxane). Specific receptors for a number of coagulation factors are exposed on the platelet surface. In addition, platelets contain a number of coagulation factors, such as von Willebrand factor, factor XIII, factor X and factor V, as well as inhibitors of fibrinolysis, which obviously play an important role in the haemostatic process.

For durable haemostasis, a fibrin plug has to be formed. Fibrin formation occurs on the surface of the aggregated platelets. It is regulated essentially by three plasma systems: the coagulation cascade, the protein C-dependent system, and the fibrinolytic system. These systems consist of circulating pro-enzymes, undergoing activation when attached on the receptor sites of the platelet surface. The last enzyme to be formed in the coagulation cascade is thrombin, which converts fibrinogen to fibrin. According to current concepts of haemostasis, a burst of thrombin is initiated through the exposure of tissue factor at the site of injury, with formation of a complex between tissue factor and factor VII/VIIa (Nemerson 1988). The complex of factor VIIa and tissue factor is capable of activating the final pathway of the clotting cascade, thereby forming the first burst of thrombin. This route of haemostasis is then blocked by a special inhibitor, the so-called extrinsic pathway inhibitor (Rapaport 1989; Rao and Rapaport 1990). However, through thrombin formation, the rest of the coagulation cascade is activated, ensuring continued haemostasis.

Diagnosis of haemostatic defects

The most important consideration which should apply to all patients before surgery is a detailed patient history, including inquiries relating to any bleeding problems, particularly in connection with tooth extraction or previous surgery or trauma, as well as bleeding problems in other family members. Laboratory tests should not be used for screening purposes but only for confirmation of suspicion of a haemostatic defect and to analyse further the nature of this disorder (Eika and Godal 1978; Eisenberg, Clarke, and Sussman 1982).

Laboratory tests

Defects within the initial phase are diagnosed by measuring platelet count and bleeding time. The Duke bleeding time, performed in the ear lobe, should be less than 5 minutes. The Ivy bleeding time is performed on the front of the forearm with a simplate II lancet, and should be less than 12 minutes. Bleeding time is prolonged when there are too few platelets or when there is a defect of platelet function such as in uraemia or in von Willebrand's disease.

The overall coagulation potential is measured by whole blood coagulation time or by measuring the activated partial thromboplastin time (APTT).

The APTT is prolonged in the most important of the congenital bleeding disorders, haemophilia A and B, in patients with acquired antibodies against factor VIII, and in patients undergoing treatment with heparin or oral anticoagulants.

Prothrombin time measures the final common pathway of the coagulation cascade. It is prolonged in pataients with decreased levels of vitamin K-dependent clotting factors, synthesized in the liver. The prothrombin complex is usually measured with one of the commercially available kits such as Stargo prothrombin assay (SPA). A prolonged prothrombin time may indicate severe liver disease, or treatment with oral anticoagulation drugs such as warfarin or antiprothrombin. The commercially available assays used for adjusting oral anticoagulation are standardized using a standard thromboplastin, and the result should be given in the international normal ratio (INR). The therapeutic range is between 2.0 and 4.0.

By a careful patient history and by using the coagulation tests mentioned, when indicated, it should be possible to identify all defects in coagulation and haemostasis caused by a deficient platelet count or platelet function, or by defective plasma clotting factors, including the prothrombin complex.

Types of bleeding disorders

For practical purposes, bleeding disorders caused by coagulation defects can be divided into two main groups: congenital and acquired disorders. The acquired disorders are of two types: they may be drug induced or caused by various diseases. In addition, bleeding may be caused by an abnormal proteolytic fibrinolysis, usually secondary to some serious disorders.

Congenital bleeding disorders

The most common types of congenital disorder are haemophilia A and B, and von Willebrand's disease.

Haemophilia A and B are clinically identical but caused by lack of one of two different coagulation proteins: factor VIII in haemophilia A, and factor IX in haemophilia B. Von Willebrand's disease is due to a defect in the factor VIII complex, resulting in deficient platelet function. Haemophilia A and B are clinically different in all respects from von Willebrand's disease, as seen in Table 5.1. Haemophilia, being a disorder of plasma coagulation factors, has normal platelet function and therefore normal bleeding time but prolonged coagulation time (Nilsson, Hedner, Ahlberg, Larsson, and Bergentz 1977). Von Willebrand's disease, being a disorder in platelet function, exhibits a prolonged bleeding time but usually has a normal coagulation time (Nilsson, Bergentz, and Larson 1979). This explains why haemophilia is dominated by bleeding into major joints and muscles while

Table 5.1. Clinical differences in haemophilia and von Willebrand's disease.

	Haemophilia	von Willebrand's disease
Heredity	Sex linked	Autosomal dominant
Course	Constant	Spontaneous improvement
Platelet function	Normal	Impaired
Bleeding time	Normal	Prolonged
Coagulation time	Prolonged	Normal (prolonged)
Type of haemorrhage	Joint and muscle bleeding	Bleeding from mucous membranes
Effect of factor VIII infusion	Immediate	Protracted

von Willebrand's disease is characterized by petechial haemorrhages and bleeding from mucous membranes.

Of even more importance for the surgeon is the knowledge of differences between severe haemophilia and mild or moderate haemophilia, as stressed by Nilsson and colleagues (1977). Severe haemophilia implies that the plasma concentration of factor VIII (IX) is less than 1 per cent of normal, which results in spontaneous haemorrhages usually starting in early infancy, leading to severe abnormalities in joints, muscles, and tendons, and often death from intracranial haemorrhage. These patients always know about their disease and are very anxious to talk about it before undergoing any type of procedure, and the bleeding problem should never come as a surprise to the surgeon. This is in marked contrast to patients with mild haemophilia, having a concentration of factor VIII (IX) of 5–25 per cent. These patients are usually not diagnosed until exposed to surgery, tooth extraction, or major trauma, and are therefore often undiagnosed even in later life. A careful history, including a family history, is important for diagnosis.

Management of patients with haemophilia and von Willebrand's disease

If the diagnosis has already been made, surgery should be performed in a hospital with a fully equipped coagulation laboratory and a team of doctors, nurses, and physiotherapists with experience of handling the problems presented by these patients. The principle for substitution therapy before and after operation is to give factor VIII in haemophilia A and von Willebrand's disease, and factor IX complex in haemophilia B, in a dose that restores coagulation to normal. It is important to continue this therapy until the wound has completely healed, and for up to 4 weeks for major surgery in severe haemophilia. In minor surgery and in mild haemophilia, this treatment period can be shortened (Nilsson *et al.* 1977).

Acquired bleeding disorders caused by drugs

The most common type of acquired bleeding disorders are iatrogenic, caused by drugs either inhibiting the platelet function or affecting the coagulation system.

Drugs inhibiting platelet function

A number of drugs interfere with platelets and their function. These include antithrombotic/analgesic drugs, antibiotics, and chemotherapeutics. In most cases the effect is without clinical significance. Acetyl salicylic acid (ASA) and dextran are, however, drugs with an effect on platelet function which is sometimes of clinical importance.

ASA causes, in some individuals, a significant prolongation of the bleeding time even when given in clinical doses (Ferraris and Swanson 1983). This prolongation is irreversible and lasts throughout the life of the platelets, which is almost 10 days. ASA inhibits the formation of thromboxane and prostacyclin by interfering with arachidonic acid metabolism. Clinical problems for the surgeon are relatively unusual, except in some cases in neurosurgery and in microsurgical procedures in the middle ear, where exact haemostasis is of utmost importance. In these cases ASA and ASA-containing tablets should be avoided for 10 days before surgery.

In most situations ASA is without any importance with regard to overall bleeding potential. Alternatively, the administration of ASA may increase the bleeding tendency in patients with other types of bleeding disorders such as that caused by heparin, or in patients with congenital bleeding disorders; in these circumstances ASA should be avoided.

Dextran interferes with the structure of the haemostatic plug (Aaberg and Rausing 1978), making it more apt to undergo fibrinolysis (Aaberg, Bergentz, and Hedner 1975). Dextran also interferes with platelet function by decreasing platelet adhesiveness with a maximal effect about 4 hours after the administration of dextran. The effect of dextran is dose dependent. In doses below about 1.5 g/kg body-weight during 24 hours, dextran does not cause bleeding problem (Bergqvist 1982), whereas with this modest dose dextran has a well-documented antithrombotic effect, decreasing in particular the incidence of pulmonary emboli and fatal pulmonary emboli. This subject had been reviewed by Bergqvist (1983).

Drug-induced thrombocytopenia is relatively common and sometimes serious. It can be immunogenic or due to cytotoxic effects. Examples of drugs which may cause thrombocytopenia are kinins, kinidin, sulphonamides, and some antibiotics.

Drugs affecting the coagulation system

Anticoagulation drugs are used for prophylaxis against thrombosis and in the treatment of thrombotic diseases. They are given to decrease fibrin precipitation and diminish thrombotic potential, thereby also increasing bleeding tendency.

Two types of anticoagulation drugs are available: anticoagulants (vitamin K antagonists) and heparin.

Oral anticoagulants (warfarin, coumarin) interfere with the formation of prothrombin, factor IX, factor X, and factor VII, as well as protein C and protein S, resulting in the formation of defective, non-functioning coagulation factors (Stenberg and Sundqvist 1988). The gamma-carboxylation of these proteins requires vitamin K and is necessary for the function of these coagulation proteins.

Vitamin K antagonists act on the formation of new coagulation factor, and the effect on the coagulation mechanism is therefore not seen until after 2–4 days, depending on the turnover of coagulation factors. The dose is adjusted according to the prothrombin assays mentioned above; a suitable level is between 15 and 25 per cent of normal. At this level, spontaneous bleeding is relatively rare. In association with other risk factors, such as trauma or surgery, this decreased coagulation potential contributes to an increased risk of bleeding. It is important to appreciate, however, that spontaneous bleeding occurs in not fewer than 10 per cent of patients on long-term oral anticoagulants according to most reports, usually due to an accidental and temporary decrease in the prothrombin level to below 15 per cent.

Heparin or low molecular weight heparin is given intravenously or subcutaneously. Both types of heparin inhibit the coagulation cascade on several levels. A complex is formed between heparin and antithrombin III, which is normally present in plasma. This complex inhibits the final common pathway, particularly within the coagulation cascade which involves factor X and thrombin. The heparin–antithrombin III complex also inhibits over clotting factors. Low molecular weight heparin has a higher bioavailability than standard heparin. It is given once a day subcutaneously for thrombosis prophylaxis, which makes it easier to administer than standard heparin (Bergqvist, *et al.* 1988).

Standard heparin prolongs the coagulation time as measured with the APTT assay. The effect on APTT is much less marked for low molecular weight heparin, and therefore this drug cannot be monitored by recording the APTT.

For treatment of thrombo-embolic diseases, heparin is given at the so-called full dose. For prophylaxis, heparin is given at lower doses. When full dosage is given, there is a marked defect in the coagulation system, causing excessive haemorrhage following even minor trauma, tooth extraction, or minor surgery. Low-dose heparin, used for thrombosis prophylaxis, does not cause such bleeding problems. It has frequently been discussed whether epidural anaesthesia is safe in patients given low-dose heparin. Although the data presented are somewhat difficult to interpret, most reports now seem to indicate that epidural anaesthesia can be used in patients on low-dose heparin without an increased risk for haematoma formation (Löfström 1988).

Management of patients with drug-induced bleeding disorders

ASA and dextran in clinical doses rarely cause bleeding problems except in special circumstances where the success of the operation depends on perfect haemostasis. In emergency surgery in patients who have already received ASA, the use of antifibrinolytic drugs (tranexamic acid) may decrease the risk of bleeding problems.

Vitamin K antagonists may cause problems for surgeons either after temporary overdose, causing spontaneous bleeding, or in emergency surgery in patients on long-term anticoagulation treatment. In these situations, withdrawal of the drugs will result in formation of new, normal, coagulation factors but it will take between 2 and 4 days for haemostasis to become normal. Extra vitamin K can be given but will not speed up the process markedly. In critical situations, when it is important to establish normal coagulation as soon as possible, plasma can be given. Another possibility is to give factor IX complex. This contains a concentrate of all the vitamin K-dependent coagulation factors and is usually administered in severe cases of haemophilia B as described earlier. Factor IX complex should be used only in critical situations because there is a significant risk of transferring blood-borne virus infection, such as hepatitis.

When bleeding problems occur in connection with treatment with heparin or low molecular weight heparin, the first step is to stop heparin therapy. Protamine sulphate can be given as an antidote to standard heparin. Overdose of protamine may, however, produce complications such as an increased bleeding tendency or hypotension (Lindblad 1989). Protamine sulphate can also be administered as an antidote to low molecular weight heparin, but the exact dose depends on the type of low molecular weight heparin given. The dosage should therefore be tested for each drug and used as recommended by the manufacturer.

Acquired bleeding disorders caused by disease

Liver disease

In parenchymatous liver disorders such as severe hepatitis, liver cirrhosis, or after prolonged cholestasis, the concentration of vitamin K-dependent coagulation factors will decrease, resulting in a deficiency in the final common pathway of haemostasis, as indicated by a prolonged prothrombin time. This contra-indicates surgical procedures and may even cause spontaneous haemorrhages.

In addition to vitamin K-dependent coagulation factors, antithrombin III is also synthesized in the liver. A decreased concentration of antithrombin III is therefore an early sign of deficient liver function. Theoretically, a marked decrease of antithrombin III should decrease the bleeding tendency and/or cause thrombosis, but this does not seem to be a problem in clinical practice.

Uraemia

Patients with marked kidney dysfunction always have a bleeding tendency (uraemic bleeding), mostly characterized by bleeding from mucosal membranes. These patients have a normal platelet count, but deficient platelet function, which is considered to be caused by toxic substances accumulating in renal failure or possibly by defects in the von Willebrand factor (Larsson 1971).

Platelet disorder

Thrombocytopenia may be caused by impaired production of platelets in the bone marrow or by increased destruction of platelets (Stenberg and Sundqvist 1988). Impaired production occurs in leukaemia, myeloma, myelosclerosis, and other haematological disorders. Widespread cancer metastases in bone marrow may also impair platelet production.

Increased destruction of platelets in the circulating blood may be immunogenic and caused by a virus infection such as rubella, rubeola, or influenza. In these situations thrombocytopenia is usually temporary. Another disorder is so called idiopathic thrombocytopenic purpura (morbus Werlhof) which is caused by antibodies against platelets and is usually irreversible.

Management of patients with acquired bleeding disorders caused by disease

Liver disease

The deficiency in the prothrombin complex can be substituted by plasma infusion, which does not have to be fresh or fresh frozen. In critical situations, with very marked defects, when the prothrombin complex in plasma approaches zero, factor IX complex can be given with the restrictions mentioned.

Since fibrinolytic activators are normally metabolized in the liver, severe liver disease also causes an increased fibrinolytic tendency. Fibrinolytic inhibitors, such as tranexamic acid, should therefore be given.

Uraemia

Active treatment of the uraemia is important. We have found that kidney transplantation is by far the most effective, but repeated treatments with dialysis may also be of value (Ljungqvist, Bergentz, Leandoer, and Nilsson 1969). Antifibrinolytic drugs can be given to inhibit the lysis of the haemostatic plugs formed. The antifibrinolytic drugs are, however, excreted via the kidney, and the amount given should therefore be restricted and adjusted according to renal function. Drugs interfering with platelet function, such as ASA and dextran, should be avoided or given in reduced doses to uraemic patients.

Platelet disorders

Platelet transfusions are the most commonly used mode of treatment. The recipients of a platelet transfusion, however, soon become immunized after a few transfusions. Platelet transfusion should, therefore, not be advocated merely because of a low platelet count, but solely because of persistent bleeding which cannot be controlled by other means.

When there is an increased destruction of platelets of immunogenic origin, such as in idiopathic thrombocytopenic purpura, steroids can be given. In children, gamma-globulins have also been tried with some success. In chronic cases in adults, a splenectomy should be performed in addition to administration of steroids.

Increased proteolytic activity

Increased proteolytic activity occurs following extensive tissue damage after major trauma, fractures, or burns. All cells contain a number of proteolytic enzymes which are released into the circulation following cellular injury. There are cellular enzymes which primarily activate the fibrinolytic system, as well as pro-coagulant enzymes activating the coagulation cascade, resulting in the formation of thrombin. Some cells are especially rich in fibrinolytic enzymes and other cells predominantly produce pro-coagulant enzymes. Accordingly, episodes characterized by a release of an abundance of fibrinolytic enzyme or episodes dominated by thrombin formation may develop, depending on which organ is traumatized. In most cases, however, both systems are activated and the picture is characterized by proteolytic activity, including both fibrinolytic and pro-coagulant enzymes.

The body has a potent defence mechanism against a systemically increased proteolytic activity, including specific inhibitors, as well as a detoxification mechanism by the reticulo-endothelial system. Therefore, free proteolytic activity seldom occurs, and is in most cases transient. In patients with systemically increased fibrinolytic activity, however, serious bleeding may occur. Such patients have an increased bleeding tendency, characterized by diffuse haemorrhages, particularly from wounds and other sites of injury. Such fibrinolytic–proteolytic episodes are usually transient. Treatment should first of all be directed against the underlying disorder. Single doses of an antifibrinolytic drug, such as tranexamic acid, can result in immediate cessation of the bleeding.

A predominant activation of the coagulation system typically occurs in septic states. This situation may result in disseminated intravascular coagulation (DIC). In these conditions it is important to direct the treatment towards the underlying disease.

Surgical principles in treating patients with bleeding disorders

The surgical management of patients with bleeding disorders is often difficult, requiring the experience of a senior surgeon and preferably a surgeon with a special interest in this type of patient. Surgical judgement regarding these patients is often critical. Surgical symptoms are sometimes caused by the bleeding disorder, or are markedly influenced by such a disorder. Spontaneous submucosal bleeding in the intestinal tract may cause intestinal obstruction, retroperitoneal haematoma may obstruct the duodenum and the common bile duct causing jaundice, or recurrent subcutaneous haematoma may give rise to pseudo-tumours (Nilsson *et al.* 1977). When a surgeon is evaluating a patient with a known bleeding disorder, it is essential always to consider that the bleeding disorder may be causing the surgical problem.

For pre-operative evaluation of patients with bleeding disorders, non-invasive diagnostic techniques are recommended whenever possible. It is particularly important to remember that angiography, performed with intra-arterial catheterization, may give rise to massive haematoma and pseudo-aneurysms. Arterial puncture should therefore not be performed until the bleeding disorder has been corrected.

For surgical procedures, an atraumatic technique with careful haemostasis should be employed. Certain types of surgery, such as gastric resection, mastectomy, and thyroid or parathyroid operations, involve a greater than average risk of post-operative haemorrhage (Bergqvist and Källerö 1985). The use of drains does not seem to help provide information on bleeding complications, nor does it facilitate the decision to reoperate. Of 5518 patients undergoing cholecystectomy, 41 required reoperation for bleeding, but in only seven was the drain helpful in making the decision for further surgery (Truedson 1982). The most important sign of bleeding after intra-abdominal surgery is shock. Very early reoperation is important to minimize the consequences of bleeding. Nevertheless, post-operative bleeding requiring reoperation increases the risk of a number of further complications, including repeated bleeding requiring a second reoperation (Bergqvist and Källerö 1985).

Patients with a marked bleeding disorder, such as severe haemophilia, should also be managed carefully in the post-operative period. It is recommended that the patient stay slightly longer in bed after operation, that operative physiotherapy be given with greatest care, and that sutures be left in place somewhat longer than in patients with normal haemostasis.

Summary

A bleeding disorder is a relatively rare cause of post-operative haemorrhagic complications. In most cases such complications are due to errors in surgical technique and their cause often remains unknown. If the patient suffers from a bleeding disorder, it is, however, important to be aware of the problem before surgery. This is best accomplished by a careful patient history which, if positive, should be supplemented with a limited number of laboratory analyses. We have reviewed the most common types of congenital and acquired bleeding disorders, giving recommendations for precautions that should be taken when surgery is necessary.

References

Aaberg, M. and Rausing, A. (1978). The effect of dextran 70 on the structure of *ex vivo* thrombi. *Thromb. Res.* **12**, 1113–22.

Aaberg, M., Bergentz, S.-E., and Hedner, U. (1975). The effect of dextran on the lysability of *ex vivo* thrombi. *Ann. Surg.* **181**, 342–5.

Bergentz, S.E. (ed.) (1987). Hemotherapy. World Progress Symposium. *World J. Surg.* **11**, 1–124.

Bergqvist, D. (1982). Dextran and haemostasis. A review. *Acta Chir. Scand.* **148**, 633–40.

Bergqvist, D. (1983). *Postoperative thromboembolism. Frequency, etiology, prophylaxis.* Springer-Verlag, Berlin.

Bergqvist, D. and Källerö, S. (1985). Reoperation for postoperative haemorrhagic complications. *Acta Chir. Scand.* **151**, 17–22.

Bergqvist, D., Mätzsch, T., Burmark, U.S., *et al.* (1988). Low molecular weight heparin given the evening before surgery compared with conventional low-dose heparin in prevention of thrombosis. *Br. J. Surg.* **75**, 888–91.

Eika, C.H. and Godal, H. (1978). The value of preoperative haemostatic screening. *Scand. J. Haematol.* **21**, 349–54.

Eisenberg, J., Clarke, J., and Sussman, S. (1982). Prothrombin and partial thromboplastin times as preoperative screening tests. *Arch. Surg.* **117**, 48–51.

Ferraris, V. and Swanson, E. (1983). Aspirin usage and perioperative blood loss in patients undergoing unexpected operations. *Surg. Gynecol. Obstet.* **156**, 439–42.

Larsson, S.O. (1971). On coagulation and fibrinolysis in renal failure. *Scand. J. Haematol. Suppl.* **15**, 1–59.

Lindblad, B. (1989). Protamine sulphate: a review of its effects: Hypersensitivity and toxicity. *Eur. J. Vasc. Surg.* **3**, 348–52.

Ljungqvist, U., Bergentz, S.E., Leandoer, L., and Nilsson, I.M. (1969). Coagulation and fibrinolysis after renal transplantation. *Scand. J. Urol. Nephrol.* **3**, 23–9.

Löfström, B. (1988). Regional anaesthesia and anticoagulant therapy. In *Bleeding and thrombotic disorders in the surgical patient* (ed. H. Renck) pp. 107–12. Appleton and Lange, Norwalk.

Nemerson, Y. (1988). Tissue factor and hemostasis. *Blood* **71**, 1–8.

Nilsson, I.M. (1979). *Haemorrhage and thrombotic diseases*. John Wiley, London.

Nilsson, I.M., Bergentz, S.-E., and Larsson, A. (1979). Surgery in von Willebrand's disease. *Ann. Surg.* **190**, 746–52.

Nilsson, I.M., Hedner, U., Ahlberg, Å., Larsson, A., Bergentz S.-E. (1977). Surgery of hemophiliacs — 20 years experience. *World J. Surg.* **1**, 55–66.

Rao, L.V.M. and Rapaport, S.I. (1990). Factor VIIa-catalyzed activation of factor X independent of tissue factor: its possible significance for control of hemophilic bleeding by infused factor VIIa. *Blood* **75**, 1069–73.

Rapaport, S.I. (1989). Inhibition of factor VIIa/tissue factor-induced blood coagulation: with particular emphasis upon a factor Xa-dependent inhibitory mechanism. *Blood* **73**, 359–65.

Salo, M. (1988). Immunosuppressive effects of blood transfusion in anaesthesia and surgery. *Acta Anaesthesiol. Scand.* **32** (Supplement 89), 26–34.

Stenberg, P. and Sundqvist, S.B. (1988). Drug-induced bleeding disorders. In *Bleeding and thrombotic disorders in the surgical patient* (ed H. Renck) pp. 37–44. Appleton and Lange, Norwalk.

Truedson, H. (1982). *Cholecystectomy with prophylactic intraperitoneal drain. Clinical studies on the discharge, consequence and necessity of prophylactic drainage.* Thesis. Umeå University.

6. Screening for breast cancer

Roger W. Blamey

Breast cancer is a common disease in the Western world. One in every 12–13 women in the UK will suffer from breast cancer during her lifetime, and 50 per cent of these will die from the disease. The mortality rate from breast cancer remains static, despite the introduction of new therapeutic agents. Breast cancer screening has been shown in several population studies to diminish the mortality rate from breast cancer, and appears to be a major advance. Breast cancer screening is therefore now being implemented for all women between the ages of 50 and 65 years in the UK.

The evidence from trials

The first trial on breast cancer screening to be established was the New York Health Insurance Plan (HIP) study (Shapiro 1989). This trial relied upon clinical examination and two-view mammography, carried out on four annual occasions. Forty-one thousand women were invited for these screening procedures and a further 31 000 were identified and followed up but were not invited for screening. The study began in the 1960s and compliance was poor: only 65 per cent attended even one screening and only 40 per cent attended all four. Nevertheless, the trial demonstrated a clear reduction in the mortality rate from breast cancer in the group invited for screening, and this benefit (Fig. 6.1) has been maintained for up to 18 years.

Despite the publication of this reduction in the mortality rate in the 1970s, little notice had been taken of the study from the point of view of establishing breast cancer screening world-wide. In the late 1970s the Swedish Screening Trials commenced their study. Four groups were involved based on Malmö, the 'Two Counties', Stockholm, and Göteborg. Studies varied a little in the age groups included, in the numbers of women studied, in the number of mammographic views taken, and in the interval between screens, which varied from 18 to 33 months. However, they had several points in common. First, clinical examination was not involved as a routine. Second, the studies were largely based on the single view/oblique mammogram designed and shown by Lundgren (1976) as being an effective way of inspecting the breast. The screening methods used were therefore more cost effective than that of the HIP study, since the abandonment of clinical examination, fewer mammographic views, and a longer interval between screens all saved on cost.

The first of the Swedish studies to report was the Two Counties study; at 7

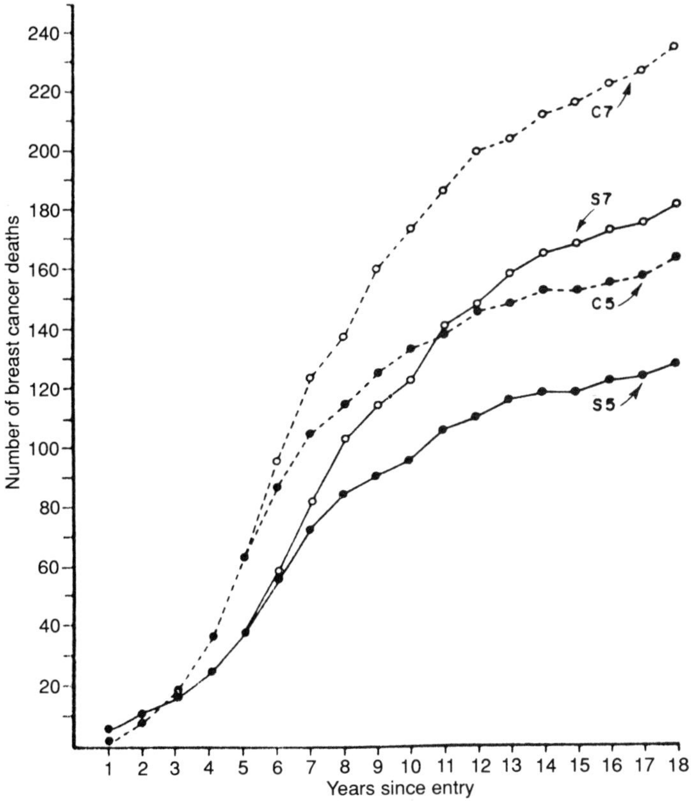

Fig. 6.1. Cumulative mortality rates from breast cancer in the New York Health Insurance Plan study. S, study group invited for mammography; C, control group. A lower mortality rate is seen in the study group, the difference being seen a few years after the study commenced and maintained up to 18 years later despite the fact that screening was carried out only for the first 4 years. [Reproduced from Shapiro (1989) by kind permission of *Cancer*.]

years it was appreciated that the mortality rate was lower in the population offered screening than in the control population not offered screening (Tabar, Fagerberg, Duffy, and Day 1989). The scale of the difference was similar to that seen at 7 years in the HIP study, despite the different method used for screening; it amounted to a one-third diminution of the mortality rate in the study group. The Two Counties trial has been reanalysed at a later date, and by 9 years the difference in the mortality rate between study and control group is even wider. The method of randomization meant that more women were deliberately entered to the study arm and an adjustment has to be made for this in comparing the results of these two arms. Once this adjustment has been made it is seen that the number of observed deaths at 9 years in the women invited for screening was 160; the number that would have been expected in a population of similar size calculated from the observed deaths in the control group was 217. Thus, 57 women who might have expected to die from breast cancer by 9 years had not done so in the study group. Analysis of the Two Counties trial shows that the relative risk reduction was restricted to women aged over 50 years; there was a 40 per cent relative risk reduction in women aged between 50 and 59 years, and a reduction of similar magnitude in women aged between 60 and 69 years. The 40–49 year olds, however, had only a 0.92 relative risk of dying from breast cancer, and this very small reduction is far from being statistically significant.

As the results of the other randomized trials of screening have emerged it is apparent that similar results have been obtained, even though attendance has been less in the other trials; the attendances for the prevalent (first) screen in the trials were: Malmö 74 per cent, Stockholm 80 per cent, Göteborg 84 per cent, the Two Counties study 89 per cent. The only other group to carry out a randomized controlled trial at much the same time as the Swedish centres was in Edinburgh, where trial attendance was only 60 per cent in the initial screening round. Nevertheless all of these groups have demonstrated a relative risk reduction in the mortality rate in the post-menopausal age groups. The Malmö study, at 8 years, showed 2.6 deaths per 1000 women in the study group of women aged between 55 and 70 years, and 3.3 per 1000 in the appropriate age control group (Andersson, Aspegren, Janzon, Landberg, Lindholm, Linell, Ljungberg, Ranstam, and Sigfusson 1988). The Edinburgh study showed three deaths per 1000 women in the study group aged 55–65, years and 4.2 deaths per 1000 women in the control group of the same age (Roberts, Alexander, Anderson, Chetty, Donnan, Forrest, Hepburn, Huggins, Kirkpatrick, Lamb, Muir, and Prescott 1990), and the Stockholm study (Frisell, Eklund, Hellstrom, Glas, and Somell 1989) showed a relative risk reduction of 40 per cent in the 50–64 year olds. All the randomized trials of breast cancer screening, therefore, have given results in the same direction; the population mortality rate from breast cancer is reduced by mammographic screening in women aged over 50 or 55 years, that is, in effect, in post-menopausal women only.

In addition to these randomized trials there has been a British trial on the early detection of breast cancer, which was not randomized but was carried out between different areas of the country — some with mammographic screening, some with education for breast self-examination, and some with no intervention. Two case–control studies have been reported from Holland (Verbeek, Hendricks, and Holland 1987) and one from Italy (Palli, Turco, Buiatti, Ciatto, Crocetti, and Paci 1989). All have shown similar results to the randomized trials: that there is a reduction in risk of dying from breast cancer in the older age groups identified by mammographic screening.

The really important figure is the reduction in mortality rate demonstrated in randomized trials. The mortality rate from breast cancer is a very hard statistic; it is not affected by biases such as lead time (falsely lengthening the apparent survival time) or length bias (which relies on the detection at a small size of cancers that would in any case do well because of their biological nature). A reduction in the mortality rate means that the number of women dying from the disease has been cut by the intervention and can be attributed only to the intervention itself.

How does breast screening work?

Breast screening has its effect, as would be anticipated, by detecting cancers at a small size, possibly before they have metastasized. Perhaps ultimate prognosis depends on the number of metastases, rather than whether metastasis has occurred or not, but this is an academic point. Possibly screening also works by detecting ductal carcinomas *in situ* (DCIS) and treating these; DCIS account for about 4 per cent of the cancers diagnosed in women referred to breast clinics from the non-screened population, but in the screened population in the first screen this figure is about 20 per cent. DCIS left untreated means that there is a one in two chance of an invasive carcinoma appearing later in the breast; intervention to prevent this occurring must ultimately have an effect on the mortality rate from breast cancer. The main effect of screening seems to lie in the detection and treatment of invasive cancers at an early stage. The earliness of their detection is illustrated by Figure 6.2, from the study of screening carried out in Guildford in the UK (Thomas and Price 1987), which shows the average annual incidence of breast cancer and the numbers detected at the prevalent screen and later at the first incident screen. At both screens the numbers of cancers picked up at screening are higher than those that would have been expected to have been seen in any one year. In the years between mammographic screens the numbers of cancers diagnosed are below the number that would have been expected in any one year. This indicates that cancers are being picked up perhaps 2 years ahead of the time at which they would normally be expected to present. The figures from the HIP study (Shapiro 1989) indicated that tumours detected by mammographic screening have a better prognosis than those that are detected by clinical examination at screening, those that occur at the interval between screening, or those that occur in the control group. This amelioration in the prognosis of cancers picked up at screening eventually translates into improved mortality figures.

Mammographic screening and age

The trials of mammographic screening have so far failed to demonstrate a reduction in the mortality rate in women under the age of 50 years. The

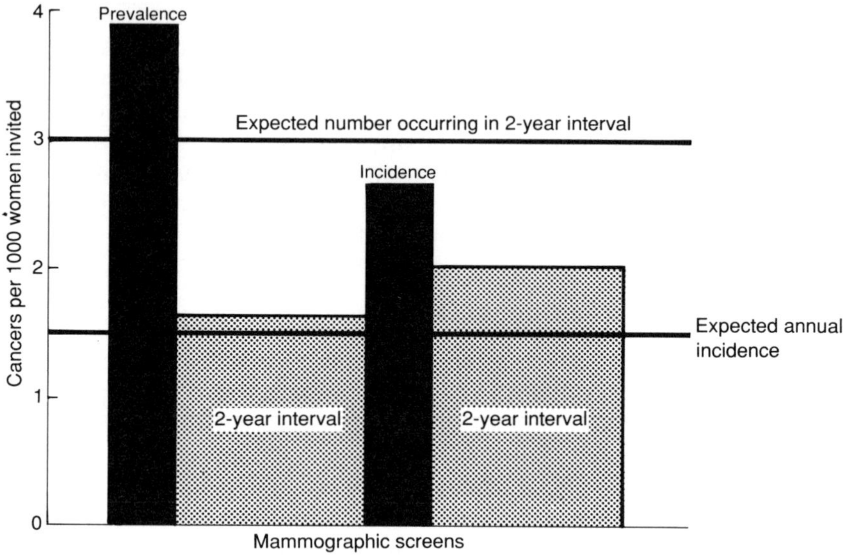

Fig. 6.2. Detection of cancers in the Guildford screening project. [Reproduced from Thomas and Price (1987) by kind permission.]

Two Counties study reported a relative reduction of 0.92 in this age group, in the Stockholm study the relative risk for a 40–49-year-old woman was 1.0, and the Edinburgh and Malmö studies both failed to show a reduction in the breast cancer mortality rate in women under the age of 55 years. The most likely explanation is the relative density of the mammogram in the pre-menopausal woman compared with the post-menopausal woman. The radiologist is then attempting to find a small density against a dense background. An investigation of interval cancers in the Nijmegen programme (Peeters, Verbeek, Hendricks, Holland, Mravunac, and Vooijs 1989) led the authors to conclude that mammographic screening is relatively inefficient at this age. A multi-centre trial is being established in the UK to investigate again the effect of screening at this age.

Recommendations for national screening

As a result of the figures from these trials it was decided in the UK (and a similar decision followed shortly after that in Holland) that national mammographic screening should be introduced (Forrest Report 1987). Screening in the UK is being introduced for all women aged 50–65 years by inviting them personally to triennial screening. One hundred and twenty units have been established to cover the whole of the country. Screening is now well

Table 6.1. Prognostic factors in cancers detected in the Nottingham mammographic screening programme.

Stage	No. of patients	Grade I	Node negative
Disseminated carcinoma *in situ*	28		
Invasive			
Tubular } Tubular mixed }	51	43	49
Ductal NOS	30	6	21
Lobular	17	1	13
Other	10	4	8
Locally advanced (> 5 cm)	8		

advanced and the majority of units involved has now carried out half of their prevalent screen. The prevalent screen is, as might have been expected from the outcome of the other trials, detecting cancers at a small size, which tend to be very differentiated and of tumour types that would be expected to have a very good outlook, particularly tubular and tubular mixed (Table 6.1). In addition, as has been mentioned above, some 20 per cent of cancers are picked up at the *in-situ*, rather than at the invasive, stage.

Disadvantages of breast cancer screening programmes

Financial

When the programme settles into its incident rounds, approximately 1.7 cancers per 1000 women will occur each year; this means that the maximum number possible for detection at triennial screening is about 5 per 1000 women. The proportion of these expected to be picked up at the incidence screening examinations is only about 50 per cent. Therefore, for every 1000 mammograms carried out in the incidence rounds, some 997 will not detect a breast cancer. This has obvious cost implications. However, the essential financial calculation is that approximately 2000 women per annum will have their lives extended who would normally have been expected to die from breast cancer at about the age of 60–70. If a similar calculation is made for women who contract other normally fatal disease at between 55 and 60 years of age, and are kept alive for 10–15 years by medical means, we see that the cost of prolonging the woman's life by breast cancer screening comes to around £20 000 sterling (since the total screening programme will cost around £40 million sterling per annum); in comparison, the cost of extending a woman's life by dialysis and transplantation for renal failure for a 10-year period would be about £300 000 sterling; the costs of extending a woman's life by coronary artery bypass surgery (calculated for the whole of the coronary artery bypass programme) would probably be around £30–40 000 sterling. The costs of breast cancer screening per life year gained are, therefore, in line with other health care procedures.

Open biopsy

Once an abnormality has been detected by mammographic screening, it has to be investigated, and this may lead to open operative biopsy. About 10 women in very 100 screened in the prevalent round do have some kind of abnormality on their radiograph. Radiological experience can bring this down to approximately five women being brought back for investigation of the abnormality. If all five of these women were to receive open biopsy, this would mean that 50 women per 1000 would be biopsied. In the prevalence round, the approximate cancer detection rate lies between 6 and 8 per 1000. Therefore, many more women would need biopsy for benign lesions than the number having cancers detected. By careful assessment (which will be described below) it is possible to equate the number of open benign biopsies to the number of cancers detected in the prevalence round; in the incidence rounds this ratio should be approximately one benign biopsy to every six cancers detected.

Anxiety

The third possible disadvantage is that by inviting women for breast cancer screening a degree of anxiety is generated in the population. This has to be acknowledged, for no programme of health prevention can ever be entirely devoid of giving rise to anxiety. However, I do not believe that high levels of anxiety have been generated in the population. Women called back for assessment are anxious, and the methods of keeping this anxiety to a minimum are described below.

Other possible methods for the early detection of breast cancer

Education for breast self-examination was tested in Nottingham as part of the UK multi-centre trial on the early detection of breast cancer. Women between the ages of 40 and 65 years were invited to education by personal invitation from their general practitioner (GP) or family doctor, and education was carried out by non-medical staff (specially trained nursing sisters and radiographers). Of the 89 010 women invited, 37 788 attended after the first invitation and a further 7 per cent responded to a second round of invitation. After attendance at the lecture if a woman discovered an abnormality in her breast she was able to reattend a self-referral clinic, and in the period between 1979 and 1986 a total of 6862 women were self-referred. At self-referral the women were examined clinically by the same nurses or radiographers who had given the lectures, and by mammography. During the 7 years after the commencement of education, 751 breast cancers were

Table 6.2. Size of breast cancers detected in the Nottingham health district before (control) and after (study) commencement of the Nottingham education for breast self-examination project.

	In situ and < 2 cm	2.1–5 cm and advanced	Not known
Study (n = 751)	351 (47)	348 (46)	52 (7)
Control (n = 751)	281 (37)	402 (54)	68 (9)

Values in parentheses are percentages.
$\chi^2 = 11.46$; 1 d.f.; $p < 0.001$ (tumour size, study versus control group).

Table 6.3. Nottingham breast self-examination project case–control study*.

	Relative risk	95 per cent confidence limits
Pre-menopausal	0.85	0.45–1.60
Post-menopausal	0.66	0.45–0.97
Both	0.70	0.50–0.97

* One hundred and eighty women who had died from breast cancer were each paired with three women who had not died from breast cancer and compared with respect to attendance at breast self-examination lectures. The relative risk of dying from breast cancer was significantly lower in those women who had attended for education.

diagnosed in the population that had been invited. Historical comparison was undertaken of the features of these cancers with the 751 cancers that had occurred in the same population immediately before the education commenced (Locker, Caseldine, Mitchell, Blamey, Roebuck, and Elston 1989). The size of the tumours in these two groups is compared in Table 6.2; it may be seen that the tumours in the study group are significantly smaller than the tumours in the historical controls. Within the invited population a case–control study was also carried out; this showed that women who attended for education had a significantly lower chance (relative risk reduction of 0.66) of dying from breast cancer, in comparison with women who had not attended for education. Interestingly, the advantage was, as with mammographic screening, confined to women aged 50 years and over (Table 6.3).

It would seem from these figures that breast self-examination does reduce the size at which tumours present and, together with the amelioration of the other prognostic factors (grade and lymph node stage), makes it likely that there will be a small impact on the survival rate in the population. However, the number of *in-situ* cancers detected did not increase and the well-differentiated tumours of opproximately 1 cm in diameter, which are detected in the mammographic screening programmes, were also not seen. Nevertheless, breast self-examination is highly cost effective in terms of the cost of diagnosis of a breast cancer. Certainly, from our experience in Nottingham, we feel that breast self-examination should still be advocated to women who are receiving mammographic screening, for with a 3-year interval some 50 per cent of breast cancers will continue to present between screenings and should be detected as early as possible.

Establishment of a breast screening programme

The breast screening programme relies on women being invited to a basic screening examination. In the UK, the invitation is sent out by the patient's GP for the woman to attend for mammographic screening only, without clinical examination. The mammographic screening takes the form of a single-view, oblique mammogram, although many centres are using the conventional two-view mammography (cranio-caudal and oblique) at the first (or prevalent) round.

A delivery point has then to be determined for the screening programme, that is the point at which the woman is released from the screening programme. There are four possible such points: the first of these is for a screening unit to simply send a report that an abnormality has been found to the GP who is responsible for seeing that this is investigated. This is highly unsatisfactory from many points of view. It results in the longest period of anxiety for the woman whilst she is undergoing referral from the doctor and awaiting an appointment in the hospital; also inappropriate referral to a surgeon not used to dealing with screen-detected problems may occur.

The second delivery point is after the breast screening unit has decided whether there is a significant lesion which requires biopsy or whether the woman has no abnormality. This has the advantages that the patient is fully evaluated before being seen by the surgeon; it is possible to obviate the delay in referral in these circumstances by asking the GP to nominate the surgeon, before screening is carried out, to whom he or she would like the cases referred, and inviting this surgeon to the assessment session for patients from the practice. However, this requires that one surgeon is a regular member of the team dealing with screen-detected cases.

The third delivery point is that adopted by the majority of screening programmes in the UK: a surgeon is nominated who takes a full part in the screening unit and its management. This surgeon is expected to attend the assessment sessions in order that he or she may carry out clinical examination and give a clinical opinion on any women found to have significant lesions on their mammograms. This carries the advantage that only one or two surgeons on each unit are attending patients called back for assessment, and this implies that they will gain the necessary experience in dealing with these problems. The surgeons should carry out palpation before any needling procedures are carried out, since they will otherwise be palpating what is essentially a bruise and will not know whether a palpable lesion was present before needling or how large it was. These are important findings in deciding the way in which patients are managed. Organized consultant surgeons should carry out this work themselves and not deputize to clinical assistants or to 'breast care physicians'. The role of the latter would be relegated simply to seeing women who had no significant lesion; women who have a significant lesion have to be seen by the surgeon in any case, and should be seen (as has been pointed out) before any invasive procedures are undertaken. If only one or two surgeons working with the team are operating on the patients, histological specimens will be sent to only one pathologist who similarly will gain expertise on the diagnosis of these rather difficult borderline lesions. Needless to say, the decisions of the pathologist are most important in determining the way in which detected cancers and borderline lesions are managed.

The fourth delivery point is simply to state that the surgeon who is the member of the team will undertake treatment on all cases detected by the unit. The majority of units have adopted the third delivery point, since a consensus of opinion is more easily agreed with GPs and other surgeons on that level.

Assessment

The last three delivery points all require an assessment process to be established within the screening units to investigate mammographic abnormalities. The aims of assessment are to diagnose cancer but also to minimize anxiety during the diagnosis and (as has already been discussed) to keep the benign biopsy rate down to an acceptable level.

The minimization of anxiety during diagnosis is achieved by keeping the interval between the receipt of the letter and the time for a woman to attend at assessment down to the minimum possible (probably 2 days), by establishing a 'hot line' which is staffed by the counselling sister who should be a member of the screening team. Of course, the obvious means of avoiding anxiety is to invite as few people back as possible to assessment; several units are therefore using two mammographic views for their prevalent screen, thereby avoiding calling women back for summation shadows, for example. A further way to avoid women being recalled is to ensure that the film is technically adequate; in static units the radiographer should see the film before the patient leaves the unit and take further views if necessary. The Royal College of Radiologists (1990) has suggested that not more than 10 women per 100 screened should be called back to the assessment clinic on the prevalence round, and probably about 5 per 100 can be achieved.

The benign biopsy rate is determined by the decisions of radiologist, pathologist, and surgeon working together. It is essential that these three individuals confer over each case rather than work separately. By conference over cases it is certainly possible to keep the benign biopsy rate down to one benign open biopsy to one cancer detected in the prevalence round, and in fact several units are running at rates rather lower than this, about 0.8 benign to 1 malignant. The number of benign biopsies carried out in the incidence rounds should be very much lower, because there are previous mammograms with which the incidence films may be compared.

Assessment is for women who have screen-detected lesions but the facility should also be there for the radiographer to call back women with clinical abnormalities, which have been noticed or drawn to the radiographer's attention by the woman when the basic screening mammogram was carried out. For this reason radiographers should spend time in the symptomatic breast clinics so that they can familiarize themselves with abnormalities such as lump, skin tethering, nipple eczema, or nipple discharge. The finding of a clinical abnormality by the radiographer should result in the woman being called back for assessment, even if the mammogram shows no abnormality. As was discussed under breast self-examination, in our own unit women who have discovered a clinical abnormality in the interval between screens are also seen at the assessment clinic.

The assessment *team* consists of radiologist (obviously a skilled radiographer who is able experienced in techniques such as cone views, magnification, and possibly ultrasonography); the surgeon; the pathologist, who also reads the cytological tests; and the counselling sister. Not all of these individuals need to be present for the whole of the assessment clinic. For example, the radiologist at a reading of the basic screen can separate cases into those called back because of a probable technical problem (not all the breast on the mammogram, or a lesion that is likely to be due to summation shadows which needs further mammographic views before being declared normal) and cases likely to need a clinical examination for a genuine lesion. The pathologist would not find it cost effective to attend to give only three or four cytological diagnoses in the whole session, but as long as they are batched this is possible. The counselling sister does not need to see every woman called back for assessment but she could be on call, because some women are very distressed at having been called back, despite being assured that there is no abnormality present; the counselling sister is also needed to talk to women given the diagnosis of cancer. Surgeon and counselling sister together should give this news, since it must be mandatory to discuss with the patient the exact operation to be performed and give the date of admission.

The unit must have the *equipment and expertise* to carry out special radiological views, to carry out fine needle aspiration cytology, and to use stereotactic and ultrasonographic techniques for impalpable lesions.

The assessment team must have clear policies for the *management* of a palpable lump. Impalpable lesions need further assessment and exact interpretation of cytology.

The only *decisions* that can be made for any one woman are that there is no abnormality, that there is a carcinoma present, or thirdly that the lesion is probably normal although this cannot definitely be stated. For example, in this last category are women with small areas of microcalcification, thought likely, but not certainly, to be benign; they are advised to have another mammogram at 1 year before being declared normal.

After diagnosis the assessment team must discuss the management of any cancers discovered. They have the necessary information and the necessary expertise, and it surely should be the team who had these skills who manages, or at least recommends the appropriate management, of the cancers. Furthermore the surgeon and the counselling sister have already achieved same rapport with the woman.

Quality assurance in the screening programme

To ensure that breast cancer screening is being successfully implemented, a number of quality assurance measures must be carried out. In the UK several groups have been recognized which are responsible for making recommendations on quality assurance and providing means of auditing these. These bodies are groups from the Royal College of Radiologists, the British Association for Surgical Oncology on behalf of the Royal College of Surgeons, the Royal College of Pathologists, and the College of Radiographers. The membership of each group is agreed both by the nominating bodies and by the health regions, and the groups are termed 'the Big 18s' (indicating the number of regions concerned).

These groups have laid down guide-lines as to how the various professionals should work within breast cancer screening. They have specified the equipment and resources that units need and have laid down targets on performance. Several of these have been referred to previously in this chapter. Performance indicators have been set on subjects such as compliance, waiting times, number of biopsies, cosmetic effect of the biopsies, accuracy of the diagnosis, numbers of *in-situ* and invasive cancers detected, and their size and treatment. Quality assurance groups are established in each health region in the UK, and are able to monitor whether the targets are being achieved. Indicators also exist for the individual disciplines: for radiographers on matters of mammographic technique; for radiologists on the correct reading of radiographs; for pathologists on the interpretation of borderline lesions; and for surgeons on the methods of treatment adopted. In order to maintain quality assurance an audit programme has been similarly introduced for each discipline (BASO Breast Screening Group 1990; Royal College of Pathologists 1990; Royal College of Radiologists 1990).

Table 6.4. The 'borderline' between benign disease with no increased cancer risk and breast cancers regularly presenting symptomatically.

	Increasing risk
Atypical hyperplasia	↓
Lobular carcinoma *in situ*	
carcinoma *in situ*	
Ductal	
Cribriform	
Comedo	
Micro-invasive carcinoma	
Invasive carcinoma	
Tubular	
Mucoid	
Ductal NOS grade I	
Tumour < 1 cm in diameter	

NOS: not otherwise specified.

Management of screen-detected lesions

The lesions diagnosed at prevalent screen are comprised of carcinoma *in situ*, small invasive carcinomas, or benign lesions with epitheliosis or atypia. These lesions represent a small minority of the breast cases seen before the advent of screening; they are the borderline (Table 6.4) between totally benign disease and symptomatic breast cancer.

In addition to these, a number of clearly benign lumps are discovered, such as fibro-adenomas. Lesions in the breast with all the radiological characteristics of malignancy (smooth regular surface, homogeneous) are usually declared benign by the radiologist and are not necessarily called back to assessment. A number of women are called back who have some slight radiological abnormality around these lumps, and they may be found clinically to have a breast lump. Until recently all palpable lumps, especially in the age group being screened, were removed for full histological examination. However, recently we have changed our policy towards clinically benign lumps. As long as the lump appears to be benign on clinical examination, on imaging by mammography and ultrasonography, and two fine needle aspirates taken 6 weeks apart show sufficient numbers of cells for diagnosis and these cells are benign epithelial cells, then we are prepared to declare the lump benign, leave it *in situ*, and return the woman to screening; a lump showing any of these abnormalities is excised.

Borderline lesions

The 'borderline' lesions are entities that are rarely encountered in symptomatic breast clinics and, therefore, present a new challenge to the surgeon in their management; clinical trials of treatment are being established in these conditions.

Atypical hyperplasia

The finding of atypical hyperplasia does indicate a degree of risk, although without a coincident family history this is not high, giving a relative risk of around five times (Dupont and Page 1985). The risk is akin to that of a woman with a first-degree relative with breast cancer, and these women should receive screening rather more frequently than that of the programme as a whole.

Lobular carcinoma *in situ*

Lobular carcinoma *in situ* is usually an incidental finding made during the biopsy of some other lesion. It does indicate a significantly raised chance of contracting breast cancer over the following 10–20 years, although the cancer may not be at the site nor in the breast that has been biopsied. It is our policy to follow these women closely with annual clinical examination and mammography.

Ductal carcinoma *in situ* (DCIS)

Although the incidence of breast cancer in the UK is about 1.7 per 1000 women per annum, the prevalent screen is at present detecting between six and eight cancers per 1000 women screened. About 20 per cent of these are DCIS. Of the invasive cancers detected, some 40 per cent are small and very well differentiated, usually of the tubular or tubular mixed type. These tumours have an extremely good prognosis and by their primary treatment may be considered as having been cured.

DCIS gives the woman a high chance, probably greater than one in two, of developing cancer, which is usually close to the site of the biopsy. In this case intervention is indicated. The previous results of treatment of DCIS (Schnitt, Silen, Sadowsky, Connolly, and Harris 1988) indicate that whilst mastectomy is not unexpectedly curative in these lesions, lesser operations than mastectomy, whether with radiotherapy added or not, do give a high chance over subsequent years of a further carcinoma, which is likely to be invasive carcinoma, in the affected breast. Work by Holland, Hewndricks, Verbeek, Mravunac, and Schuurmans Stekhoven (1990) indicates that in some 40 per cent of women the disease is widespread within the breast.

It is our policy, therefore, to try to detect those DCIS which are diffuse before surgery. We carry out magnification mammography and any woman considered to have diffuse disease is offered a mastectomy or subcutaneous mastectomy with prosthetic reconstruction. However, in women with lesions that appear to be localized, with excision only is offered. If, on pathological examination of the specimen, several margins are involved and the disease appears to be diffuse, then the patient is readmitted for mastectomy, but if excision seems complete with a minimum of 1 cm clear around the edge of the tumour, then the patient is simply followed up with regular clinical examination and mammography of the treated breast.

There is a clinical trial under the auspices of the UK Co-ordinating Committee on Cancer Research (UKCCCR) on localized DCIS which compares wide excision alone with the addition of tamoxifen or the addition of radiotherapy or the addition of both treatments. For DCIS with diffuse disease, there is a clinical trial under the auspicies of the British Association for Surgical Oncology (BASO) which compares mastectomy with mastectomy and the addition of tamoxifen, looking at any effect in diminishing cancer risk in the opposite breast over the succeeding years.

Small well-differentiated tumours

Small well-differentiated tumours (tubular and tubular mixed) are less often diffuse or multi-centric than DCIS; their management therefore appears easier. These tumours have an extremely good prognosis (Dixon, Page, Anderson, Lee, Elton, Stewart, and Forrest 1985). Mastectomy seems to be over-treatment of these tumours and, indeed, the addition of radiotherapy may well be unnecessary. It has been our policy simply to excise these lesions and to check that a sufficient histological margin has been achieved as for DCIS. There is a clinical trial under the auspices of BASO on these lesions, which compares wide excision alone with wide excision with the addition of tamoxifen, wide excision plus the addition of radiotherapy, or wide excision plus the addition of both.

Conclusion

Screening for breast cancer has been shown to save years of life in women who would have otherwise have died from the disease. The cost of doing so appears to be in line with other health care procedures. However, it is a difficult task and has to be undertaken with care and with the assurance of quality if it is to achieve its aim and if it is not to cause side-effects. Screening is bringing to light a number of lesions at the 'borderline' which the surgeon is not accustomed to meeting. The end-point of breast screening is the correct treatment of these lesions, and suggested therapeutic options have been described.

References

Andersson, I., Aspegren, K., Janzon, L., Landberg, T., Lindholm, K., Linell, F., Ljungberg, O., Ranstam, J., and Sigfusson, B. (1988). Mammographic screening and mortality from breast cancer: the Malmo mammographic screening trial. *Br. Med. J.* **297**, 943–8.

BASO Breast Screening Group (1990). Quality assurance and the assurance of quality in the management of cancers detected in breast cancer screening: the role of BASO. *Eur. J. Surg. Oncol.* **16**, 532–5.

Dixon, J.M., Page, D.R., Anderson, T.J., Lee, D., Elton, R.A., Stewart, H.J., and Forrest, A.P.M. (1985). Long term survivors after breast cancer. *Br. J. Surg.* **72**, 445–8.

Dupont, W.D. and Page, D.L. (1985). Risk factors for breast cancer in women with proliferative breast disease. *N. Eng. J. Med.* **312**, 146–51.

Forrest Report (1987). *Breast cancer screening*. Report to the Health Ministers of England, Wales, Scotland, and Northern Ireland by a Working Group chaired by Sir Patrick Forrest. Her Majesty's Stationery Office, London.

Frisell, J., Eklund, G., Hellstrom, L., Glas, U., and Somell, A. (1989). The Stockholm breast cancer screening trial — 5 year results and state at discovery. *Br. Cancer Rest. Treat.* **13**, 79–87.

Holland, R., Hewndricks, J.H.C.L., Verbeek, A.L.M., Mravunac, M., and Schuurmans Stekhoven, J.H. (1990). Extent, distribution and mammographic/histological correlations of breast ductal carcinoma *in situ*. *Lancet* **335**, 519–22.

Locker, A.P., Caseldine, J., Mitchell, A.K., Blamey, R.W., Roebuck, E.J., and Elston, C.W. (1989). Results from a seven-year programme of breast self-examination in 89,010 women. *Br. J. Cancer* **60**; 401–5.

Lundgren, B. (1976). The oblique view mammography. *Br. J. Radiol.* **50**, 625–8.

Palli, D., Turco, M.R., Buiatti, E., Ciatto, S., Crocetti, E., and Paci, E. (1989). Time interval since last test in a breast cancer screening programme. A case–control study in Italy. *J. Epidemiol. Community Health* **43**, 241–8.

Peeters, P.H.M., Verbeek, A.L.M., Hendricks, J.H.C.L., Holland, R., Mravunac, M., and Vooijs, G.P. (1989). The occurrence of interval cancers in the Nijmegen screening programme. *Br. J. Cancer* **59**, 929–32.

Roberts, M.M., Alexander, F.E., Anderson, T.J., Chetty, U., Donnan, P.T., Forrest, P., Hepburn, W., Huggins, A., Kirkpatrick, A.E., Lamb, J., Muir, B.B., and Prescott, R.J. (1990). Edinburgh trial of screening for breast cancer: mortality at seven years. *Lancet* **335**, 241–6.

Royal College of Pathologists Working Group (1990). *Guidelines for pathologists in breast cancer screening*. Screening Publications, Oxford.

Royal College of Radiologists Working Group (1990). *Quality assurance guidelines for radiologists*. Screening Publications, Oxford.

Schnitt, S.J., Silen, W., Sadowsky, N.L., Connolly, J.L., and Harris, J.R. (1988). Ductal carcinoma *in situ* (intraductal carcinoma) of the breast. *N. Eng. J. Med.* **318**, 898–903.

Shapiro, S. (1989). Determining the efficacy of breast cancer screening. *Cancer* **6**, 1873–80.

Tabar, L., Fagerberg, G., Duffy, S.W., and Day, N.E. (1989). The Swedish two-country trial of mammographic screening for breast cancer: recent results and calculation of benefit. *J. Epidemiol. Community Health* **43**, 107–14.

Thomas, B.A. and Price, J.L. (1987). The Guildford breast screening project: 6 year assessment. *Recent Results Cancer Res* **105**, 67–72.

Verbeek, A.L.A., Hendricks, J.H.L.C., and Holland, R. (1987). Mammographic screening and breast cancer mortality: age-specific effects in the Nijmegen project 1975–82. *Lancet* **i**, 865–6.

7. Soft tissue sarcomas of the extremities

Riad N. Younes, Man Hei Shiu, and Murray F. Brennan

'Any fool can cut off a leg, it takes a surgeon to save one' [George G. Ross (1834–92)].

Soft tissue sarcomas are rare tumours accounting for no more than 1 per cent of all malignancies diagnosed in the US, representing more than 5000 new cases per year (Silverberg, Boring, and Squires 1990) (Fig. 7.1). Soft tissue sarcomas occur in any location in the body. They arise from connective tissues, representing approximately 50 per cent of the body-weight, derived from the embryonic mesoderm.

In this chapter we will address extremity soft tissue (extra-skeletal) sarcomas, which comprise 60 per cent of all sarcomas, with the majority (75 per cent) occurring in the lower extremity (Fig. 7.2). They occur in all age groups and present no sex predilection.

Aetiology

The aetiology of soft tissue sarcoma is not clear. Some tumours develop at the site of previous local trauma, e.g. a desmoid tumour in the scar of a caesarean section. This is a rare occurrence, being identified in only 6 per cent of tumours arising in the abdominal wall (Shiu, Flancbaum, Hajdu, and Fortner 1980).

Exposure to radiation is associated with a higher incidence of soft tissue sarcomas. In a retrospective study performed at Memorial Sloan-Kettering Cancer Center (MSKCC) (1935–85) 16 patients had developed Hodgkin's disease following irradiation. Most were irradiated after 1974 and this recent increase in incidence was attributed to more aggressive radiotherapy regimens and to improved patient survival (Smith 1987). A majority (35 per cent) of post-irradiation sarcomas are osteosarcomas, 22 per cent being soft tissue malignant fibrous histiocytoma, usually developing 10 or more years after therapy. Lymphangiosarcoma is described in organs with chronic lymphoedema due to filariasis (Muller, Hajdu, and Brennan 1987) or to mastectomy with lymph node dissection (Stewart and Treves 1948; Woodward, Ivins, and Soule 1972), with or without post-operative radiotherapy.

On rare occasions, soft tissue sarcoma can occur in patients exposed to

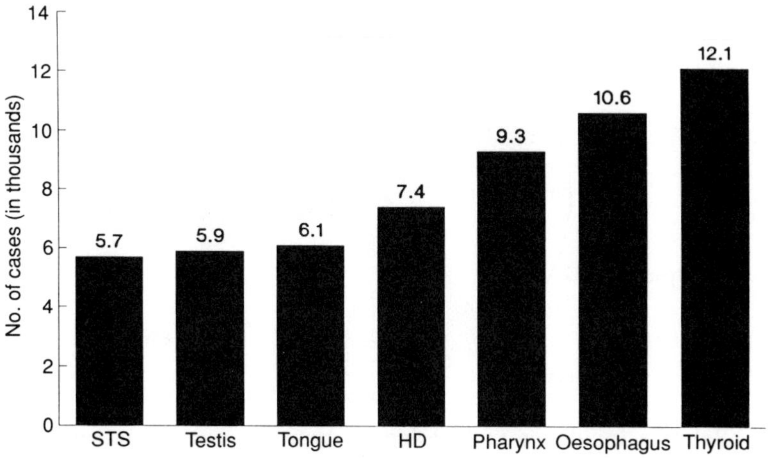

Fig. 7.1. Estimated incidence of new cancers in the US (1990). STS, soft tissue sarcoma: HD, Hodgkin's disease. [Reproduced from Silverberg *et al.* (1990).]

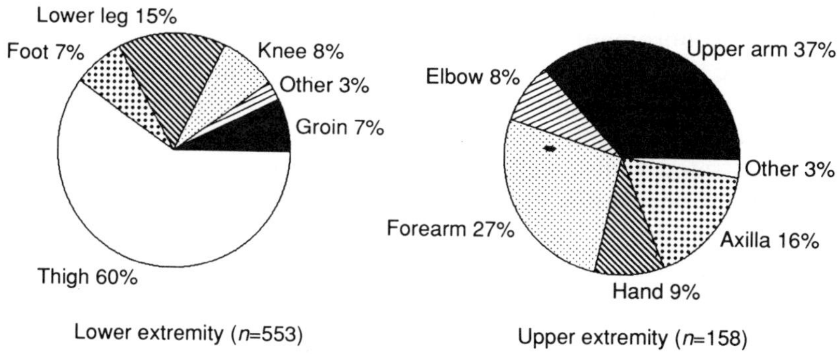

Fig. 7.2. Distribution of soft tissue sarcomas of the extremities in 711 patients admitted to, the Memorial Sloan-Kettering Cancer Center, 1982–9.

known carcinogens (such as polyvinyl chloride and arsenic), as well as to the radiology contrast medium, Thorotrast (colloid suspension of radioactive thorium dioxide). These latter patients develop hepatic hemangiosarcomas (Horta, Motta, Abbatt, and Roriz 1965; Falk, Creech, Heath, Johnson, and Key 1974; Falk, Herbert, Edmonds, Heath, Thomas, and Popper 1981). Active debate continues concerning the role of dioxins in the aetiology of soft tissue sarcomas. Studies have failed to show convincing evidence for a correlation between exposure to dioxins and an increased likelihood of sarcomatous change (Greenwald, *et al.* 1984; Kang, *et al.* 1987).

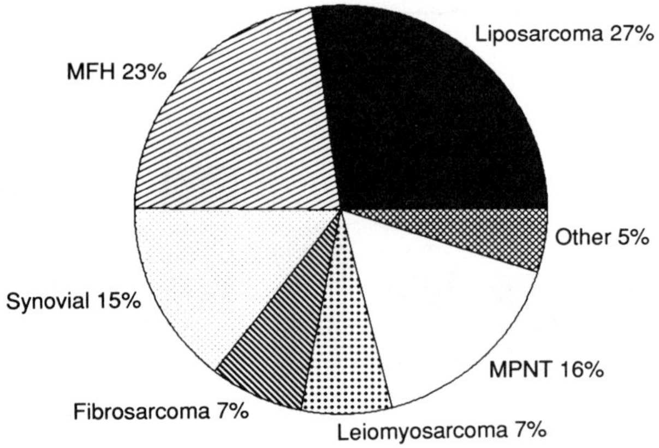

Fig. 7.3. Relative incidence of histological types of soft tissue sarcoma of the extremities in 711 patients admitted to the Memorial Sloan-Kettering Cancer Center between July 1982 and July 1989. MFH, malignant fibrous histiocytoma; MPNT, malignant peripheral nerve tumour.

Some inherited disorders exhibit an increased incidence of soft tissue tumours. Neurofibromatosis and Gardner's syndrome are associated with the occurrence of malignant peripheral nerve and desmoid tumours respectively. Non-random chromosomal alterations occurring in synovial cell sarcoma (Karakousis, Dalcin, Turc-Carel, Limon, and Sandberg 1987) have been demonstrated whilst preliminary reports define genetic abnormalities, the presence of oncogenes, and, more recently, expressivity of the neuroblastoma gene product (Cance, Brennan, Dudas, Huang, and Cordon-Cardo 1990).

Pathological features

Soft tissue sarcomas vary in size, shape, and consistency. Most tumours appear to be well circumscribed by a pseudo-capsule of compressed normal tissues. Extension of tumour beyond the pseudo-capsule is common, either visible or invisible to naked-eye examination. Large, poorly differentiated tumours often show evidence of haemorrhage and necrosis.

Liposarcoma, malignant fibrous histiocytoma, malignant peripheral nerve tumour, tendosynovial sarcoma, fibrosarcoma, and leiomyosarcoma are the commonest types of sarcoma occurring in the lower limb (Fig. 7.3). Most of these tumours (60 per cent) are high grade on presentation (Collin, Hajdu, Godbold, Friedrich, and Brennan 1986). In our institution, such tumours are classified by the pathologist, as showing histopathological evidence of high- or low-grade malignancy, depending on assessment of histological features of histogenesis, differentiation, cellularity, degree of nuclear pleomorphism, mitosis, necrosis, and stromal contents.

The grade of a tumour has been found to be a useful predictor of the risk of metastasis and recurrence. Various investigators have examined other tumour characteristics that may offer additional prognostic information. Ueda, Aozasa, Tsujimoto, Ahsawa, Uchida, Aoki, Ono, and Matsumoto (1989) reported that reactivity of tumour cells with monoclonal antibody Ki-67 might represent a significant prognostic marker in patients with soft tissue sarcomas. DNA ploidy has also been studied as a potentially useful indicator of recurrence and metastasis in soft tissue sarcomas (Kreicberg, Tribukait, Willems, and Bauer 1987).

Clinical evaluation of the patient

Clinical presentation

The most common clinical presentation is with a painless mass whose size varies according to the site of the tumour. More superficial tumours are usually detected earlier, whereas deeply located lesions are discovered only after more extensive growth has occurred. Although usually painless, soft tissue sarcoma can present as an acutely painful tumour, secondary to trauma or spontaneous intra-tumoural bleeding, or with chronic, insidious pain due to necrosis or neural involvement.

Diagnostic evaluation

The patient requires a comprehensive history, the emphasis being on predisposing diseases or exposure to carcinogens and physical examination. The primary tumour is assessed regarding size, site, and depth. Relationships to, and possible invasion of, major arteries, nerves, veins, or bone are noted. Bone invasion in primary extremity sort-tissue sarcomas can occur but is uncommon. Imaging studies by computed tomography (CT) or magnetic resonance imaging (MRI) should be performed for accurate anatomical delineation of the tumour. All patients require chest radiography and should also have a thoracic CT scan if metastasis is suspected, or it the lesion is high grade and large, because the lung is the major site of metastatic spread.

Lymph node involvement occurs in fewer than 3 per cent of all extremity sarcomas. The potential for lymph node involvement is more frequently associated with rhabdomyosarcoma, epithelioid synovial sarcoma, and more rarely in other lesions.

Staging of soft tissue sarcoma

Although comprising a large number of heterogeneous tumours originating from varying cell types, soft tissue sarcomas present some common clinico-

Table 7.1. AJC Staging System for soft tissue sarcomas (American Joint Committee Staging Manual 1988).

T Primary tumour		
	T_1	Tumour less than 5 cm in diameter
	T_2	Tumour 5 cm or greater in diameter
G Histological grade of malignancy		
	G_1	Low
	G_2	Moderate
	G_3	High
N Regional lymph nodes		
	N_0	No histologically verified metastases to regional lymph nodes
	N_1	Histologically verified regional lymph node metastasis
M Distant metastasis		
	M_0	No distant matastasis
	M_1	Distant metastasis
Stage I		
Stage IA	G_1 T_1 N_0 M_0	
Stage IB	G_1 T_2 N_0 M_0	
Stage II		
Stage IIA	G_2 T_1 N_0 M_0	
Stage IIB	G_2 T_2 N_0 M_0	
Stage III		
Stage IIIA	G_3 T_1 N_0 M_0	
Stage IIIB	G_3 T_2 N_0 M_0	
Stage IV		
Stage IVA	G_{1-3} T_{1-2} N_1 M_0	
Stage IVB	G_{1-3} T_{1-2} N_{0-1} M_1	

pathological patterns that allow their grouping and staging in a broader fashion. Proper staging permits a rational formulation of the therapeutic approach and prediction of the prognosis of patients with soft tissue sarcoma. Factors that significantly affect the outcome of these patients include grade, size, and depth of invasion of the primary tumour upon presentation, as well as the presence of regional or distant metastatic disease. High-grade, poorly differentiated sarcomas, of diameter greater than 5 cm, deeply invasive tumours, and the presence of metastases each correlates with an ominous prognosis (Collin *et al.* 1986).

The American Joint Committee Staging System for soft tissue sarcoma (1988) is shown in Table 7.1. A slightly different scheme, utilized at the Memorial Sloan-Kettering Cancer Center, was advocated by Hajdu in 1985, and is depicted in Table 7.2. We have found the latter to be simple to apply in clinical management, and accurate for the prediction of outcome.

Table 7.2. Memorial Sloan-Kettering Cancer Center staging system for soft tissue sarcomas.

Prognostic factors	Favourable	Unfavourable
Size (diameter)	Small (< 5 cm)	Large (> 5 cm)
Site	Superficial	Deep
Grade	Low	High

	Stage
3 Favourable factors	0
2 Favourable and 1 unfavourable	I
1 Favourable and 2 unfavourable	II
3 Unfavourable	III
Metastasis	IV

Management (Fig. 7.4)

Biopsy

Biopsy of a potentially malignant tumour in the extremities should be carefully planned and executed, in order that sufficient pathological information will be obtained without seriously interfering with the eventual therapeutic approach. In that sense the biopsy must encompass an adequate, representative fragment of viable neoplastic tissue (Fig. 7.5).

A variety of techniques can be employed, depending on the clinical setting. Needle biopsy is simple and reliable, especially for superficial, circumscribed lesions without extensive necrosis. Incisional or excisional biopsies are regarded as being superior in the provision of adequate tissue to facilitate planning of definitive therapy.

Under local anaesthesia, the use of a trocar-type needle is preferred, as it yields a larger fragment of tissue for pathological characterization. This may sometimes be insufficient for definitive diagnosis, requiring further needle or open biopsy. It is advisable that, if possible, definitive treatment should not be undertaken on the strength of needle biopsy alone.

An alternative diagnostic procedure is excisional biopsy. Tumour cell shedding and spillage during excision must be minimal, with avoidance of dissection into normal surrounding tissues or organs. In performing such a biopsy, orientation of the skin incision is of paramount importance, bearing in mind the scope of possible definitive and more extensive surgery. The incision on the extremities should be made longitudinally, parallel to the long axis of the limb, in such a way that an *en-bloc* excision of the entire scar, together with the tumour, can subsequently be performed.

Meticulous haemostasis is important, as accumulation and extravasation

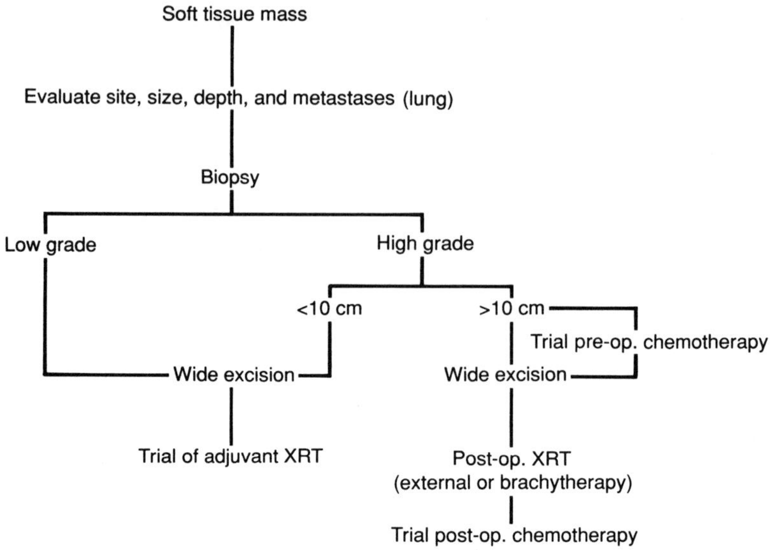

Fig. 7.4. Management of patients with soft tissue sarcoma of the extremities. XRT, X-ray therapy.

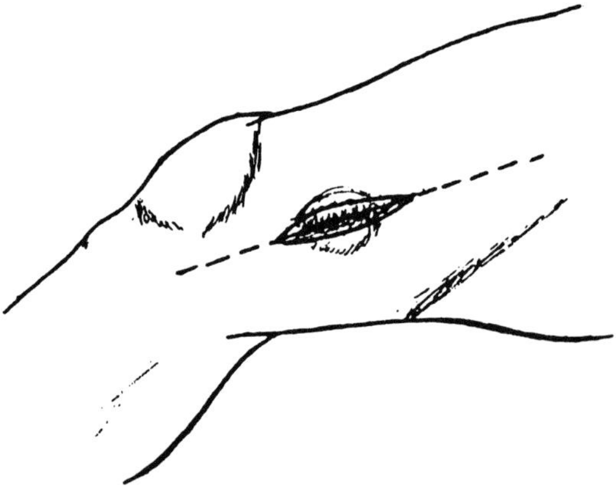

Fig. 7.5. Incision for biopsy of a mass in the extremities, preferentially performed along the longitudinal axis of the limb.

of blood or serosanguinous fluid may result in higher infection rates, and risk the potential spread of tumour cells carried through adjacent tissues by the accumulating fluid. If adequate haemostasis is difficult to attain, the insertion of drains, through the incision, is indicated.

Excisional biopsy is the method of choice for small superficial tumours. For large superficial or deep sarcomas, incisional biopsy is preferred so that dissection is minimal, with less risk of violating deep tissue planes. Careful haemostasis is required and the orientation of the skin incision is similar to that for excisional biopsy.

The anatomical location of the tumour and extent of invasion of adjacent organs must be adequately assessed pre-operatively, in order to plan operative strategy and consider the likelihood of complete resection with wide margins, or the necessity for adjuvant therapy. Patients presenting with tumours abutting or invading important structures (blood vessels, nerves, bones, etc.) must be evaluated, with an assessment made of the relative risks and benefits of conservative versus radical ablation of the tumour. These problems are magnified when one encounters neoplastic involvement of proximal segments of the extremities, shoulders, or pelvic girdles, or of the axial skeleton.

The surgical approach to a locally recurrent tumour usually requires an extensive resection of the recurrence and all the anatomical planes violated by surgery undertaken for the primary neoplasm, often including skin flaps, fascia, and drain tracts. In such circumstances adjuvant supplementary local, and in many cases, systemic treatment is frequently required.

Once the diagnosis and histological characterization of the tumour have been established, a treatment plan can be formulated.

Treatment planning

Three treatment modalities are commonly used in the management of soft tissue sarcoma: surgery, radiation therapy, and chemotherapy. These modalities may be used singly or in combination depending on the anatomical location of the tumour, and whether or not metastatic disease is present, or likely. A knowledge of the pattern of recurrence in patients treated for soft tissue sarcoma is of importance in the design of appropriate management strategy of these tumours.

In a report of 307 patients with complete resection of localized high-grade soft tissue sarcomas treated at the National Cancer Institute, the authors showed a recurrence rate of 35 per cent, with a median disease-free interval of 18 months. Isolated pulmonary metastasis was the most common pattern of initial recurrence (52 per cent) followed by isolated local recurrence (20 per cent).

The outcome of patients with recurrent disease was dependent upon the site of recurrence, rather than on the site of the primary sarcoma. Sixty-two

Table 7.3. Predictors of local recurrence in soft tissue sarcomas of the extremity (multi-variate analysis — Memorial Sloan-Kettering Cancer Center.

Factor	*p*-value
Pathology	
Embryonal rhabdomyosarcoma	0.001
Neurofibrosarcoma	0.002
Presentation with recurrent disease	0.001
Age > 53 years	0.002
Inadequate margins	0.01
High grade	0.04

per cent of patients with a first recurrence were subsequently rendered disease free at surgery. Thirty of these patients (35 per cent) remained free from disease at median follow-up of 28 months after the resection of a first recurrence. An aggressive surgical approach may further salvage 11 per cent of patients with subsequent isolated metastatic disease, but a majority of these patients eventually die with widespread, unresectable sarcoma (Potter, Glenn, Kinsella, Glatstein, Lack, Restrepo, White, Seipp, Wesley, and Rosenberg 1985).

Through extensive studies evaluating patients with soft tissue sarcomas, several factors were shown to be correlated with the prognosis of the patients. Depending on the presentation of the lesion, its location, size, and grade, the prognosis of the patient can be predicted and, therefore, appropriate planning can be undertaken. Some features at presentation are associated with a greater likelihood of local recurrence (Table 7.3), whereas other variables are predictors of survival (Table 7.4). These factors ought to be borne in mind when planning treatment in each individual case.

Surgical excision is the mainstay of therapy for soft tissue sarcoma of the extremities when there is no evidence of distant metastases, complete resection offering the best chance of a long-term, disease-free survival. Management requires careful planning in order to reduce the risk of local recurrence and distant metastases, and yet preserve maximum function and anatomical integrity. The high frequency of local recurrence (42 per cent) after simple excision of the tumour (Cantin, McNeer, Chu, and Booher 1968), and the controversial fact that further treatment of a recurrent tumour is often futile, suggest efforts must be made to achieve a wide margin of resection beyond tumour boundaries during the initial definitive surgical excision.

Both surgeon and patient must realize that the extent of functional loss and the risk of recurrence are closely related to how far the scope of resection exceeds the confines of the sarcoma, i.e. the margins of resection. The size and anatomical relationships of the tumour to vital structures

Table 7.4. Prognostic factors related to survival of patients with soft tissue sarcoma of the extremity (multi-variate analysis) — memorial Sloan-Kettering Cancer Center.

Factor	p-value
Painful mass	0.04
Age > 53 years	< 0.0001
High grade	< 0.0001
Proximal site	0.02
Size > 10 cm	< 0.0001
Positive regional lymph nodes	0.02
Amputation	< 0.0001
Inadequate margins	< 0.0001

obviously dictate the nature of the resection. A margin of tissue of normal appearance must be included to encompass microscopic tumour extensions. The width and adequacy of this margin of resection, as planned and executed, will ultimately determine the degree of functional loss and the risk of recurrence.

When the margin is inadequate and the risk of local recurrence is high, advantage may be taken of adjuvant therapeutic modalities such as radiation therapy for optimal radical excision, with minimal anatomical mutilation. Radiation therapy by external beam or interstitial techniques has been shown to be highly efficacious in ablating minimal gross or microscopic residual sarcoma.

Another issue arising during planning for surgical treatment of soft tissue sarcoma is the necessity or otherwise of regional lymphadenectomy. The low overall incidence of regional lymph node involvement (3 per cent) and the morbidity associated with lymph node excision mitigate against elective lymphadenectomy in the standard treatment of soft tissue sarcoma of the extremities. Nevertheless, biopsy of clinically suspicious regional lymph nodes should be performed and pathologically involved nodes excised. Soft tissue sarcomas that have a predilection for lymph node involvement include rhabdomyosarcoma and epithelioid synovial sarcoma.

The extent of surgical resection can be considered in three categories (Table 7.5). These vary according to the width of the margins of adjacent tissues resection beyond the tumour pseudo-capsule. The size of the tumour or of the anatomical structures removed do not necessarily relate in a direct fashion to this classification. If, for example, high amputation is performed for a tumour that invades the trunk, the procedure might still be considered as a limited margin resection if this margin is inadequate and consequently residual disease is visible or suspected.

Table 7.5. Categories of surgical procedures for resection of soft tissue sarcomas.

Type of excision	Surgical procedures	Surgical margins
Limited margin	Intra-capsular excision Enucleation Excisional biopsy 'Shell-out'	Positive
Wide	> 5-cm margin beyond pseudo-capsule	Negative
Compartmental	Excision of all major compartments involved by the tumour	Negative

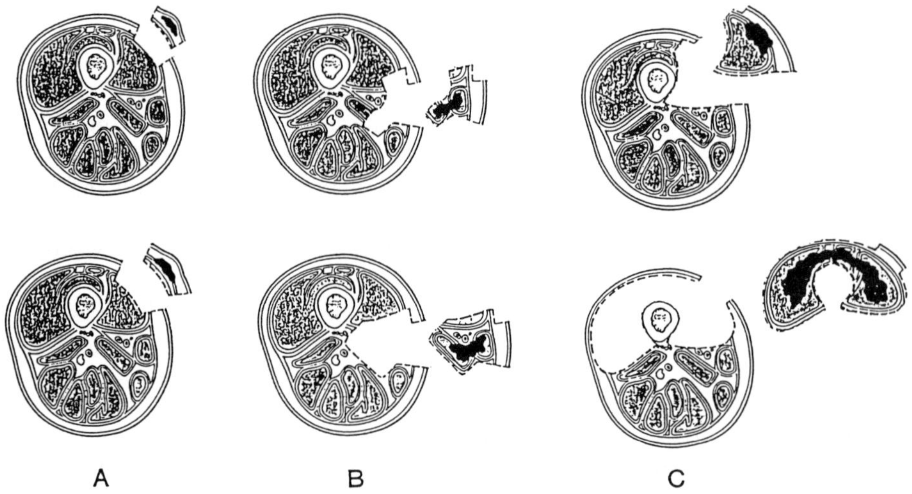

Fig. 7.6. Extent of resection of soft tissue sarcoma (cross-sectional view). A, limited margin resection; b, wide-margin resection; C, compartmental resection.

Limited margin excision (Fig. 7.6A)

Limited margin excision is indicated for sarcomas in close vicinity to vital organs intended to be spared, or in cases where the operative procedure is regarded as palliative. Examples are tumours growing into the popliteal or antecubital areas along neurovascular structures. On preservation of these structures, resection of the tumours will leave residual neoplastic cells at the surgical margins. Such a resection cannot be considered sufficient treatment for soft tissue sarcoma and should be accompanied by adjuvant therapy in the form of radiotherapy or chemotherapy.

Wide margin excision (Fig. 7.6B)

This is the minimum procedure considered adequate for the treatment of soft tissue sarcoma. In this category, tumour is removed with a wide margin of normal adjacent tissues. The specimen is excised *en bloc* without exposing the tumour, or its pseudo-capsule, at any time during the operative manoeuvres.

Although there is no defined adequate margin most surgeons resect a 5-cm width of normal tissues around circumscribed small sarcomas 5-cm in diameter, while extending the resection over wider margins for ill-defined or large 5-cm sarcomas.

Muscle group or compartmental resection (Fig. 7.6C)

This technique consists of completely resecting a musculo-fascial compartment, or a group of muscles containing the tumour. It is usually performed for sarcomas confined within muscle bundles without invasion to adjacent structures. In a recent report, compartmental excision comprised 15 per cent of operations for soft tissue sarcomas of the extremities (Stotter, Fallowfield, Mott, Fisher, and Westbury 1990*a*).

Surgical incisions for the management of soft tissue tumours should be well planned in advance. These should be placed over the sarcoma, in the longitudinal axis of the extremity. In this manner adequate exposure of the tumour, muscles, and neurovascular structures adjacent to the neoplasm is obtained. Incisions for biopsy of suspicious lesions should also be placed longitudinally in order to be encompassed in the definitive resection of the tumour without the unnecessary sacrifice of extensive areas of skin.

After incision of the skin, the tumour should be palpated under the cover of adjacent normal tissues, its extension and boundaries assessed, and the scope of the resection, as well as the planes of surgical dissection determined. Great care must be taken not to expose the tumour or its pseudo-capsule at any time during the dissection, in order to avoid seeding of malignant cells in the resection bed.

The muscle bundles and the tumour should be resected *in toto* and *en bloc* if possible. In many situations, however, the lesion is in contact with neurovascular bundles which, if resected, would result in incapacitating or undesirable disability. A decision must then be made whether to proceed with the resection, or to accept a reduced tumour-free margin in the interests of minimizing loss of limb function. The width of the resected margin and the likelihood of residual disease dictate the necessity for adjuvant local therapy such as radiotherapy.

It is now becoming increasingly popular to perform a limb-sparing resection followed by radiotherapy. The results of several prospective studies show that with this approach the frequency of local recurrence, and the overall survival rate, are comparable to those of patients treated by radical limb amputation.

Difficulties with would healing have often prevented successful treatment of soft tissue sarcomas of the extremities in the past. Today many of these problems may be prevented by the judicious use of reconstructive procedures for skin coverage and prosthetic replacement of blood vessels, bones, and joints. These techniques permit wider tissue excision, better tolerance to radiotherapy, and better aesthetic and functional results. Modern rehabilitation programmes can further enhance function of the extremity following both amputation and limb-sparing procedures.

Results of treatment

Historical developments

The recognition that sarcoma cells tend to spread widely within fascial barriers, which form the compartments of a limb, led to the advocacy of radical resection of the entire involved muscle compartment or, alternatively, amputation. Satellite lesions may sometimes be found in surrounding muscles at a considerable distance from the main tumour mass, and this may explain the high rate of local recurrence in patients treated with marginal excision of the lesion. A report from our institution showed that local recurrence following surgical treatment alone occurred in 18 per cent of patients submitted to amputation, 30 per cent with wide excision, and 42 per cent of patients after simple excision of the tumour (Cantin *et al.* 1968). Other studies have reported local recurrence rates ranging from 48 to 77 per cent (Enterline, Culberson, Rochlin, and Bradey 1960; Martin, Butler, and Albores-Saavedra 1965; Brennhovd 1966). It was thus evident that local excision as sole treatment is inadequate for the control of local tumour growth and recurrence.

Clinical studies have demonstrated that wide excision with adjuvant radiotherapy can result in rates of local control that are equivalent to those obtained with radical resection, without the morbidity that accompanies amputation.

While adjuvant radiation therapy was evolving, outcome in patients who underwent amputation led to the realization that loss of the limb did not guarantee cure. In a series of 139 soft tissue sarcomas of the lower extremity treated by amputation at MSKCC, only 45 per cent of patients survived 5 years (Shiu and Hajdu 1981). Many patients develop distant metastases despite successful local control by amputation. Others survived free from disease and begged the question whether a resection short of amputation could have achieved the same results.

In a randomized study undertaken by Rosenberg, Tepper, Glatstein, Costa, Baker, Brennan, DeMoss, Seipp, Sindelar, Sugarbaker, and Wesley (1982) at the National Cancer Institute (NCI), patients with soft tissue

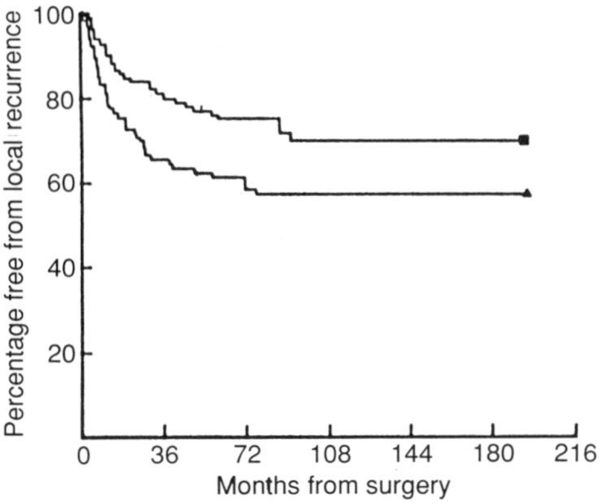

Fig. 7.7. Local recurrence according to the histological grade of the sarcoma. ■, Low grade (n = 116); ▲, high grade (n = 183); p = 0.008.

sarcoma treated by limb-sparing operation plus radiotherapy were compared with those undergoing amputation. The 5-year disease-free survival was 78 per cent in the conservative surgery and radiation group, compared with 81 per cent in patients subjected to amputation; the actuarial overall survival rates were 89 and 88 per cent respectively.

These results and later experience with combined treatment modalities indicate that local surgical excision associated with radiotherapy is effective for local tumour control of many soft tissue sarcomas of the limb and that such combined therapies can produce survival rates comparable to radical limb amputation. Obviously, not all patients need radiation therapy. Small superficial sarcomas can be treated by excision alone without irradiation, provided a wide margin of resection can be achieved. On the contrary, there are patients whose disease is so advanced that it can be extirpated only by amputation.

Survival, local control, and prognostic factors

The outcome in 423 patients treated for localized soft tissue sarcoma of the limb between 1968 to 1978 at MSKCC have recently been reviewed. The 5 and 10-year survival rates after surgical treatment were, respectively, 64 and 54 per cent for the upper limb, 60 and 53 per cent for the lower limb. Important clinicopathological characteristics that adversely affected survival were identified (see Table 7.4), and rates of local recurrence and mortality are shown in Figures 7.7 and 7.8, respectively. Local tumour recurrence in the amputation stump with or without metastases developed in 15 per cent of amputees, whereas 35 per cent of patients treated by limb-sparing resections developed local tumour recurrence.

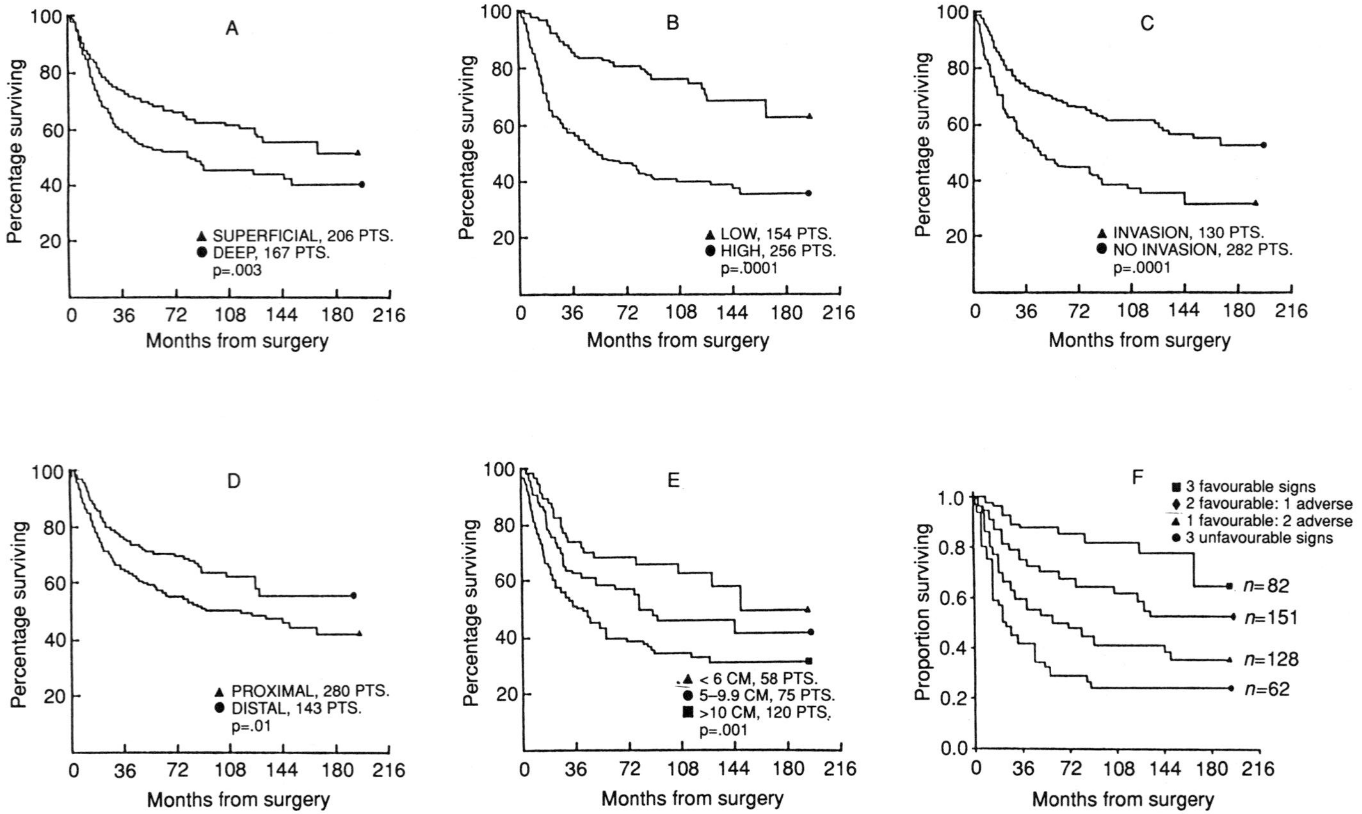

Fig. 7.8. Survival of patients with soft tissue sarcomas according to various prognostic factors: A, depth; B, histological grade; C, neurovascular invasion; D, site; E, size; F, Memorial Sloan-Kettering Cancer Center grading system (see Table 7.2).

Multivariate analysis of clinicopathological factors showed that multiple factors were significantly associated with a shorter survival period following limb-sparing surgical treatment (see Table 7.4). These results heightened interest in multimodality therapy for these patients.

The role of radiotherapy in the control of the local recurrence rate after resection of a soft tissue sarcoma has been previously evaluated (Shiu, Turnbull, Nori, Hajdu, and Hilaris 1984; Shiu, Collin, Hilaris, Nori, Manolatos, Anderson, Hajdu, Lane, Hopfan, and Brennan 1986). Prospective studies demonstrated that a combination of radiation to the anatomical site of the tumour, with a limb-sparing resection, produced similar disease-free and overall survival rates when compared with amputation. Conventional radiation therapy of soft tissue sarcoma of the limb requires the administration of 6000 cGy over a wide field, coning down to a narrower field where gross tumour is sited. These treatments require 5–7 weeks of out-patient attendance whilst control rates of 60–95 per cent have been reported, depending on the size, grade, and other characteristics of the sarcoma. Complications such as wound breakdown, lymphoedema, and bone fracture may arise occasionally.

At the MSKCC, we have developed an alternative technique of radiation therapy in which the tumour bed is treated several days after surgery by brachytherapy (e.g. with iridium-192), through pre-place catheters (Shiu *et al.* 1984). This technique offers several theoretical and practical advantages, including higher precision in the dose distribution and a very short duration of treatment, with only 4–5 days in hospital.

In order to determine the efficacy and potential morbidity of such treatment we performed a prospective randomized study at the MSKCC comparing the effect of adjuvant radiotherapy delivered by brachytherapy in patients who underwent resection of extremity or superficial truncal tumours. Patients were randomly assigned to brachytherapy versus no brachytherapy, provided all grossly visible tumour was removed, irrespective of the width of the resection margin. The local recurrence rate was significantly lower in the brachytherapy group (4 per cent) than in the non-irradiated group (14 per cent). No survival benefit has yet been observed, even though retrospective studies have shown that patients presenting with locally recurrent tumours have a significantly decreased survival rate when compared with the outcome for primary tumours. This might be due to the relatively short follow-up period, 16 months, in the study.

An important observation from this study is that optimal benefit from brachytherapy was seen in those patients with high-grade tumours (Brennan, Hilaris, Shiu, Lane, Magill, Friedrich, and Hajdu 1987*b*). Adjuvant brachytherapy resulted in an unacceptable wound complication rate (48 per cent), when the catheters were loaded with radioactive material between the first and fifth post-operative days (Arbeit, Hilaris, and Brennan 1987). When catheters were loaded 5 or more days after operation, there was a significantly lower frequency of wound complications (14 per cent). We now load irradiation sources on or after the sixth post-operative day, and have markedly reduced the likelihood of serious wound complications (Ormsby, Hilaris, Nori, and Brennan 1989). This policy is consistent with previous observations in the laboratory investigation of wound healing and irradiation (Devereux, Kent, and Brennan 1980).

Adjuvant chemotherapy

The high frequency of lung metastases in patients with resected soft tissue sarcoma directed attention towards the evaluation of systematic adjuvant regimens, in order to decrease the possibility of distant spread. Several studies of adjuvant chemotherapy for patients with soft tissue sarcoma have been reported, the benefits of which are still controversial.

With a single-agent response rate ranging from 20–40 per cent, doxorubicin has been shown to be the drug of choice because of its efficiency against metastatic soft tissue sarcomatous disease (Blum 1975). A correlation between doxorubicin dosage and tumour response has been shown in randomized studies (Schonfeld, Rosenbaum, Horton, Wolfer, Falkson, and DeConti 1982; Pezzi, Pollock, Evans, Lorigan, Pezzi, Benjamin, and Romsdahl 1990). Cardiac toxity, with occasional deaths due to intractable heart failure, is a well recognized, major disadvantage. Several clinical trials have documented significant improvements in disease-free status (Rosenberg, Tepper, Glastein, Costa, Young, Baker, Brennan, DeMoss, Seipp, Sindelar, Sugarbaker, and Wesley 1983; Chang, Kinsella, Glatstein, Baker, Sindelar, Lotze, Danforth, Sugarbaker, Lack, and Steinberg 1988), as well as overall survival (Rosenberg *et al.* 1983) in the patients receiving adjuvant chemotherapy, not confirmed in other studies (Eilber, Giuliano, Huth, and Morton 1986; Wilson, Wood, Lerner, Antman, Amato, Corson, Proppe, Harmon, Carey, and Greenberger 1986; Alvegard, Sigurdsson, Mouridsen, Solheim, Unsgaard, Ringborg, Dahl, Nordentoft, Blomqvist, Stener, and Ranstam 1989).

Recently, in a retrospective analysis of a randomized pre-operative chemotherapy (CYVADIC) trial of patients with large tumours (> 5 cm) and unfavourable histological features, Pezzi and colleagues reported a significant increase in disease-free and overall survival rates in patients who responded to chemotherapy (Pezzi *et al.* 1990). Alterations in the standard regimens were shown to lessen the cardiotoxic side-effects of doxorubicin administration in patients with localized, high-grade, soft-tissue tumours (Brennan, Friedrich, Almadrones, and Magill 1987*a*). Adjuvant trials using drugs other than doxorubicin are currently in progress.

Intra-arterial infusion chemotherapy

A multi-disciplinary approach for the treatment of high-risk, soft-tissue sarcoma with combined pre-operative regional chemotherapy and radiotherapy followed by limb-sparing surgery has been proposed by Eilber, Morton, Eckardt, Grant, and Weisenburger (1984). This regimen resulted in low local recurrence (4 per cent) and high survival rates (65 per cent).

In a recently reported multi-centre study evaluating the effects of combined regional therapy in extremity soft tissue sarcomas, the authors administered intra-arterial infusion with doxorubicin, followed by radiotherapy. Disease-free and overall survival rates at 48 months were 47 and 56 per cent, respectively (Wanebo, Temple, Popp, Douvill, and Yablonski 1990). Eilber and his colleagues are continuing further studies to determine whether similar results can be obtained with intravenous, as opposed to intra-arterial, infusion.

Hyperthermia

The presence of multiple areas within large tumours which are significantly underperfused limit the efficacy of radiotherapy. Hyperthermia is theoretically advantageous when used concomitantly with radiation, whereby an increase in local temperature enhances perfusion of the tumour, and hence its sensitivity to radiotherapy.

A phase II trial has been documented recently, showing an advantage, as measured by the degree of histopathological changes, to twice-weekly when compared with weekly hyperthermia combined with conventional radiation therapy in patients with soft tissue sarcomas treated preoperatively (Leopold, Harrelson, Prosnitz, Samulski, Dewhirst, and Oleson 1989). Whether this will translate into significant impact on response rates or on patient survival rates is still uncertain.

References

Alvegard, T.A, Sigurdsson, H., Mouridsen, H., Solheim, O., Unsgaard, B., Ringborg, U., Dahl, O., Nordentoft, A.M., Blomqvist, A., Stener, B., and Ranstam, J. (1989). Adjuvant chemotherapy with doxorubicin in high-grade soft-tissue sarcoma: a randomized trial of the Scandinavian Sarcoma Group. *J. Clin. Oncol.* **7**, 1504–13.

Arbeit, J.M., Hilaris, B.S., and Brennan, M.F. (1987). Wound complications in the multimodality treatment of extremity and superficial truncal sarcomas. *J. Clin. Oncol.* **5**, 480–8.

Blum, R.H. (1975). An overview of studies with Adriamycin (NSC 123127) in the United States. *Cancer Chemother. Rep.* **6**, 247–51.

Brennan, M.F. (1989). Management of soft-tissue sarcoma. *Am. J. Surg.* **158**, 71–8.

Brennan, M.F., Friedrich, C., Almadrones, L., and Magill, G. (1987*a*). Prospective randomized trial examining the cardiac toxicity of adjuvant doxorubicin in high-grade extremity sarcomas. In *Adjuvant therapy of cancer* (ed. S. Salmon) pp. 745–51. Grune & Stratton, New York.

Brennan, M.F., Hilaris, B., Shiu, M.H., Lane, J., Magill, G., Friedrich, C., and Hajdu, S.I. (1987*b*). Local recurrence in adult soft-tissue sarcoma. *Arch. Surg.* **22**, 1289–93.

Brennhovd, I.O. (1966). The treatment of soft-tissue sarcomas — a plea for a more urgent and aggressive approach. *Acta Chir. Scand.* **131**, 438–42.

Cance, W.G., Brennan, M.F., Dudas, M.E., Huang, C.M., and Cordon-Cardo, C. Altered expression of the retinoblastoma gene product in human sarcomas: biological and clinical correlations. (submitted for publication).

Cantin, J., McNeer, G.P., Chu, F.C., and Booher, R.J. (1968). The problem of local recurrence after treatment of soft-tissue sarcoma. *Ann. Surg.* **168**, 47–53.

Chang, A.E., Kinsella, T., Glatstein, E., Baker, A.R., Sindelar, W.F., Lotze, M.T., Danforth, D.N., Sugarbaker, P.H., Lack, E.E., and Steinberg, S.M. (1988). Adjuvant chemotherapy for patients with high-grade soft-tissue sarcomas of the extremity. *J. Clin. Oncol.* **6**, 1491–500.

Collin, C., Hajdu, S.I., Godbold, J., Friedrich, C., and Brennan, M.F. (1986). Localized operable soft-tissue sarcoma of the lower extremity. *Arch. Surg.* **121**, 1425.

Devereux, D.F., Kent, H., and Brennan, M.F. (1980). Time dependent effects of Adriamycin and X-ray therapy on wound healing in the rat. *Cancer* **45**, 2805.

Eilber, F.R., Giuliano, A.E., Huth, J.F., and Morton, D.L. (1986). Adjuvant Adriamycin in high-grade extremity soft-tissue sarcoma: a randomized prospective trial. *Proc. Am. Soc. Clin. Oncol.* **5**, 488.

Eilber, F.R., Morton, D.L., Eckardt, J., Grant, T., and Weisenburger, T. (1984). Limb salvage for skeletal and soft-tissue sarcomas: multidisciplinary preoperative therapy. *Cancer* **53**, 2579–84.

Enterline, H.T., Culberson, J.D., Rochlin, D.B., and Bradey, L.W. (1960). Liposarcoma: a clinical and pathological study of 53 cases. *Cancer* **13**, 932–50.

Falk, H., Creech, J.L., Heath, C.W., Johnson, M.N., and Key, M.M. (1974). Hepatic disease among workers at a vinyl chloride polymerization plant. *JAMA* **230**, 59.

Falk, H., Herbert, J.T., Edmonds, L., Heath, C.W., Thomas, L.B., and Popper, H. (1981). Review of four cases of childhood hepatic angiosarcoma-elevated environmental arsenic exposure in one case. *Cancer* **47**, 382.

Greenwald, P., Kovasznay, B., Collins, D.N., *et al.* (1984). Sarcomas of soft tissue after Vietnam service. *J. Natl. Cancer Inst.* **73**, 1107.

Hajdu, S.I. (1985). *Differential diagnosis of soft tissue and bone tumors*. Lea and Febiger, Philadelphia.

Horta, J.S., Motta, L.C., Abbatt, J.D., and Roriz, M.L. (1965). Malignancy and other late effects following administration of Thorotrast. *Lancet* **ii**, 201.

Kang, H., Enzinger, F., Breslin, P., *et al.* (1987). Soft tissue sarcomas and military service in Vietnam: a case–control study. *J. Natl. Cancer Inst.* **76**, 693.

Karakousis, C.P., Dalcin, P., Turc-Carel, C., Limon, J., and Sandberg, A.A. (1987). Chromosomal changes in soft-tissue sarcoma: a new diagnostic parameter. *Arch. Surg.* **122**, 1257–60.

Kreicberg, A., Tribukait, B., Willems, J., and Bauer, H.C.F. (1987). DNA flow analysis of soft tissue tumors. *Cancer* **59**, 128.

Leopold, K.A., Harrelson, J., Prosnitz, L., Samulski, T.V., Dewhirts, M.W., Oleson, J.R. (1989). Preoperative hyperthermia and radiation for soft tissue sarcomas: advantage of two vs one hyperthermia treatments per week. *Int. J. Radiat. Oncol. Biol. Phys.* **16**, 107–15.

Martin, R.G., Butler, J.J., and Albores-Saavedra, J. (1965). Soft tissue tumors:

surgical treatment and results. In *Tumors of bone and soft tissue*. Year Book Medical, Chicago.

Muller, R., Hajdu, S.I., and Brennan, M.F. (1987). Lymphangiosarcoma associated with chronic filarial lymphedema. *Cancer* **59**, 179.

Ormsby, M.V., Hilaris, B.S., Nori, D., and Brennan, M.F. (1989). Wound complications of adjuvant radiation therapy in patients with soft-tissue sarcomas. *Ann. Surg.* **210**, 93–9.

Pezzi, C.M., Pollock, R.E., Evans, H.L., Lorigan, J.G., Pezzi, T.A., Benjamin, R.S., and Romsdahl, M.M. (1990). Preoperative chemotherapy for soft-tissue sarcomas of the extremities. *Ann. Surg.* **211**, 476–81.

Potter, D.A., Glenn, J., Kinsella, T., Glatstein, E., Lack, E.E., Restrepo, C., White, D.E., Seipp, C.A., Wesley, R., and Rosenberg, S.A. (1985). Patterns of recurrence in pts with high grade soft-tissue sarcomas. *J. Clin. Oncol.* **3**, 353–66.

Rosenberg, S.A., Tepper, J., Glatstein, E., Costa, J., Baker, A., Brennan, M.F., DeMoss, E.V., Seipp, C., Sindelar, W.F., Sugarbaker, P., and Wesley, R. (1982). The treatment of soft-tissue sarcoma of the extremities: prospective randomized evaluations (1) limb sparing surgery plus radiotherapy compared with amputation and (2) the role of adjuvant chemotherapy. *Ann. Surg.* **196**, 305–15.

Rosenberg, S.A., Tepper, J., Glastein, E., Costa, J., Young, R., Baker, A., Brennan, M.F., DeMoss, E.V., Seipp, C., Sindelar, W.F., Sugarbaker, P., and Wesley, R. (1983). Prospective randomized evaluation of adjuvant chemotherapy in adults with soft-tissue sarcomas of the extremities. *Cancer* **52**, 424–34.

Schonfeld, D., Rosenbaum, C., Horton, J., Wolfer, J.M., Falkson, G., and DeConti, R.C. (1982). A comparison of Adriamycin versus vincristine and Adriamycin, and cyclophosphamide for advanced sarcoma. *Cancer* **50**, 2757–62.

Shiu, M.H. and Hajdu, S.I. (1981). Management of soft-tissue sarcoma of the extremity. *Semin. Oncol.* **8**, 172.

Shiu, M.H., Flancbaum, L., Hajdu, S.I., Fortner, J.G. (1980). Malignant soft-tissue tumors of the anterior abdominal wall. *Arch. Surg.* **115**, 152.

Shiu, M.H., Turnbull, A.D., Nori, D., Hajdu, S., and Hilaris, B.S. (1984). Control of locally advanced extremity soft-tissue sarcomas by function saving resection and brachytherapy. *Cancer* **53**, 1385–92.

Shiu, M.H., Collin, C., Hilaris, B.S., Nori, D., Manolatos, S., Anderson, L.L., Hajdu, S.I., Lane, J.M., Hopfan, S., and Brennan, M.F. (1986). Limb preservation and tumor control in the treatment of popliteal and antecubital soft-tissue sarcomas. *Cancer* **57**, 1632–9.

Silverberg, E., Boring, C.C., and Squires, T.S. (1990). Cancer statistics, 1990. *CA* **40**, 9–26.

Smith, J. (1987). Postradiation sarcomas of bone in Hodgkin's disease. *Skeletal Radiol.* **16**, 524–32.

Stewart, F.W. and Treves, N. (1948). Lymphangiosarcoma in postmastectectomy lymphedema: a report of six cases of elephantiasis chirurgica. *Cancer* **1**, 64.

Stotter, A., Fallowfield, M., Mott, A., Fisher, C., and Westbury, G. (1990) Role of compartmental resection for soft-tissue sarcoma of the limb girdle. *Br. J. Surg.* **77**, 88–92.

Ueda, T., Aozasa, K., Tsujimoto, M., Ahsawa, M., Uchida, A., Aoki, Y., Ono, Y., and Matsumoto, K. (1989). Prognostic significance of Ki-67 reactivity in soft-tissue sarcomas. *Cancer* **63**, 1607–11.

Wanebo, H.J., Temple, W.J., Popp, M.B., Douvill, C.E., and Yablonski, M.

(1990). Combination regional therapy for extremity sarcoma. *Arch. Surg.* **125**, 355–9.

Wilson, R.E., Wood, R.C., Lerner, H.L., Antman, K., Amato, D., Corson, J.M., Proppe, K., Harmon, D., Carey, R., and Greenberger, J. (1986). Doxorubicin chemotherapy in the treatment of soft-tissue sarcoma: combined results of two randomized trials. *Arch. Surg.* **121**, 1354–9.

Woodward, A.M., Ivins, J.C., and Soule, E.M. (1972). Lymphangiosarcoma arising in chronic lymphedematous extremities. *Cancer* **30**, 562.

8. Surgery of the parotid: how I do it

Na'il Al-Naqeeb

The parotid is the largest of the salivary glands and many of its pathological disorders require special expertise for their management. Although inflammatory disorders are the most common condition, operations on the gland are more frequently performed for neoplasia. Successful operative procedures require identification and preservation of the facial nerve and avoidance of rupture of the tumour capsule in neoplastic lesions. Thus, superficial or partial parotidectomy should be the minimal undertaking for lesions of the parotid.

Surgical anatomy

Early anatomical studies described the parotid gland as a bi-lobed structure consisting of a larger superficial and a smaller deep lobe connected by an isthmus, with the facial nerve lying in a connective tissue plane separating the two lobes. Later studies refuted the bi-lobar theory and demonstrated the presence of numerous salivary connections bridging the gap between nerve branches (McKenzie 1948, Winsten and Ward 1956).

Facial nerve

The facial nerve emerges from the skull at the stylomastoid foramen, just posterior to the base of the styloid process, and passes downwards, giving off post-auricular and digastric branches before curving anterolaterally to enter the posterior border of the parotid gland very shortly after leaving the foramen. The nerve, once within the parotid, divides into two main trunks. The major division, temporo-facial and cervico-facial, continue forward and subdivide into a variable number of terminal branches, which innervate the muscles of facial expression. These are generally categorized as five branches (temporal, zygomatic, buccal, mandibular, and cervical) In most adults the exit of the facial nerve from the stylomastoid foramen is at a point about 1 cm above the tip of the mastoid process and 1–1.5 cm deep to its anterior border.

Greater auricular nerve

This sensory nerve is the largest branch of the cervical plexus. Arising posterior to the sternocleidomastoid, it crosses the anterior border of this muscle dividing into anterior and posterior branches at the inferior pole of the parotid gland. The posterior branch, which supplies both surfaces of the lower part of auricle, is usually sacrificed during parotidectomy.

Parotidectomy

Indications

Neoplasia is the main indication for parotidectomy. Fewer than 3 per cent of head and neck neoplasms occur in the salivary glands and, of these, 80 per cent affect the parotid (Skolink, *et al.* 1977; Martis 1983; Friedman, *et al.* 1986). Seventy to ninety per cent of parotid tumours are benign, being either pleomorphic or monomorphic adenomas, while about 3–12 per cent have been reported to be malignant (Bardal and Hall 1970; Rakow 1973; Nigro and Spiro 1977; Baker and Coloney 1979; Heeneman and Maran 1979; Som, Biller, and Lawson 1981; Miamaris and Ball 1986).

Inflammatory lesions, namely sialectasis, also merit resection. This latter disease is characterized by abnormal ductal dilatation with areas of stenosis and stasis of secretions. It causes recurrent painful attacks of sialadenitis. The management of this painful disorder is largely conservative but total parotidectomy may become necessary if the condition becomes resistant to medical therapy.

Congenital lesions such as lymphangioma, haemangioma, or periauricular sinuses may require surgical management. Parotidectomy may also be indicated for exposure and resection of tumours which are located adjacent to or in contact with the parotid gland. Metastases in the parotid lymph nodes may require removal with block dissection of the neck when there is malignant involvement of drainage areas of primary tumours.

Objectives of parotidectomy

Radical resection entails complete removal of the lesion with safety margins to prevent implantation and tumour recurrence. Total removal of the parotid is also required for treatment of sialectasis for prevention of further attacks of sialoadenitis. Preservation of function, by avoidance of facial nerve injury, is imperative unless there is direct involvement by the tumour. Cosmetic incisions must be properly planned in order to give an acceptable scar.

Types of resection

Superficial parotidectomy

The constitutes removal of all parotid tissue superficial to the facial nerve, with the dissection and preservation of the nerve and its branches. It is the procedure of choice for excisional biopsy and for all benign tumours of the superficial lobe.

Total conservative parotidectomy

The operation comprises removal of both lobes of the parotid with preservation of the facial nerve and its branches. This procedure is usually undertaken for sialectasis, benign tumours of the deep lobe, recurrent pleomorphic adenoma (in which lesions are multiple or involve a considerable part of the gland), and for all malignant tumours that do not involve the facial nerve.

Total radical parotidectomy

Removal of both lobes of the parotid sacrifices the facial nerve. This technique is recommended for malignant tumours with clinical evidence of facial palsy. The extent of resection is determined according to the histopathological diagnosis and extent of involvement of surrounding tissue (Guillamondegui, Byers, *et al.* 1975; Shidnia, *et al.* 1977; McNancy, *et al.* 1983). At operation the whole gland is resected with the facial nerve and the involved surrounding tissues. A radical block neck dissection is performed for all malignant lesions when lymph nodes are clinically and/or cytologically involved.

Enucleation

This option is not advisable for parotid lesions as it carries the risks of facial nerve injury and tumour implantation. It can, however, be practised for removal of a lymph node in the superficial parotid lobe and for Warthin's tumour. It is very rarely undertaken in our own practice.

Partial (limited) parotidectomy

The removal of part of the parotid containing the tumour is occasionally advocated. This technique of parotidectomy is suitable for the tumours in the inferior part of the parotid lateral to the lower branch of the facial nerve, and particularly for Warthin's tumour.

Pre-operative investigations

An accurate pathological diagnosis of a mass in the parotid region should be obtained before parotidectomy.

Clinical assessment

Neoplastic lesions

A painless mass is the usual clinical finding in the majority of patients. Presentation with a painful swelling is likely to be due to inflammation or malignant infiltration but facial palsy almost invariably indicates malignancy. Facial nerve involvement by parotid cancer is evident in approximately 15 per cent of patients (Saunders, Hirata, and Jacques 1986). Tumours of the deep lobe may occasionally present as a parapharyngeal mass and can be detected by bi-manual examination of the pharynx.

Inflammatory lesions

Patients with chronic sialoadenitis may experience recurrent attacks of painful diffuse salivary swelling. Cases of localized sialoadenitis are sometimes difficult to distinguish from parotid neoplasms.

Investigations

Plain radiology

Sixty per cent of parotid stones are radiopaque and can be demonstrated by lateral and oblique radiological examination (Hugh 1986).

Sialography

Sialography is helpful for confirmation of the inflammatory nature of parotid swellings by verifying the characteristic ductal pattern with areas of narrowing, dilatation, or expansion. It may demonstrate the extent of damage to acini and ducts and detect a fistula and/or diverticulum as well as being of value in deep-seated tumours by delineating identification of the duct system. Sialography is, however, unrewarding in the evaluation of tumour.

Ultrasonography

Ultrasonography is helpful for the evaluation of neoplasms (Carr and Bowerman 1986). It is operator dependent and can, in experienced hands, be 100 per cent accurate for the detection of tumours. It may be possible to distinguish between benign and malignant lesions by documentation of a characteristic border, being well defined in benign tumours (Watson 1989). Ultrasonography can also identify a lymph node outside the main capsule of the parotid gland and may be of value in localizing the lesions for cytological examination.

Computed tomography (CT)

CT is very sensitive for detection of salivary gland tumours and can easily identify extra-glandular masses (Bryan, *et al.* 1982). It cannot distinguish between benign disease, early malignancy, and an area of focal sialadenitis (Watson 1989). CT is essential for assessment of the extent of infiltration of surrounding tissues by malignant tumours.

Radio-isotope scanning

Radio-isotope scanning is not an accurate diagnostic procedure. It is more valuable and specific for diagnosis of an inflammatory process (acute and chronic sialoadenitis), in which uptake is higher than in tumours. Warthin's tumour is the only neoplastic lesion to show uptake of the isotope.

Decreased salivary gland function occurs in certain connective tissue diseases such as rheumatoid arthritis, Sjögren's syndrome, systemic lupus erythematosus, sarcoidosis, or scleroderma. Following radiation therapy and chronic sialoadenitis, there is also decreased function.

Increased technetium-99m concentration in salivary glands occurs in acute sialadenitis of bacterial or viral causes, following acute salivary gland obstruction, Mikulicz disease, or in Warthin's tumour.

Magnetic resonance imaging (MRI)

This procedure distinguishes the parotid gland from its neighbouring structures and may provide a direct image of the facial nerve within the parotid gland (Mandelblatt, *et al.* 1987; Teresi, *et al.* 1987*a*; Teresi, *et al.* 1987*b*).

Fine needle aspiration biopsy (FNAB)

FNAB is the most sensitive, rapid, inexpensive, and painless procedure for the diagnosis of parotid lesions. It distinguishes accurately between benign and malignant lesions within the parotid region (Eneroth, Jakobsson, and Zajick 1965; Eneroth, Jakobsson, and Zajick 1969; Eneroth, Jakobsson, and Zajick 1971; Frable and Frable 1977; Behbehani, *et al.* 1990).

In our experience, the diagnostic sensitivity of FNAB for malignant tumours is 93 per cent and the diagnostic specificity is 100 per cent (i.e. no false-positive diagnosis of malignancy).

Open biopsy

Open biopsy of a parotid tumour is not advisable since it carries a controversial risk of implantation and recurrence. In the majority of our patients, the principal method of investigation is limited to accurate clinical assessment followed by FNAB.

Despite all the above investigations, the final diagnosis of a parotid mass may rest with surgical exploration and superficial parotidectomy plus frozen section.

Superficial parotidectomy

Anaesthesia

General anaesthesia with endotracheal intubation is necessary. Hypotensive anaesthesia can greatly reduce the bleeding during operation, allowing a dry field for easy identification of the facial nerve and its branches. We use either trimetaphan or sodium nitroprusside for controlled hypotensive anaesthesia.

Position of the patient

The patient is placed in the supine position, with the head of the table elevated 15° to reduce venous engorgement. The shoulder is elevated by keeping a soft pillow beneath it and the head is turned to the opposite side, exposing the face. The eyes are protected with application of antibiotic ointment and closed, using soft medical tape. The ipsilateral shoulder, chest, neck, face, forehead, and entire ear are exposed and antiseptic solution is applied. The area is draped to expose the operative field. A suture is placed through the earlobe so the latter can be elevated during the operation. A wick of wool is inserted into the ear. A transparent polyurethane incise drape, to cover the cheek, allows the inspection of the angle of mouth and eye contraction if the facial nerve is irritated.

Exposure of the facial nerve

All forms of parotidectomy begin by exposing the facial nerve. However, a variety of methods to expose the facial nerve have been advocated. My own preference is for parotidectomy with exposure of the main trunk of the facial nerve (Janes 1940; Martin 1944). Alternative procedures are:

1. *Parotidectomy with exposure of mandibular branch of facial nerve* (Sistrunk 1921; Adson and Ott 1923; Baily 1941). The mandibular branch is exposed as it crosses the posterior facial vein, just anterior to the lower pole of the parotid gland where it lies on the masseter muscle above the angle of the mandible. The branch is traced posteriorly through the parotid until the main trunk of the facial nerve is identified. This technique is useful for small tumours lying in the tail of the parotid, or for bulky lesions which make identification of the main trunk difficult.

2. *Parotidectomy with exposure of peripheral branches of the facial nerve* (McCormack, Cauldwell, and Anson 1945; State 1949). Here the individual branches of the facial nerves are identified at the anterior border of the gland. Each individual branch is traced from before backward, elevating the superficial part of the gland until an area free of tumour is reached.

3. *Parotidectomy with exposure of Stensen's duct* (Ulin, Ehrlich, and Smith 1957). The dissection starts at the parotid duct, which has a constant position anterior to the parotid gland. It is closely related to the buccal branch of the facial nerve which is then followed posteriorly. More branches of the facial nerve are then identified and similarly delineated. A modification of this procedure is carried out by injection of methylene blue through the parotid duct. After raising a flap, the identification of the buccal branch is facilitated by identification of the parotid duct (Wang, Jun, Donoff, and Guralnick 1985).

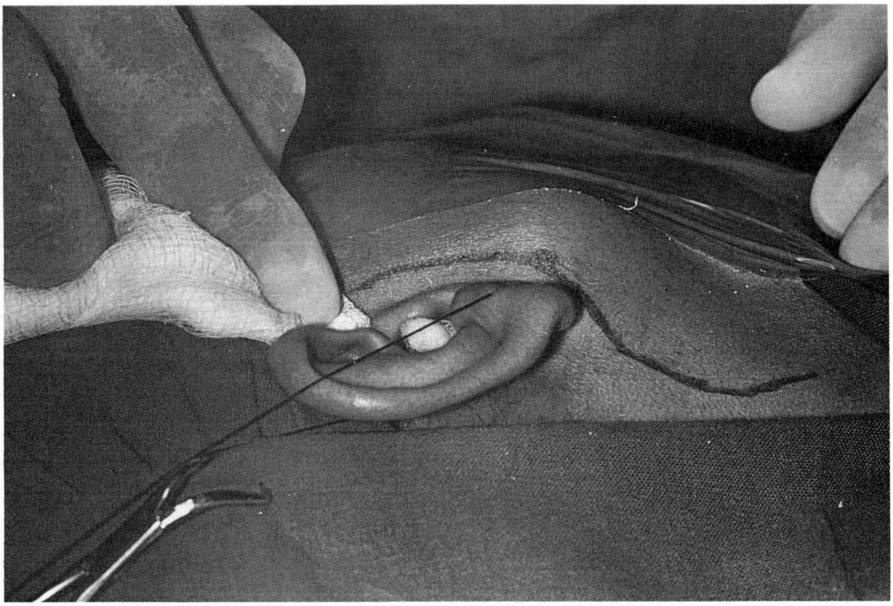

Fig. 8.1. Skin incision.

4. *Parotidectomy starting at the zygomatic arch* (Reissner 1952). Dissection of the nerve can begin by exposing the upper two branches of the facial nerve, the temporal and zygomatic. These two branches are large and more constant in position, and it is unusual for parotid tumours to occur at the level of the zygoma. These branches are exposed above the parotid at the zygoma where they lay directly over the periosteum and are then followed to the upper division of the trunk and the main trunk.

Skin incision (Fig. 8.1)

A smooth S-shaped incision is made, beginning in the peri-auricular skin crease at the level of zygoma, cutting downwards and curving smoothly below the pinna and extending forward below the mandibular angle. The skin incision is deepened to the subcutaneous tissue level, leaving only the parotid capsule intact. The skin incision can be extended upward or downward as required.

Raising the skin flaps (Fig. 8.2)

The anterior skin flap is raised superficial to the capsule, to expose the superficial lobe of the parotid gland. This is done by use of cutting diathermy and the dissection is carried out anteriorly, short of the anterior border of the gland so that the branches of the facial nerve are not injured.

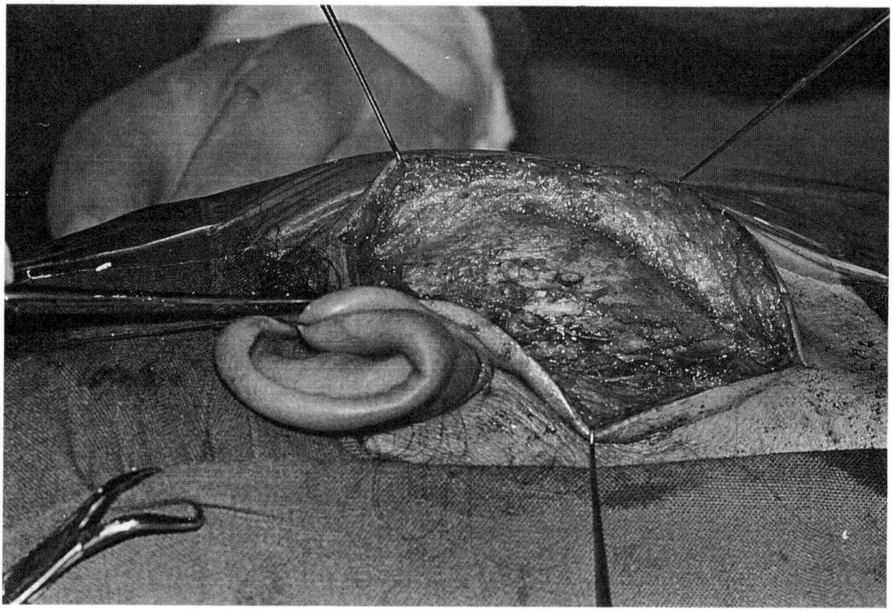

Fig. 8.2. Dissection and raising of the skin flaps.

The posterior skin flap is raised in the same manner to expose the cartilaginous meatus, mastoid process, and the sternomastoid muscle, posterior to the tail of the parotid which lies on this muscle. The dissection is performed using cutting diathermy with the tail of the gland lifted by a small clamp and pulled forward. I identify the facial vein below the inferior edge of the parotid with careful dissection since it lies in a plane deep to the neural structures.

The great auricular nerve is also encountered at the inferior pole of the parotid, running superiorly and anteriorly over the sternomastoid muscle, and is almost inevitably divided at this stage. The branches to the ear lobe may be preserved in order to prevent post-operative anaesthesia in this area. This is possible only in anteriorly located tumours because of the fear of tumour penetration of lesions at other sites.

The dissection of the parotid is begun posteriorly by separating the sternocleidomastoid muscle. Sharp dissection is needed to incise the dense fascia between the parotid gland and mastoid process and sternomastoid muscle, keeping close to these latter structures. The plane between the posterior border of the parotid and the cartilaginous meatus is an areolar one and can be easily opened using blunt dissection to enter the parotid space. Care should be taken not to enter parotid gland tissue so that the operative field can be kept free of blood. The dissection is carried out into a

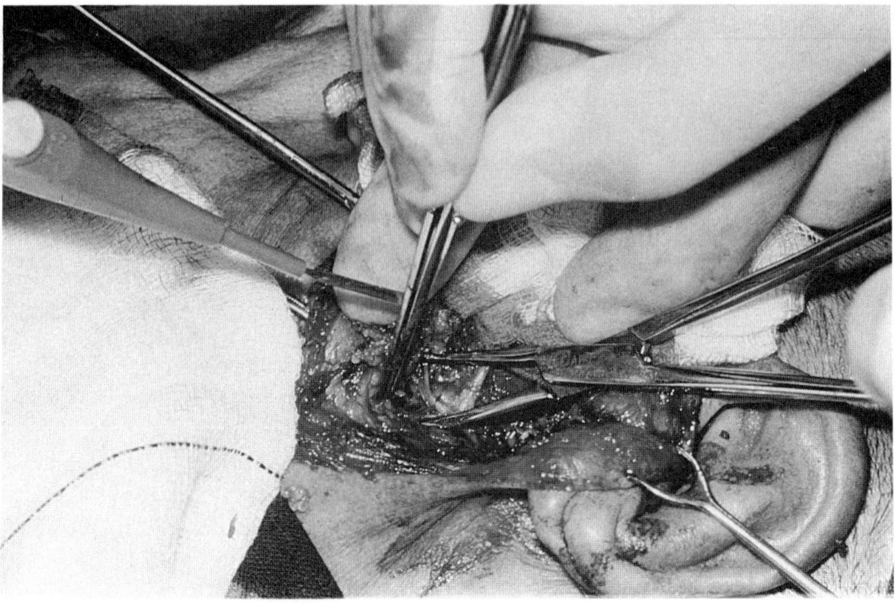

Fig. 8.3. Early identification of the nerve.

deeper plane until the bony meatus, which can be felt by the tip of the finger, is encountered. Liberal use is made of diathermy to stop bleeding from small blood vessels during this process.

Facial nerve and its branches

The search for the main trunk of the facial nerve now begins by retraction of the parotid gland with some tension anteriorly. I search for the nerve using a haemostat to dissect the tissue between the bony meatus and the mastoid process. It is usually found just below and deep to a horizontal, imaginary plane that bisects the bony meatus (Fig. 8.3). Not infrequently, bleeding from the stylomastoid artery, which accompanies the nerve, warns of its close proximity. This vessel is diathermied and divided. The facial nerve is a thick cord-like structure and identification of the styloid process, and of the underlying posterior belly of digastric muscle, may help to identify the trunk which usually emerges between them. I have discontinued use of the nerve stimulator for nerve identification.

After visualization of the trunk of the facial nerve, the operation proceeds with blunt dissection along the nerve trunk to identify its main division into superior and inferior branches (Fig. 8.4). The dissection is continued with a haemostat along the individual branches. An artery forceps is introduced in a horizontal plane just superficial to the nerve and gently opened, elevating

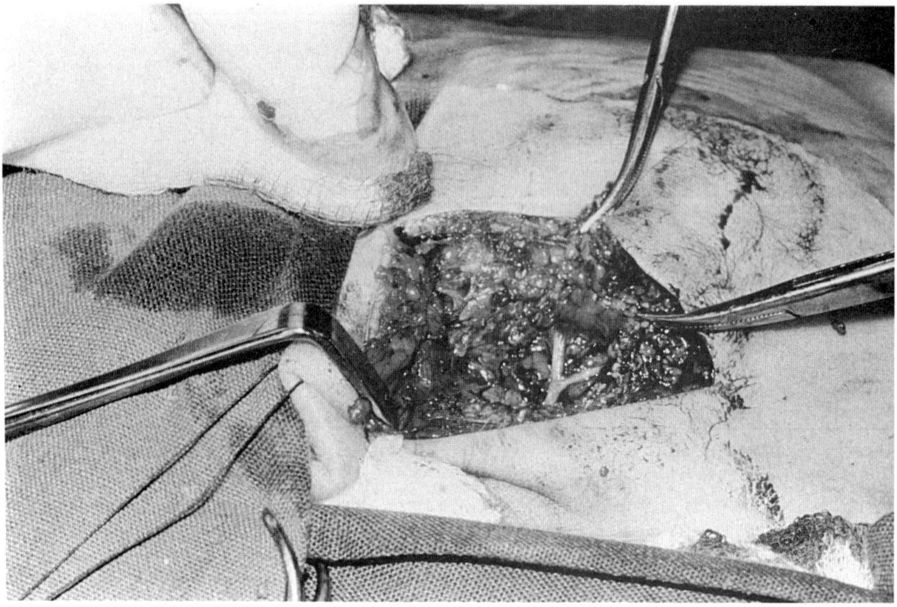

Fig. 8.4. Trunk of the facial nerve and its main divisions.

the overlying parotid tissue which is divided carefully under direct vision using scissors or scalpel. During this procedure various bleeding points are secured using ligatures or diathermy, keeping clear from the nerve branches. Occasionally the use of magnifying glasses to follow the course of branches of the facial nerve is helpful. This manoeuvre is continued until the superficial lobe of the parotid is separated from the branches of the facial nerve. The facial vein is usually preserved except for tributaries that drain the superficial lobe.

The parotid gland is then incised along its anterior border with no attempt to identify and ligate the parotid duct. This is accomplished only when it comes in the field (Fig. 8.5).

Haemostasis using unipolar diathermy is carefully undertaken after blood pressure has been raised and the wound is then closed over a suction drain (Fig. 8.6).

Limited superficial parotidectomy

This is a suitable technique for small pleomorphic adenomas or Warthin's tumours when they are located in the lower pole of the parotid. The lower posterior part of the parotid containing the tumours is excised leaving the upper portion intact. This may be performed without exploring the nerve, as

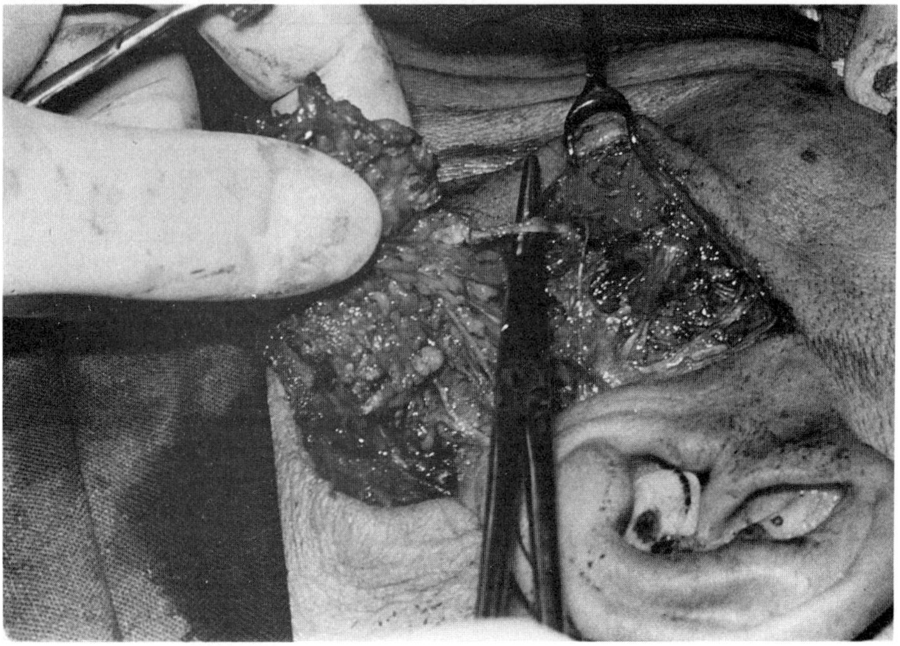

Fig. 8.5. Identification of the parotid duct.

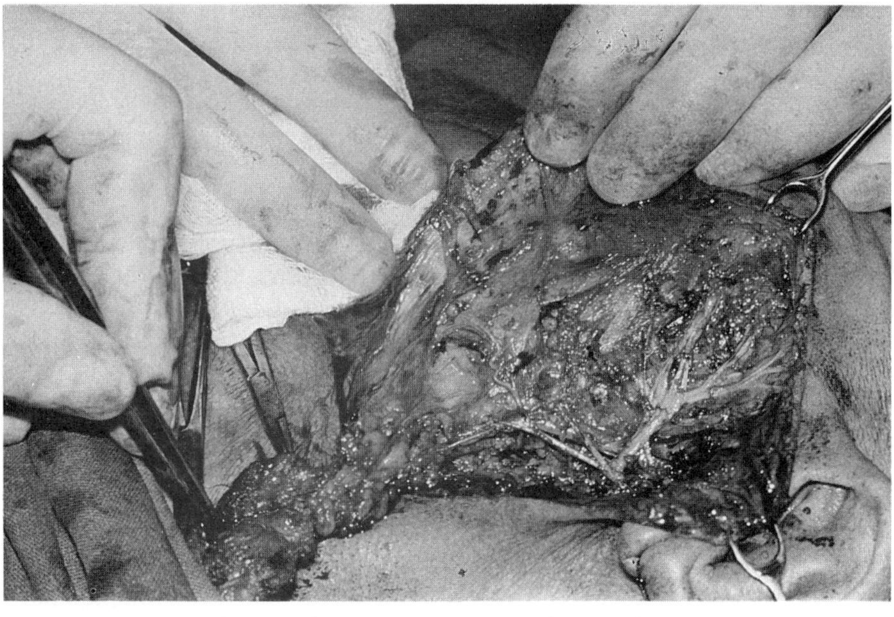

Fig. 8.6. Superficial parotidectomy at the completion of operation.

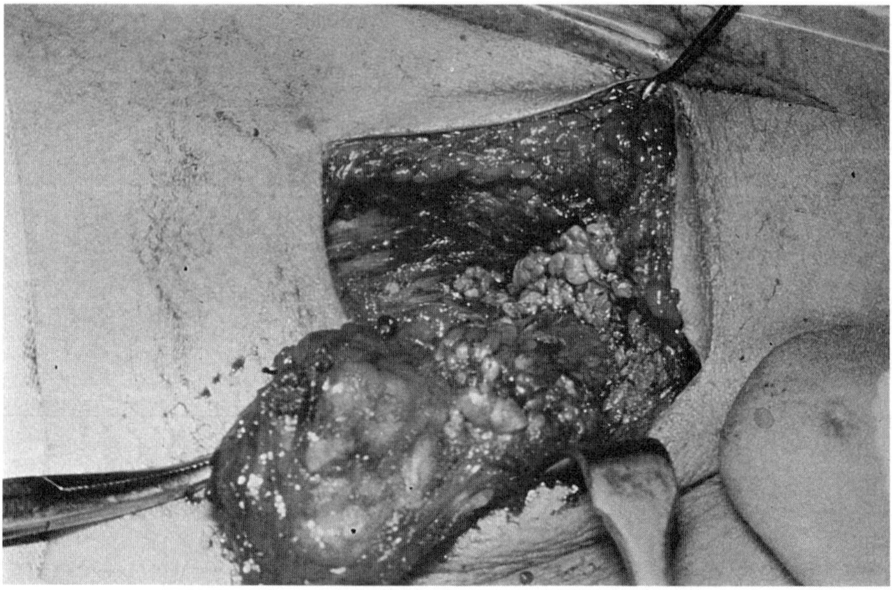

Fig. 8.7. Limited parotidectomy.

described by Martis (1983) (Fig. 8.7), but in our opinion this method does not ensure the safety of the facial nerve from accidental injury. A safer approach is facilitated by identification of the cervofacial division of the facial nerve with excision of the portion of the parotid lying superficially and inferiorly. This can be done by identifying the mandibular nerve as it crosses the facial vein (Sistrunk 1921) or more carefully by tracing the main trunk of the nerve along its lower division.

Total conservative parotidectomy

This operation is advocated for benign tumours of the deep lobe, malignant tumours which do not involve the facial nerve, recurrence of pleomorphic adenoma, and for sialectasis.

The superficial lobe is removed as described earlier and the diagnosis confirmed by frozen section. The facial nerve and its branches are dissected from the underlying parotid gland by blunt dissection with an artery forceps; sharp dissection is also used for complete separation from the deep parotid lobe. The nerve may be lifted using rubber bands to facilitate the dissection of the deep lobe. Although I do this frequently, I make sure that no undue tension is applied (Fig. 8.8). The posterior facial vein runs longitudinally deep to the parotid and has to be ligated both superiorly and inferiorly to

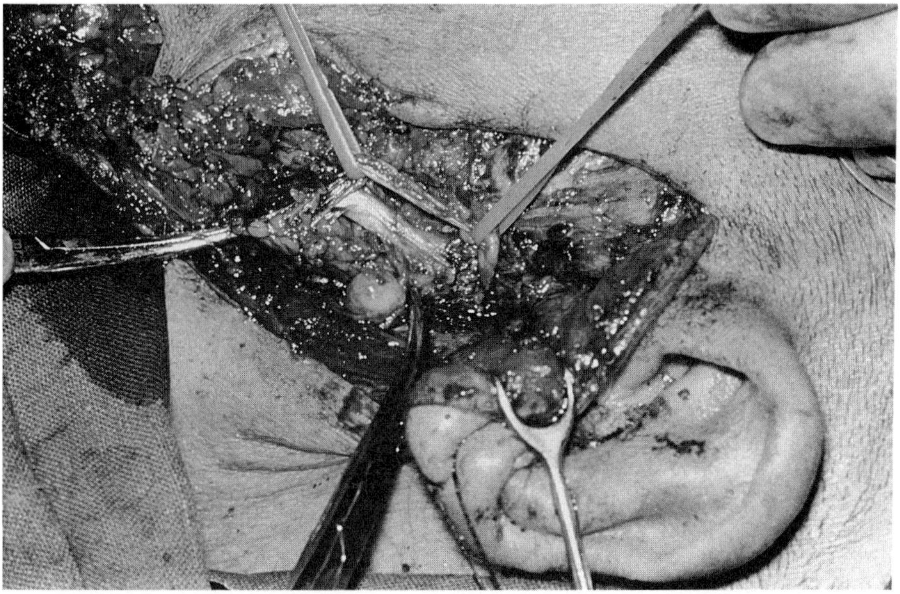

Fig. 8.8. Deep lobe dissection.

the deep parotid lobe. The external carotid artery and its two terminal branches, the superficial temporal and internal maxillary, are encountered and usually ligated. The deep lobe is then carefully raised from the underlying deeper structures and delivered from between the two main divisions of the facial trunk. The whole deep lobe can be elevated, leaving the nerve intact with no surrounding parotid tissue (Fig. 8.9). The wound is then closed over a suction drain.

The procedure is usually difficult in recurrent pleomorphic adenoma. The use of magnifying glasses is necessary to identify the facial nerve and its branches in areas of fibrosis which make damage more likely. At the end of the procedure I usually make use of a microscope to check the integrity of the nerve and its branches.

Total radical parotidectomy

This procedure is indicated only for extensive malignant tumours with clinical involvement of the nerve and facial palsy. The resection is planned according to the extent of the tumour. If the tumour is judged to be localized to the gland itself and not extending into the surrounding tissues, attempts are made to preserve the terminal branches of the nerve beyond the parotid margin and to identify and preserve the nerve trunk.

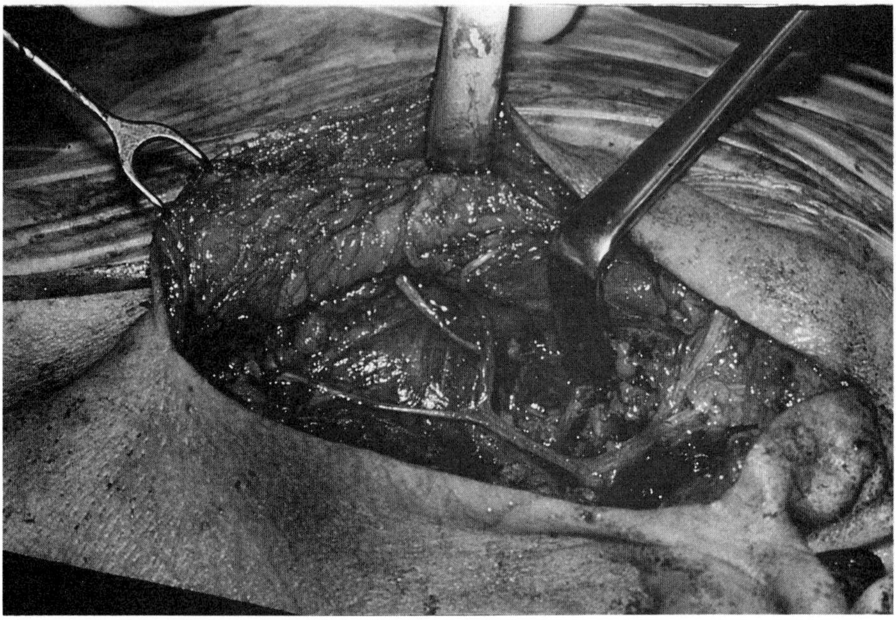

Fig. 8.9. Total conservative parotidectomy.

A cable nerve graft is used to bridge the gap between the main trunk and the terminal branches. This may not be possible if the malignant tumour has exceeded the confines of the parotid gland and invaded the surrounding structures, thus demanding a more extensive resection of the facial nerve trunk, particularly in cases of adenoid cystic carcinoma, known for its peri-neural spread, where the whole trunk of the nerve has to be sacrificed. Some authors have described excision of the mastoid process to visualize an uninvolved part of the trunk, but in my experience this has not been practicable. If only the terminal branches of the nerve are preserved, then a hypoglossal nerve cross-over graft is performed. When the tumour is so extensive that no terminal branches can be secured during the radical excision, the resulting facial palsy is subsequently managed by other reconstructive procedures, e.g. a facial sling or muscle interdigitation.

Technique of total radical parotidectomy

The skin incision is pre-auricular, curving below the mandible and extending further forward to the submandibular region. This skin incision is modified to avoid any areas of cutaneous involvement (Fig. 8.10).

I begin the procedure by a suprahyoid block dissection of lymph nodes,

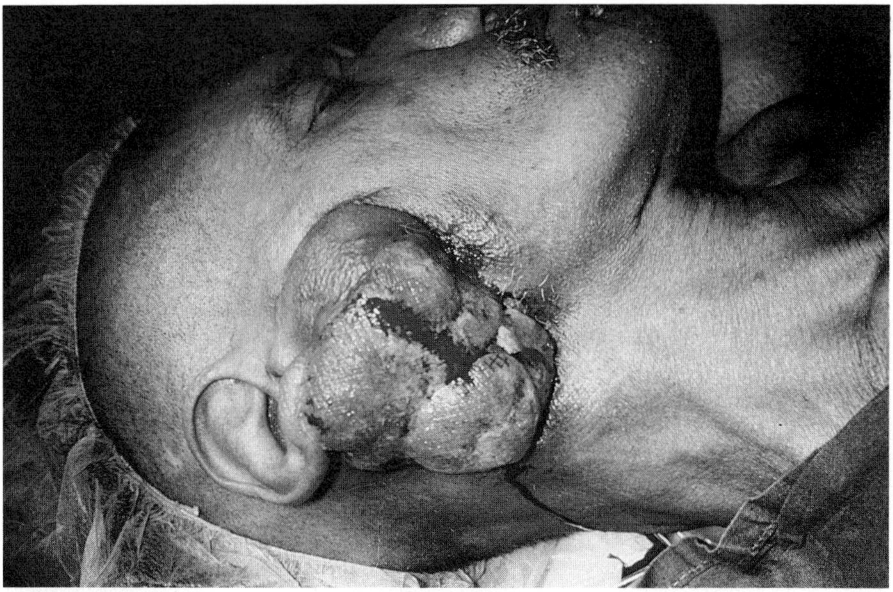

Fig. 8.10. Malignant extensive parotid tumour.

ligating the external carotid artery in continuity. This will minimize blood loss when the area of the tumour is dissected. Tumour adherent to the cartilaginous portion of the external auditory canal requires removal of a portion of the canal. The whole parotid gland, the involved masseter, sternomastoid, and digastric muscle may be resected safely. The mandible may be divided to facilitate the dissection, or excised if it is involved by the tumour.

A formal block dissection of the neck is added in the presence of cervical metastasis (Fig. 8.11). This can be accomplished by extending a vertical incision from the original incision in the submandibular region. Skin defects may require flaps for closure.

Facial nerve reconstruction in parotid surgery

Cancer ablation takes priority over preservation of branches of the facial nerve or the whole nerve trunk. At the same time it is salutary to recall that reconstruction following facial nerve transection is never entirely satisfactory regarding the muscles of expression, and nerve damage is a devastating psychological trauma to both patient and surgeon.

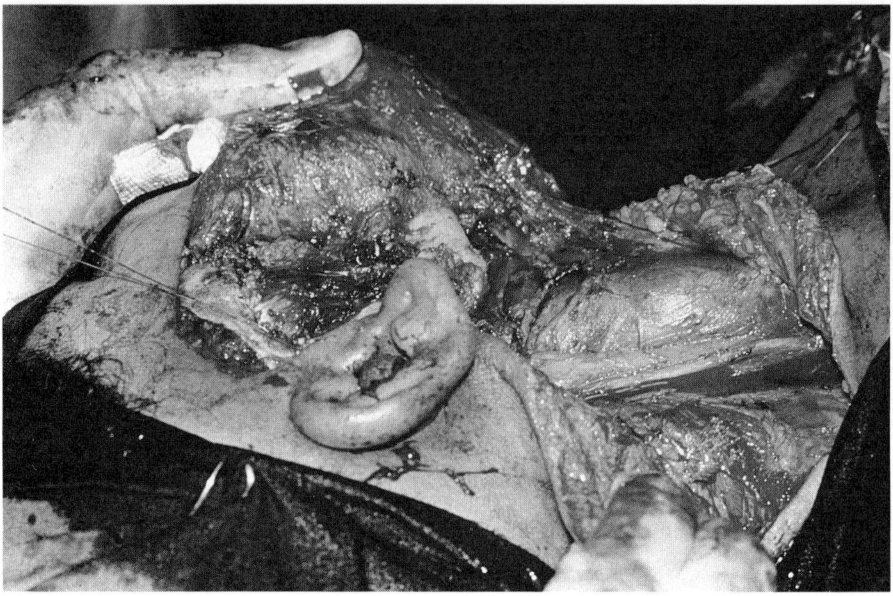

Fig. 8.11. Radical parotidectomy with block dissection.

Techniques

End-to-end suture (Fig. 8.12)

This is advised only for accidental nerve injury discovered during surgery, and gives the best functional results.

Cable nerve graft (Fig. 8.13)

This is performed to bridge the gap between the nerve trunk and its branches when the facial nerve is sacrificed in malignant tumours. The most suitable grafts are the sural and the greater auricular nerves. When the latter is used it is preferable to harvest the nerve on the contralateral side rather than the ipsilateral side, to aleviate fears of local malignant infiltration.

We prefer the use of the sural nerve which has the advantage of being of multi-branched and similar in size to the facial nerve. In order to avoid tension on the suture line, the harvested sural nerve should be of greater length than the defect to be bridged between the trunk and facial nerve branches.

The proximal end of the facial nerve is cleanly transected with a scalpel and biopsied, the proximal end of the harvested nerve also being sharply transected. The two nerve endings are sutured under the microscope using a 9-0 or 10-0 monofilament Nylon suture on a cutting needle. The sutures

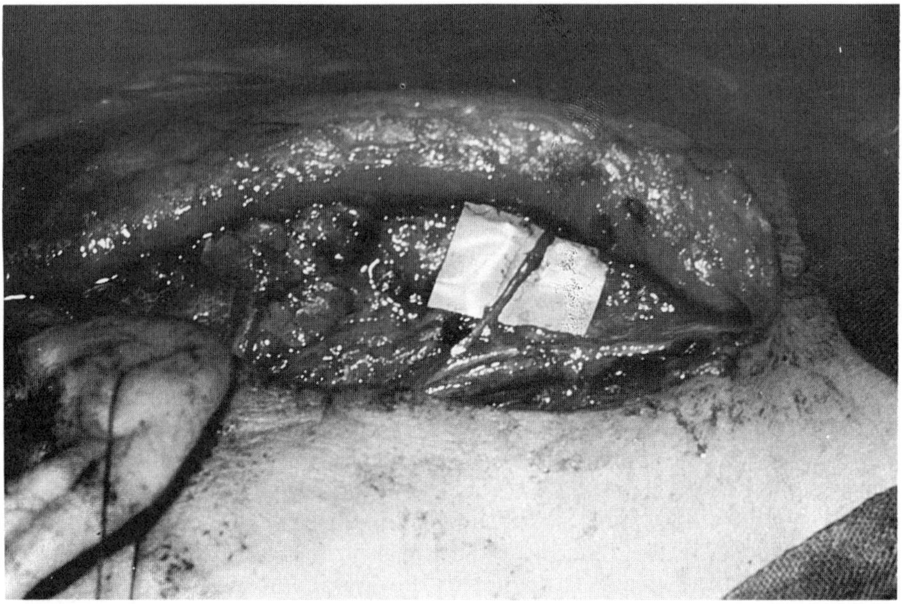

Fig. 8.12. Direct nerve suture.

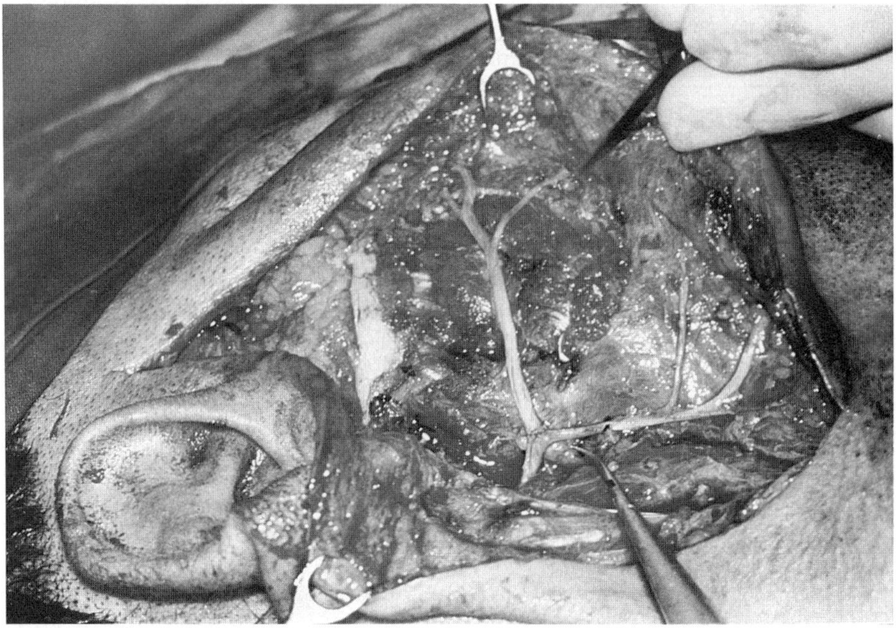

Fig. 8.13. Cable graft suture for temporofacial branch.

should pass in the nerve sheath alone, as this induces less injury to the nerve fibres. Four or five sutures are required in the main trunk to prevent axonal leakage. Similarly, the peripheral ends are sutured. If no branches have been harvested with the cable verve graft, the graft itself can be split longitudinally along its fibres into the number of branches required distally. On closure of the wound, care is taken to avoid placing a suction drain directly adjacent to the sutured nerve.

We believe that the use of silicone tubes for splintage is unnecessary. Expected return of function to the facial nerve occurs in up to 6–9 months, as the process of the nerve healing is protracted.

Nerve transposition

If the proximal facial nerve is resected with malignant tumours, a nerve cross-over graft can be performed. The hypoglossal, contralateral facial mandibular branch, spinal accessory, or phrenic nerve can be used, with the hypoglossal being the best choice because its size is similar to the facial nerve, and disability after sacrifice is minimal. The hypoglossal nerve is exposed medial to the tendon of the digastric muscle, dissected carefully, and divided before it passes deeper to the mylohyoid muscle. The cut end of the hypoglossal nerve can be split longitudinally to the desired number of branches to be anastomosed to the branches of the facial nerve, using the same technique described earlier. One can retain half of the nerve to preserve ipsilateral tongue mobility. Occasionally the facial nerve defect is long and a cable nerve graft may be used to bridge the gap between the hypoglossal nerve and the terminal branches of the facial nerve (Fig. 8.14). Good results are achieved in 90 per cent of cases. In Conley's series, 5 per cent of patients had hypertonia and excessive mass movements in the facial muscles but these recovered gradually over 10–20 years (Conley and Backer 1979).

Post-parotidectomy defect

The morbidity of the post-parotidectomy defect varies from one patient to another depending on the extent of surgery and whether superficial, total conservative parotidectomy, or radical resection, with or without resection of the underlying muscle or mandible, has been performed. Classically there are a number of methods to correct the defect:

1. For patients who have had a limited superficial parotidectomy and a large part of superficial lobe has been preserved, the remainder of the lobe can be sutured to the sternomastoid muscle.

2. The upper superficial fibres of the sternomastoid muscle may be used as a rotation flap to close relatively small defects following superficial or total conservative parotidectomy. The separated muscle fibres are fanned

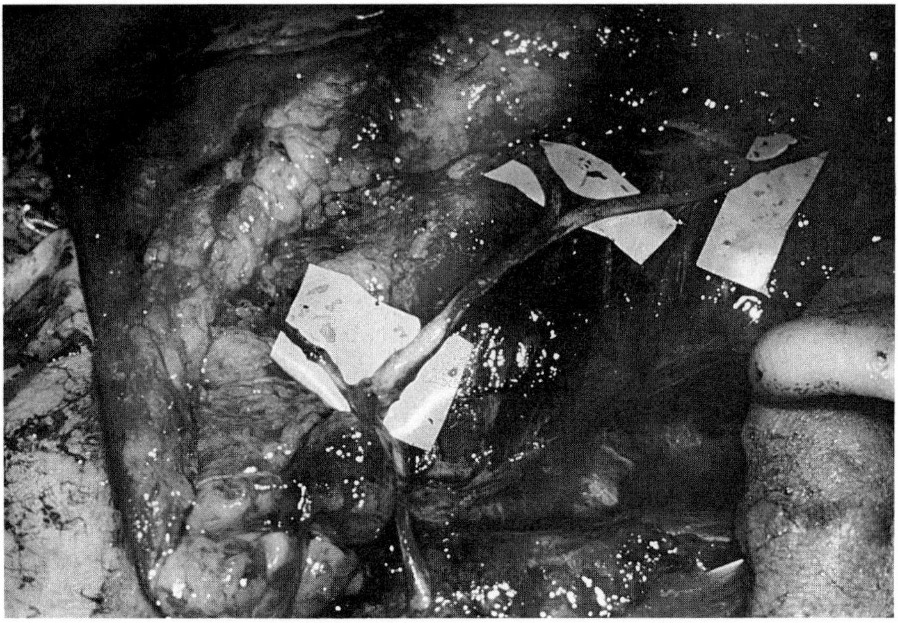

Fig. 8.14. Hypoglossal cross-over using sural nerve cable graft.

out over the main branches of the facial nerve and sutured in place to cover the defect. This is an easy, quick procedure and gives a satisfactory cosmetic result. Unfortunately, comparative studies have failed to confirm that this technique reduces the likelihood of Frey's syndrome as previously suggested (Kornblut, Wetphal, and Miehlke 1974).

3. For large defects (Fig. 8.15) when skin loss requires replacement, flaps can be either rotated or transferred as free microvascular flaps to cover the resected area (Fig. 8.16).

Complications (Fig. 8.17)

Haematoma

The parotid gland lies in a very vascular area and attention to good haemostasis is necessary to prevent haematoma formation. This complication is usually encountered in the immediate post-operative period and requires formal reopening of the wound.

Wound infection

This is uncommon in our experience. Prophylactic antibiotics are not indicated unless surgery is being carried out in an infected gland.

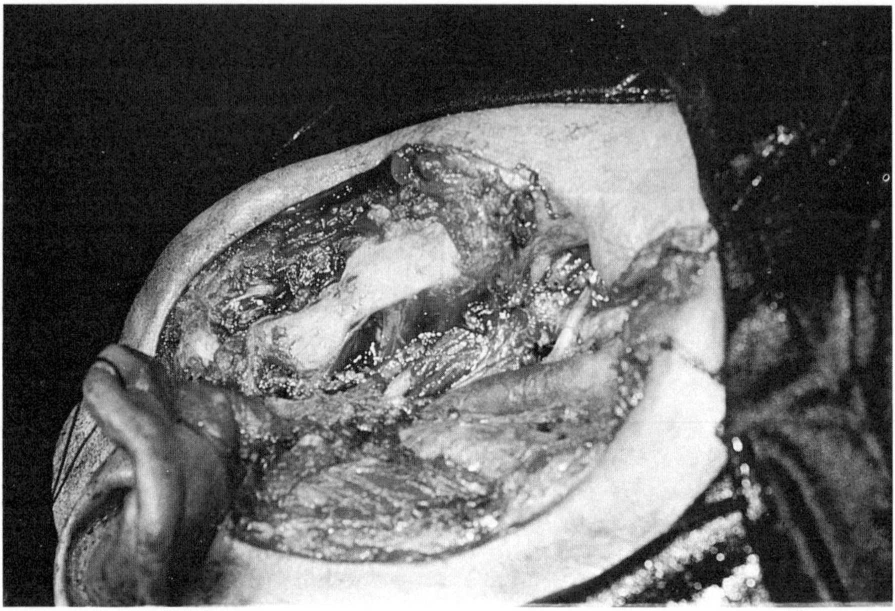

Fig. 8.15. Post-parotidectomy defect.

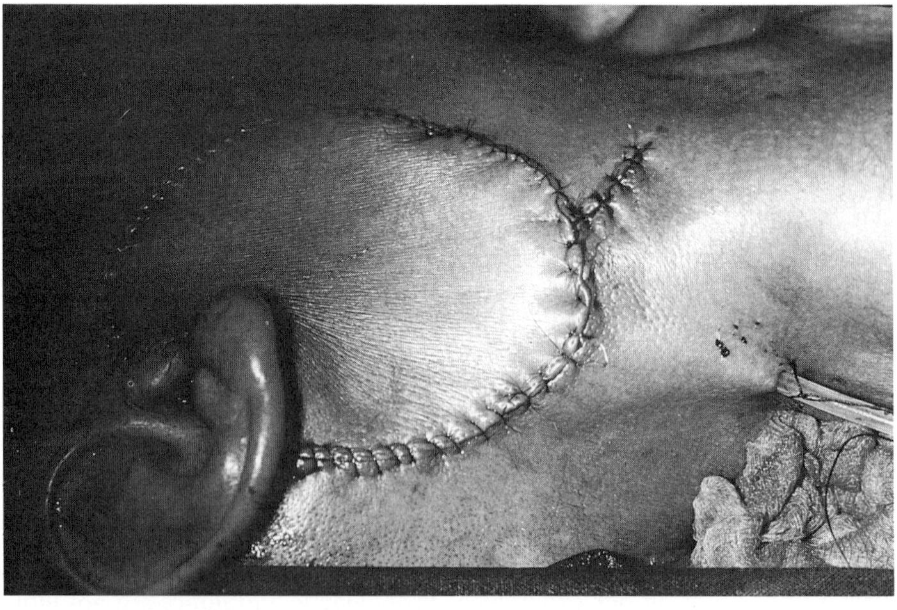

Fig. 8.16. Closure of the defect.

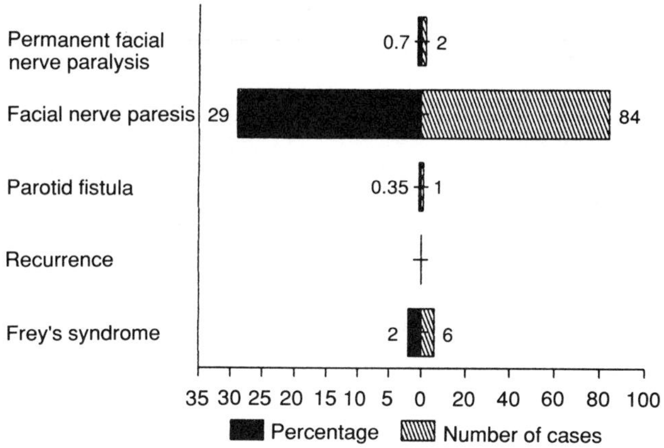

Fig. 8.17. Post-operative complications after parotidectomy.

Facial nerve injury

Temporary facial palsy may be seen after parotid surgery and, in the absence of unknown accidental transection, recovery of full function is the rule. In my experience temporary facial nerve paresis occurred in 84 of 302 cases (28 per cent) and all patients recovered within 6 months. I have observed no accidental injury of the main trunk or any of the two major branches. If the nerve is injured during parotidectomy I repair it immediately with 10-0 monofilament Prolene®. Accidental injury of one of the facial nerve branches occured in 8 of 289 parotidectomies. The branch was reanastomosed in all cases, where approximation of the epineurium was achieved with the use of surgical microscope. The function of the facial nerve returned in six of eight patients 3–6 months after surgery. Two cases (0.7 per cent) of permanant facial palsy occurred, one case involving the frontal branch to the forehead, and the second involving the mandibular branch supplying the angle of the mouth. Our results are consistent with other reports (Kidd 1968; Martis 1983; Woods 1985; Brusati, Bozzetti, and Chiapasco 1987) (Fig. 8.18).

Frey's syndrome (gustatory sweating syndrome)

This syndrome consists of redness of the skin and perspiration, related to gustatory stimuli over the region of former parotidectomy. It is due to regenerated fibres of the auriculotemporal nerve which take a wrong pathway to the sweat glands in the skin of the parotid region. Frey's syndrome is a common finding after parotidectomy, if specifically looked for, and unfortunately no preventive measures are known to avoid it. It is, however, mild in most patients and proves troublesome in only 10 per cent of cases. In our series this complication occurred in 6 of 289 patients following surgery (2 per

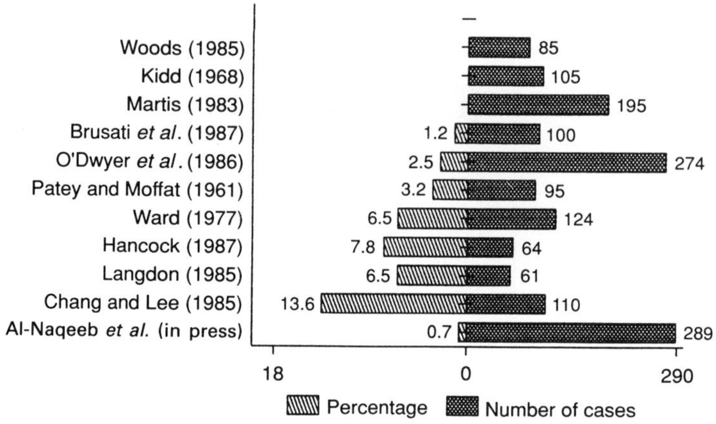

Fig. 8.18. Permanent facial nerve paralysis after parotidectomy.

cent) and was accepted as a minimal inconvenience (Fig. 8.19). If the symptoms of Frey's syndrome are distressing, it can be treated by ipsilateral tympanic neurectomy which provides relief in 80 per cent patients.

Parotid fistula

Parotidectomy is a rare cause of parotid fistula and can be successfully managed by simple pressure dressings. I have encountered this complication once only in our personal series of parotidectomies and it closed spontaneously after 7 months of conservative treatment. If a fistula persists, surgical correction consists of simple excision of the fistulous tract. Low-dose irradiation to the remaining parotid tissue can alternatively be recommended.

Sensory loss

Sensory loss to the lower half of pinna occurs due to division of the great auricular nerve. It gradually decreases with time and becomes unnoticeable. Many surgeons divide the branches of the great auricular nerve (Hobsley 1983; Woods 1983; Shaheen 1984; Saunders *et al.* 1986; Seifert, *et al.* 1986) whereas others preserve part of the great auricular nerve (Converse 1977; Strong 1986; Brown and Ord 1989). I usually sacrifice this nerve.

Recurrence rate (Fig. 8.20)

Pleomorphic adenoma

Recurrence of pleomorphic adenoma has been attributed to a number of factors, such as rupture and seeding of the tumour during surgery, multicentricity of the lesion, capsular penetration, and hypercellularity. As a rule

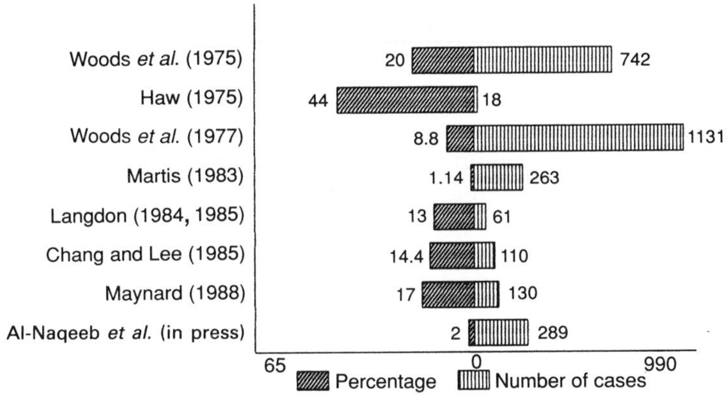

Fig. 8.19. Frey's syndrome after parotidectomy.

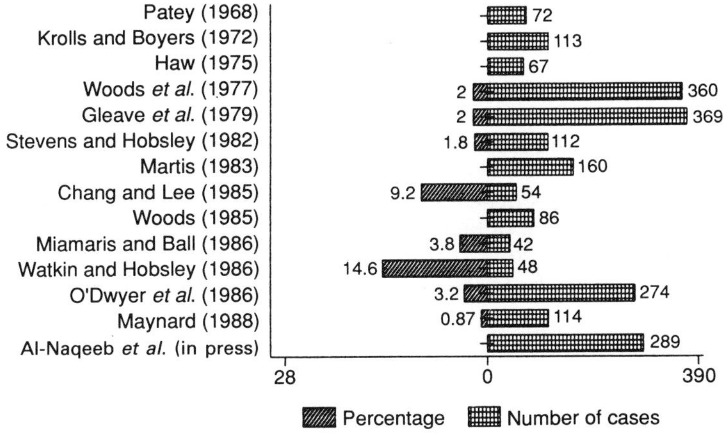

Fig. 8.20. Recurrence rate after parotidectomy.

recurrent mixed tumours are multiple and implantation in the scar of the original incision is not an uncommon finding. Recurrence is more frequent after enucleation. In a comparative study, the recurrence rate was 0 and 12 per cent after superficial parotidectomy and enuclaetion, respectively. Once a tumour recurs, the possibility of underlying malignancy should be borne in mind. In a retrospective study over 40 years, malignant change occurred in 3 of 48 cases (6 per cent) (Wennemo, Span, Emgard, and Krouthen 1988).

In our series, no recurrence was encountered following superficial parotidectomy for pleomorphic adenoma. It is important to prevent any rupture of the tumour capsule and to perform total conservative parotidectomy for tumour located in the deep lobe. Recurrence can occur after a long latent period following surgery, even as long as 20–40 years later (McFarland

1936, 1943; Krolls and Boyers 1972), and should be managed surgically by total excision of the remaining parotid tissue with removal of the overlying skin, which is often involved by recurrent nodules.

Malignant tumours

Recurrence of malignant tumour is difficult to control satisfactorily since obvious superficial tumour indicates a more aggressive recurrence in the deeper tissues, where free margins are difficult to obtain surgically. Radiotherapy alone cannot effectively control a large volume of tumour, so we usually manage these patients by radical surgical extirpation, if possible, followed by radiation therapy.

Two cases of recurrence (3.4 per cent) occurred in our series of 58 cases of malignant parotid tumours (one undifferentiated carcinoma and one muco-epidermoid carcinoma). Similar observations were recorded by other investigators (Patey 1968; Krolls and Bayers 1972; Haw 1975; Martis 1983; Woods 1985; Maynard 1988).

References

Adson, A.W. and Ott, W.O. (1923). Preservation of the facial nerve in the radical treatment of parotid tumours. *Arch. Surg.* **6**, 739.

Al-Naqeeb, N, Dashti, H., Al-Muhana, A., and Behbehani, A. Parotid gland tumours. A 15-year experience. *J. R. Coll. Surg. Edinb.* (in press).

Baily, H. (1941). Treatment of tumours of the parotid gland with special reference to surgical parotidectomy. *Br. J. Surg.* **28**, 337.

Baker, P. and Coloney, S. (1979). Retromandibular parotid tumours. *Ann. Plast. Surg.* **263**, 164.

Bardal, P. and Hall, J.B. (1970). Pharyngeal growth of parotid tumours. *Acta Otolaryngol.* **263**, 164.

Behbehani, A., Dashti, H., Al-Naqeeb, N., *et al.* (1990). The value of preoperative fine needle aspiration biopsy in planning the management of parotid gland tumours. *Med. Principle Pract.* (in press).

Brown, J.S. and Ord, R.A. (1989). Preserving the great auricular nerve in parotid surgery. *Br. J. Oral Maxillofac. Surg.* **27**, 459–66.

Brusati, R., Bozzetti, A., and Chiapasco, M. (1987). Facial nerve and parotid surgery. *J. Craniomaxillofac. Surg.* **15**, 278–80.

Bryan, R.N., Miller, R.H., Ferreyro, R.I., *et al.* (1982). Computed tomography of the major salivary glands. *AJR* **6**, 547–54.

Carr, R.J. and Bowerman, J. (1986). A review of tumours of the deep lobe of the parotid salivary gland. *Br. J. Oral Maxillofac. Surg.* **24**, 155–68.

Chang, E.Z. and Lee, W.C. (1985). Surgical treatment of pleomorphic adenoma of the parotid gland: report of 110 cases. *J. Oral Maxillofac. Surg.* **43**, 680–2.

Conley, J. and Backer, D.C. (1979). Hypoglossal–facial nerve anastomosis for reinnervation of paralysed face. *Plast. Reconstr. Surg.* **63**, 63–72.

Converse, J.M. (ed.) (1977). *Reconstructive plastic surgery. Principles and procedures in correction, reconstruction and transplantation*, Vol. 5. W.B. Saunders, Philadelphia.

Eneroth, C.M., Jakobsson, P., and Zajick, J. (1965). Aspiration biopsy of salivary gland tumours. II. Morphologic studies on smears and histologic sections from oncocystic tumours. *Acta Cytol.* **9**, 355.

Eneroth, C.M., Jakobsson, P., and Zajick, J. (1969). Aspiration biopsy of salivary gland tumours. IV. Morphologic studies on smears and histologic sections from 43 cases of adenoid cystic carcinoma. *Acta Cytol.* **13**, 59.

Eneroth, C.M., Jakobsson, P., and Zajick, J. (1971). Aspiration biopsy of salivary gland tumours. V. Morphologic investigation on smears and histologic sections of acinic cell carcinoma. *Acta Radiol. Suppl.* **315**, 85.

Frable, W.J. and Frable, M.A. (1977). Fine needle aspiration biopsy in the diagnosis of head and neck tumours. *Laryngoscope* **84**, 1069–77.

Friedman, M., Levin, B., Stovigl, T., *et al.* Malignant tumours of the major salivary glands. *Otolaryngol. Clin. North Am.* **19**, 625–36.

Gleave, E.N., Whittaker, J.S., and Nicholson, A. (1979). Salivary tumours experience over thirty years. *Clin. Otolaryngol.* **4**, 247–57.

Guillamondequi, O.M., Byers, R.M., Lung, M.A., *et al.* (1975). Aggressive surgery in treatment of parotid cancer. The role of adjuvant radiotherapy. *Am. J. Roentgenol.* **123**, 49–54.

Hancock, B.D. (1987). Pleomorphic adenoma of the parotid: removal without rupture. *Ann. R. Coll. Surg. Engl.* **69**, 293–5.

Haw, C.S. (1975). Pleomorphic adenomas of the parotid gland — review of results. *J. R. Coll. Surg. Edinb.* **20**, 25–9.

Heeneman, H. and Maran, A.G.D. (1979). Parapharyngeal space tumours. *Clin. Otolaryngol.* **4**, 57.

Hobsley, M. (1983). *A colour atlas of parotidectomy*, pp. 15–16. Wolfe Medical Publications. London.

Hugh, D.C. (1986). Assessment of salivary gland pathology. *Otolaryngol. Clin. North Am.* **21**, 547–72.

Kidd, H.A. (1968). Diseases of the parotid and Frey's syndrome. *Br. J. Hosp. Med.* **2**, 1513–22.

Kornblut, A.D., Wetphal, P., and Miehlke, A. (1974). The effectiveness of sternomastoid flap in preventing post-parotidectomy occurrence of Frey's syndrome. *Acta Otolaryngol.* **77**, 368.

Krolls, S.O. and Boyers, R.C. (1972). Mixed tumours of salivary glands. *Cancer* **30**, 276–81.

Janes, R.M. (1940). Treatment of tumours of salivary glands by radical excision. *Can. Med. Assoc. J.* **43**, 554.

Langdon, J.D. (1984). Complications of parotid gland surgery. *J. Max. Fac. Surg.* **12**, 225–9.

Langdon, J.D. (1985). Tumours of the salivary glands: clinical analysis of 68 cases. *J. Oral Maxillofac. Surg.* **43**, 688–92.

Mandelblatt, S.M., Braun, I.F., Davis, P.C., *et al.* (1987). Parotid masses: MR imaging. *Radiology* **163**, 411–14.

Martin, H. (1944). The operative removal of tumours of the parotid gland. *Surgery* **31**, 670.

Martis, C. (1983). Parotid benign tumours: comments on surgical treatment of 263 cases. *Int. J. Oral. Surg.* **12**, 211–20.

Maynard, J.D. (1988). Management of pleomorphic adenoma of the parotid. *Br. J. Surg.* **75**, 305–8.

McCormack, L.J., Cauldwell, E.W., and Anson, B.J. (1945). The surgical anatomy of the facial nerve. *Surg. Gynecol. Obstet.* **890**, 620.
McFarland, J. (1936). Mixed tumours of the salivary glands. Three hundred mixed tumours of the salivary glands of which sixty-nine recurred. *Surg. Gynecol. Obstet.* **63**, 457–68.
McFarland, J. (1943). Mysterious mixed tumours of the salivary glands. *Surg. Gynecol. Obstet.* **76**, 23–4.
McKenzie, J. (1948). The parotid gland in the relationship to the facial nerve. *J. Anat.* **82**, 183.
McNancy, D., McNeese, M.D., Guillamondegui, O.M., *et al.* (1983). Postoperative irradiation in malignant epithelial tumours of the parotid. *Int. J. Radiat. Oncol. Biol. Phys.* **9**, 1289–95.
Miamaris, C.V. and Ball, M.J. (1986). Treatment of parotid gland tumours by conservative parotidectomy. *Br. J. Surg.* **73**, 897.
Nigro, M.F. and Spiro, R.H. (1977). Lobe parotid tumours. *Am. J. Surg.* **134**, 523.
O'Dwyer, P.J., Farrar, W.B., Finkelmeir, W.R., McCabe, D.P., and James, A.G. (1986). Facial nerve sacrifice and tumour recurrence in primary and recurrent benign parotid tumours. *Am. J. Surg.* **152**, 442–5.
Patey, D.M. (1968). Tumours and other diseases of the salivary glands in relation to general physiology and pathology. *J. Laryngol. Otol.* **82**, 853–66.
Patey, D.H. and Moffat, W. (1961). A clinical and experimental study of functional paralysis of the facial nerve following conservative parotidectomy. *Br. J. Surg.* **48**, 435–40.
Rakow, R.M. (1973). Major salivary gland tumours. *Plast. Reconstr. Surg.* **51**, 514–23.
Reissner, D. (1952). Surgical procedure in tumours of the parotid gland: preservation of facial nerve and prevention of postoperative fistulas. *Arch. Surg.* **65**, 831.
Saunders, J.R., Hirata, R.M., and Jacques, D.A. (1986). Salivary glands. *Surg. Clin. North Am.* **66**, 59.
Seifert, G., Meihlke, A., Haubrich, J., *et al.* (1986). *Diseases of the salivary glands*, 332 pp. Thieme Medical Publications. Stuttgart.
Sistrunk, W.E. (1921). Mixed tumours of the parotid gland. *Minn. Med.* **4**, 155.
Shaheen, O.H. (1984). *Problems in head and neck surgery* pp. 38–00. Ballière Tindall. London.
Shidnia, H., Horback, N.C., Hamaker, R., *et al.* (1977). Carcinoma of major salivary glands. *Cancer* **40**, 2882–90.
Skolink, E.M., Friedman, M., Becker, S., *et al.* (1977). Tumours of the major salivary glands. *Laryngoscope* **87**, 873.
Som, P.M., Biller, H.F., and Lawson, W. (1981). Tumours of oropharyngeal space. *Ann. Otol. Rhinol. Laryngol. Suppl.* **90**, 3.
State, D. (1949). Superficial lobectomy and total parotidectomy with preservation of the facial nerve in the treatment of parotid tumours. *Surg. Gynecol. Obstet.* **89**, 237.
Stevens, K.L. and Hobsley, M. (1982). The treatment of pleomorphic adenomas by formal parotidectomy. *Br. J. Surg.* **69**, 1–3.
Strong, E.W. (1986). Book review. *Head Neck Surg.* **9**, 134.
Teresi, L.M., Kolin, E., Lifkin, R.B., *et al.* (1987*a*). MR imaging of the intraparotid facial nerve: nornal anatomy and pathology. *AJR* **148**, 995–1000.
Teresi, L.M., Lufkin, R.B., Wortham, D.C., *et al.* (1987*b*). Evaluation of parotid lesions by magnetic resonance imaging. *Radiology* **163**, 405–9.

Ulin, A.W., Ehrlich, E.W., and Smith, J.S. (1957). Stensen's duct, key to parotidectomy. *Arch. Surg.* **75**, 138.

Wang, D., Jun, L.S., Donoff, R.B., and Guralnick, W. (1985). A modified centripetal approach to parotidectomy. *J. Oral Maxillofac. Surg.* **43**, 14–19.

Ward, C.M. (1977). Injury of facial nerve during surgery of the parotid gland. *Br. J. Surg.* **62**, 401–3.

Watkin, G.T. and Hobsley, M. (1986). Influence of local surgery and radiotherapy on the natural history of pleomorphic adenoma. *Br. J. Surg.* **73**, 74–6.

Watson, M.G. (1989). Investigation of salivary gland disease. *Ear Nose Throat J.* **68**, 84–93.

Wennemo, C., Spandow, W., Emgard, P., and Krouthen, B. (1988). Pleomorphic adenomas of the parotid gland, superficial parotidectomy or limited excision. *J. Laryngol. Otol.* **102**, 603–5.

Winsten, J., and Ward, G.E. (1956). The parotid gland. An anatomic study. *Surgery* **40**, 585.

Woods, J.E. (1983). Parotidectomy: points of technique for a brief and safe operation. *Am. J. Surg.* **145**, 678.

Woods, J.E. (1985). Parotidectomy versus limited resection for benign parotid masses. *Am. J. Surg.* **149**, 749–50.

Woods, J.E., Chang, G.C., and Beahrs, O.H. (1975). Experience with 1,360 primary parotid tumours. *Am. J. Surg.* **130**, 460–2.

Woods, J.E., Weiland, L.H., Chong, G.C., *et al.* (1977). Pathology and surgery of primary tumours of the parotid. *Surg. Clin. North Am.* **73**, 565–73.

9. Head injury

Sira Bunyaratavej

In terms of morbidity and mortality, head injury exacts a dreadful toll on every society. For example, each year in the UK between 200 and 300 people per 100 000 of the population are admitted to hospital because of a head injury (Anderson and McLaurin 1980), and four to five times that number of patients attend hospital following a head injury but are not admitted (Jennett and McMillan 1981). Five per cent of injury is severe and it is in this group that high morbidity and mortality rates are seen; 40–50 per cent die, 10 per cent remain severely disabled or vegetative (dependent on the help of others for some or all of their activities of daily living), while the remaining 50 per cent recover to the point of being independent in terms of such functions (Miller, Butterworth, Gudman, Faulkner, Chot, Selhorst, Harrison, Lutz, Young, and Becker 1981).

From an economic standpoint, head injury also takes a substantial toll of both human and financial resources. In the US it has been extrapolated that each year there are approximately 500 000 new cases of head trauma. As many as 50 000 Americans are killed and 50 000 are disabled by head injuries each year. Tragically, the peak incidence of head injury in most patient populations is among adolescents and young adult males, who are, or are about to be, in the most productive period of life (Becker, Gade, Young, and Feuerman 1990). Apart from human costs, one estimate for the year 1977 placed the combined medical costs from head injury at over 6 billion US dollars, and lost income from head injury deaths at about 22 billion US dollars (Cooper 1982).

In almost all patient populations, road traffic accidents account for the greatest percentage of head injuries, (Caveness 1979; Kalsbeek, McLaurin, Harris, and Miller 1980; Jagger, *et al.* 1984; Whitman, Coonley-Hoganson, and Desai 1984). Most accidents can be prevented with better road building and traffic planning, for example diversion of highways away from cities or towns, more dual carriageways, and more overpass pedestrian crossings. Recognition of the importance of protecting the head from injury developed in the First World War, and led to the compulsory use of crash helmets by British army motor cyclists in 1941. The value of a satisfactorily designed helmet in minimizing the effects of head injury is now well established. It protects the skull from local injury by spreading the blow over a larger area.

It also diminishes the extent and intensity of brain damage by reducing the speed of the impact (Cairns and Holbourn 1943; Lewin and Kennedy 1950).

Other measures have also been taken during the past decade. Restraining seat belts have reduced the incidence of head and facial injury in drivers and front seat passengers (Rutherford, Greenfield, Hayes, and Nelson 1985). The use of seat belts will probably in the future universally extend to back seat passengers, and seats for children. Car manufacturers have also been active in making cars safer for occupants. Support for the back of the head and neck has been fitted for the prevention of violent extension and flexion movements. Some cars are manufactured in such a way that the front and back of the car will collapse to absorb the force on impact (Miller 1987).

There are other aspects of prevention. The association of alcohol with road traffic accidents and head injury has been studied extensively (Cairns and Holbourn 1943; National Safety Council 1976; Klauber, Barrett-Connor, and Marshall 1984), and measures to combat drunken driving should also reduce the number of road traffic accidents and head injuries. Safety precautions, including helmets for people at work, have been reported to have almost halved the number of major head injuries (Caveness 1979).

Anatomical considerations

The scalp covering the cranium has a rich vascular supply. Nerves and blood vessels are found almost entirely in the dense subcutaneous layer, and this must be borne in mind when local anaesthesia is employed. To be effective, the injection must be made into this dense layer, which is difficult to inject into, rather than in the adjacent loose areolar layer. There is free communication of the venous system, extra- and intracranially, by emissary veins, which do not possess valves and allow blood flow in both directions. This provides an excellent pressure vent, but may also be an avenue to entry for infection, if a scalp wound becomes infected.

The skull is more resilient than is often appreciated following an impact which may alter its diameter at several places. Complex deformation of the skull may also occur, causing cerebral displacement and a cavitational effect. There are many bony cavities in the wall of the skull that connect with the external atmosphere — paranasal sinuses, middle ears, and mastoid air cells. These cavities are lined with epithelium and provide a venue for leakage of cerebrospinal fluid and ascending infection.

The brain is the most fragile organ in the body. It is protected by a very hard and unyielding cranium and its stability in the cranial cavity is maintained by several structures. The brainstem joins the bulky and relatively mobile brain superior to the spinal cord, which is relatively fixed by the ligamentum denticulatum inferiorly, and is often damaged in severe head injury. All cranial nerves which emerge symmetrically from the base of the brain (except the fourth nerve which emerges from the dorsal surface of the mid-brain) also offer stability to the brain, as these become fixed to the foramen on exit from the cranial cavity.

Ramification of both arteries and veins gives strong support to the brain parenchyma. Arteries enter the base of the brain, forming the circle of Willis, giving rise to numerous tiny perforating arteries to supply the diencephalon and brainstem, which contain a reticular activating system that is necessary for normal consciousness. Other main arteries supply various cortical areas. In contrast, veins converge to the surface of the brain to empty into dural venous sinuses between the two layers of dura. The veins transverse the subarachnoid and subdural spaces obliquely to reach the sinuses. Disturbance of the stability of the brain may thus result in subdural haematoma.

Finally the meninges, especially the dura with its partitions, offer great stability to the brain. The falx cerebri prevents horizontal movement of the brain and the tentorium cerebelli supports the brain by preventing vertical movement. It is, indeed, at openings of the two partitions that two of the three well-known cerebral herniations take place when there is a mass effect in the cranial cavity, i.e. herniation across the mid-line (mid-line shift, falcine herniation) and tentorial herniation (uncal herniation). The pia and arachnoid, together with enclosed cerebrospinal fluid, also offer a great deal of stability, but more in the way of 'filling in the gap' rather than as a 'water cushion'.

At the moment of impact, with sudden acceleration of the head, there may be differential movement of the cranium and the brain. This differential movement causes strain of the structures joining the two that maintain normal stability, i.e. blood vessels, brainstem, and cranial nerves.

Mechanisms of head injury

Mechanisms of head injury are very complex, being dependent on the circumstances at the time of injury and intricate intracranial anatomical arrangements. An excellent review of this complicated subject has been documented by Gennarelli (1990). There are also many reviews of the mathematical and engineering aspects (Liu 1979; Goldsmith and Ommaya 1984; Thibault and Gennarelli 1985).

Forces may be applied to the head in two ways, static and dynamic loading. Static loading occurs when the force is relatively slowly (> 200 ms) applied to the head. This occurs in the form of a crushing or squeezing effect when there is no movement of the head involved. If the force is sufficient it results in multiple, comminuted fractures of the vault or skull base. It is very rare in real life, but in contrast to dynamic loading there is no widespread damage to the brain. Coma and severe neurological signs are, in fact, characteristically absent in this injury unless the force is strong enough to cause severe skull deformation and brain compression, which usually is fatal.

Dynamic loading is much more common and this type of injury occurs much more rapidly than static loading. It appears that the duration of loading is the critical factor in determining the type of head injury produced, and in this instance the force applied to the head acts, in most cases, in less than 20 ms. Biological tissues usually withstand strain better if deformity occurs slowly rather than quickly, and they are more brittle and will fracture at lower strain levels under rapidly applied loads.

Dynamic loading can be of two types, impulsive or impact. When head injury takes place without the head being hit directly, but by the head being set into motion or the moving head being arrested by a force applied to other parts of the body such as the chest, this is described as impulsive loading (Gennarelli 1990). Although this appears purely an academic consideration, it can occur in certain circumstances (Bakay and Glasauer 1980). A large majority of head injuries occur by impact loading which implies that the head is actually struck by an object in a very short period of time.

Mechanical effects of head injury

Impact injuries Forces acting directly on the head can produce two effects, local and remote. Local effects at the site of impact are the result of local skull deformation. The in-bending of the skull may result in fracture of the skull (linear or depressed) damage to the dura and the vessels attached to the dura, the middle meningeal artery and venous sinuses in particular, and brain contusion. If the skull does not break, but snaps back into its original position, it may produce negative pressures, contributing further to brain contusion. Remote effects are largely the result of skull distortion. When there is in-bending, the surrounding skull bends outward. The shape of the skull may alter in several places, resulting in changes in its diameter at different points. Theoretically, the out-bending skull with an increase in diameter may produce a low pressure zone in the region, and the snapping back of the skull may contribute to further injury.

Inertial injuries Dynamic loading, whether impulsive or impact, sets the head into rapid motion, be it acceleration or deceleration. Injuries inflicted by this motion are widespread and differ from impact injuries, being collectively called inertial injuries, whether resulting from acceleration, deceleration, momentum, or inertia.

Head motion results in compressive, tensile, and shear strains that cause structural damage by differential movement of the skull and the brain, and strains within the brain itself. Differential movement of the skull and the brain occurs when there is sudden acceleration of the skull and the inertia of the brain causes it to lag behind, or when there is sudden deceleration of the skull and cerebral momentum leads the brain to travel further. All factors that maintain the stability of the brain within the skull will be involved. The cortical veins may be torn and subdural haematoma may result. Cranial nerves, perforating arteries, and the brainstem may be damaged during the process. As the brain is free to move to some degree within the skull, the movement of the brain away from the skull creates regions of low pressure (tensile strain) on the contralateral side of the impact, giving rise to contra-coup contusion.

There are three kinds of acceleration. Translational acceleration occurs when the centre of gravity of the head moves in a straight line; rotational acceleration occurs when the head moves around the centre of gravity which remains stable; and angular acceleration occurs when the centre of gravity moves in more than one direction. In reality, it is angular acceleration that produces all varieties of head injury.

Pathophysiology

For the purpose of clinicopathological correlations and management, it is helpful to consider that there are two kinds of pathology following a head injury: primary and secondary lesions. Primary lesions include all injuries inflicted at the moment of impact and immediately thereafter. These encompass brain contusions and lacerations, diffuse axonal injury, and damage to blood vessels, cranial nerves, and the brainstem. Injuries of the scalp and skull may be included in this category. Secondary lesions are occasional lesions that take time to develop. Nearly all secondary lesions are expanding, space occupying, and are regarded as secondary expanding lesions. These consist of intracranial haemorrhage and brain swelling. Most patients with minor or moderately severe head injury do not develop a secondary lesion at all, whereas about half of the severely head-injured patients develop secondary lesions (Miller *et al.* 1981). At present, there are no methods available to predict the development of the lesion with any certainty.

Primary lesions

Scalp A scalp lesion usually indicates the site of impact, but the site of impact is not invariably associated with a scalp lesion. Scalp wounds may bleed excessively and in children this may be severe enough to cause hypovolaemic shock. Scalp wounds may be very deceptive in appearance. Innocent looking wounds may harbour hair, dirt, and foreign bodies which, if left unremoved, may result in infection. The infection may spread to infect bone, to extradural and subdural spaces, or, via emissary veins, to the brain itself. Bleeding into the loose areolar layer of the scalp is described as subgaleal haematoma, which may spread all over the head, crossing sutures, due to the laxity of this layer of the scalp.

Skull Skull fracture occurs as a result of deformation at the time of injury. At the site of impact, the calvarium is momentarily bent inwards, causing an abrupt rise of intracranial pressure, while at a distance, often at opposing points, there is a corresponding outward bending of the skull. Coincident with indentation of the bone at the site of impact there is also a concentric out-bending. If the object that hits the head is greater than 2 inches square and of sufficient force, skull penetration does not occur, but deformation of the skull takes place and a linear fracture may result (Gennarelli 1990). If the object is small or sharp, skull penetration may occur to result in a compound depressed fracture. The scalp wound may not be directly over the fracture site because the scalp has the capacity to slide over the skull. A depressed fracture of the skull, owing to the resilience and toughness of the bone, can also be deceptive. Once the fracture admits the objects, together with contaminating foreign bodies, such as hair, dirt, and grit, it often snaps back and the fragments lock together, giving no indication at all of penetration of the skull. If this is unrecognized it may result in potentially fatal intracranial infection.

Fracture of the skull, together with tear of the dura and arachnoid, may cause leakage of the cerebrospinal fluid from the ear or the nose, if the fracture involves paranasal sinuses, middle ear, or mastoid air cells. Structures adjacent to the fracture may also be damaged. The middle meningeal artery, which often runs in the groove on the inner table of the skull, may be torn and result in an epidural haematoma. The wall of the venous sinuses beneath the fracture may be injured, and delayed thrombosis may occur. Fracture at the cavernous region may damage the walls of the internal carotid artery and the cavernous sinus, resulting in a carotid–cavernous fistula.

Intracranial structures The brain and the structures that maintain its stability, i.e. meninges, blood vessels, cranial nerves, and brainstem, may be injured at the time of impact, particularly after dynamic loading.

Cerebral contusion Cerebral contusion may be found on the surface of the brain. These contusions consist of areas of peri-vascular haemorrhage around small blood vessels and necrotic brain. Typically, gyral crests are involved, assuming a wedge-like shape extending through the cortex to the white matter. When the pia is torn, the lesion is termed a cerebral laceration. Contusion underlying the site of impact is called coup contusion, and on the contralateral side, contre-coup contusion. Pathological and experimental studies have shown that contusions tend to occur in a characteristic distribution. These are clustered over the frontal and temporal poles and the areas between the two poles, i.e. the orbital surface of the frontal lobe and the area of cortex around the Sylvian fissure (Holbourn 1943; Adams, Mitchell, Graham, and Doyle 1977; Adams, Graham, and Gennarelli 1983). It is likely that these contusions are caused by differential movements of the cranium and brain and associated with acceleration and deceleration of the head. Irregularity of the bony surface over these areas is believed to be important in the aetiology of contusions. Movement of the skull away from the brain, opposite the point of impact, has been postulated to create a negative pressure sufficient to cause cavitation and disruption of the brain parenchyma (Gennarelli 1990).

Acute axonal injury In 1956, Strich made a notable contribution to our understanding of the pathology of head injury with a description of widespread degeneration of the white matter in the brain of patients dying many months after severe injury. In 1961, she reported the results of histopathological examination of 20 cases (Strich 1961). The widespread degeneration of the white matter described by Strich later became known as acute axonal injury. This pathology was found in post-mortem examinations of the brain of patients who had a sustained a severe head injury and never regained consciousness. Gross pathology of diffuse axonal injury consists of focal, typically haemorrhagic, lesions in the corpus callosum and dorsolateral quadrant of the mid-brain and pons. Microscopic findings, when survival time is short, are of axonal swelling or of globular ends of disrupted axons (retraction balls of Cajal) throughout the white matter of the cerebral hemispheres, brainstem, and cerebellum (Adams 1984; Graham, Adams, and Gennerelli 1987). After a period of several weeks neuroglial clusters appear around the severed axonal ends. It is believed that this type of injury is caused by inertial effect. Angular acceleration of relatively prolonged duration, especially in a coronal orientation, seems particularly harmful.

Other injuries Injuries to cranial nerves, hypothalamus, infundibulum, and pituitary stalk and gland can also occur at the time of impact and are also regarded as primary lesions. Diabetes insipidus occurs in less than 1 per cent of patients with head injury, and panpituitarism is rare (Porter and Miller 1948; McLaurin and King 1975).

Traumatic subarachnoid haemorrhage In the past, before the advent of computed tomography, this condition was undiagnosed and overlooked. Incidentally, subarachnoid haemorrhage can raise intracranial pressure to a considerable degree, depending on the source of the haemorrhage. Arterial bleeding from a large artery can markedly distend the subarachnoid space and produce brain swelling similar to that of aneurysmal rupture at operation before the arachnoid membrane is widely opened. This condition has also been overlooked and misdiagnosed as brain oedema and, of course, failed to respond to medication. Furthermore, blood in the cerebrospinal fluid may behave in much the same way as spontaneous bleeding in the subarachnoid space, i.e. to cause delayed vasospasm, and blockage of absorption of cerebrospinal fluid.

Secondary lesions

Theoretically any lesion that does not occur at the time of injury is regarded as secondary in nature. Since most secondary lesions are expanding, these may be grouped together and termed *secondary expanding lesions*.

Intracranial haematoma

Epidural haematoma This is more common in the younger age group and is less frequent later in life, because, with increasing age, the dura becomes more adherent to the inner table of the skull. A majority of epidural haematomas are found over the lateral aspect of the hemisphere, in the territory supplied by the middle meningeal vessels. It is difficult to be certain of the original site of bleeding because the haematoma separates the dura from the inner table of the skull as it increases in size and, thereby, ruptures more branches of the middle meningeal vessels that normally pass straight into the inner table of the skull. The haematoma can also arise from a bleed from dural venous sinuses, e.g. from the superior sagittal or transverse sinus. Bleeding from the latter gives rise to a posterior fossa epidural haematoma. This is uncommon, but not altogether rare, and once it occurs, failure to remove it may result in respiratory arrest.

Subdural haematoma Acute subdural haematoma is a complication of head injury, and is a result of inertial loading rather than impact force (Gennarelli 1983). Several bridging veins may rupture and bleed simultaneously to form a rapidly enlarging clot, or a subdural haematoma may be associated with brain damage, often around the Sylvian fissure. It is more commonly encountered in severe head injury than is epidural haematoma. Chronic subdural haematoma, another clinical entity altogether, occurs in the elderly and is often associated with alcoholism, brain atrophy, or other pathology. The patient does not often remember any significant head injury in the past, and those with chronic subdural haematoma do not come to hospital complaining of head injury but of chronic headache and fluctuation of consciousness. Pathologically, the haematoma is situated between two pseudo-membranes, the parietal layer which is adherent to the dura, and the visceral layer which can easily be separated from the arachnoid.

Intracerebral haematoma With the aid of computed tomography this entity is being recognized with increasing frequency in patients with closed head injury. Small intracerebral haematomas not contiguous with the brain surface may be found in several places deep in the cerebral hemisphere, but occasionally a sizeable lesion that affects intracranial pressure and displaces cerebral parenchyma is encountered. More commonly, mixed pathology with cerebral contusion and laceration is present, most often contiguous with a subdural haematoma on the surface of the brain. Delayed post-traumatic intracerebral haematomas or spat-apoplexie were reported a century ago (Bollinger 1891) and occur in about 7 per cent of serious head injuries (Gudeman, Kishore, Miller, Girevendulis, Lipper, and Becker 1979). It is not clear why haemorrhage occurs but a damaged vascular bed and defective autoregulation are proposed explanations (Gudeman *et al.* 1979).

Subdural hygroma Occasionally after injury a tear in the arachnoid acts as a flap valve and allows cerebrospinal fluid to escape into the subdural space. The collection of fluid is called subdural hygroma. Uncertainty exists as to the fate of the fluid if this is left alone; obviously, a collection interfering with the patient's normal recovery requires removal.

Brain swelling

Although there is a tendency to use the terms oedema and swelling interchangeably, it is advisable to differentiate between these in clinical practice. Brain swelling should be used to describe a non-specific increase in volume of the brain. Brain oedema is one cause of brain swelling, apart from many others, each of which has a different pathology and treatment. The most common cause of post-traumatic brain swelling is an increase in volume of the vascular compartment, when there is, for example, comprised venous return in tension pneumothorax, hyperaemia due to increased arterial carbon dioxide levels, or hypertension with impaired autoregulation of cerebral blood flow. If the cause of the swelling is rapidly eliminated the swelling may subside; alternatively this may progress to brain oedema. This subject will be discussed further under the heading of operative brain swelling.

Effects of secondary expanding lesions

These effects are the same as any associated with a space-occupying lesion, which are increased intracranial pressure or local, hydrocephalic and cerebral displacement effects.

Increased intracranial effect Secondary expanding lesions raise intracranial pressure at different rates depending on the number of bleeding points and pressure generated. The pressure/volume graph is not a straight line. After an initial period when there seems to be compensation for the rise in the volume, the pressure rises steeply. This is the danger period where delay in diagnosis and treatment may prove fatal (Fig. 9.1).

Local effect Compression on the brain by a secondary expanding lesion will produce a focal neurological deficit which is useful to localize the site of the mass lesion. Thus, a lesion of the motor area will produce weakness on the opposite side. A surface clot tends to produce hemiparesis with differential weakness of the face, arms, and leg, while a deep-seated lesion tends to produce dense hemiplegia. A deep lesion may also give rise to a deficit of the deep tracts in the brain, such as visual radiation in the temporal and parietal lobes.

Hydrocephalic effect Posterior fossa clot may compress the fourth ventricle and block drainage of cerebrospinal fluid, resulting in enlargement of, and increased pressure in, the ventricles. A rise of the intracranial pressure

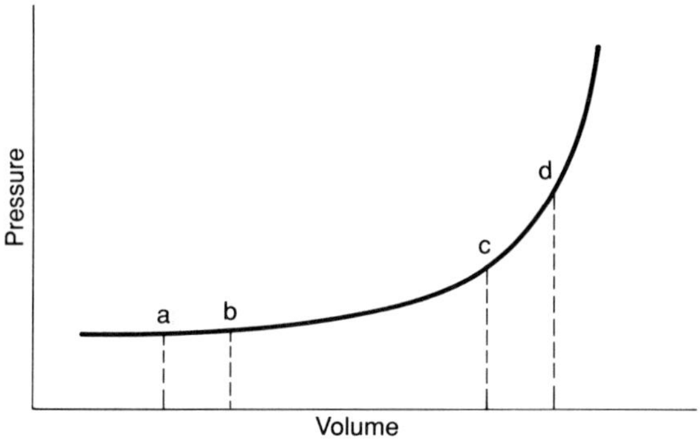

Fig. 9.1. Pressure/volume curve signifies that at a later stage (cd) the same increase in volume raises the intracranial pressure to a level much higher than that produced by the same volume in the initial stage (ab).

is dependent on the volume of the clot and the degree of secondary hydrocephalus.

Cerebral displacement effect Displacement of the brain by a mass lesion was described explicitly in Dott's 'Brain, movement and time' (Dott 1960). Secondary expanding lesions develop relatively rapidly and, therefore, displacement occurs rather early. It is evident as mid-line shift, tentorial herniation, and tonsillar herniation.

Mid-line shift Although mid-line shift may not produce established physical signs as in other forms of cerebral displacement, it is, however, very useful in clinical practice. Shift of the mid-line seen on computed tomography or on angiography indicates the effects of a mass lesion on intracranial structures, the sole exception being when mass lesions are bilateral. The cingulate gyrus actually herniates under the free edge of the falx cerebri, displacing the corpus callosum inferiorly. This is also known as subfalcine or falcine herniation. There may be some degree of diencephalic ischaemia attributable to herniation due to compression and compromise of the blood supply by stretching of the perforating arteries on shift of the mid-line, and these changes may result in deterioration in consciousness (Dott 1960).

Tentorial herniation Half a century ago this type of herniation was termed a tentorial pressure cone and firmly linked with ipsilateral oculomotor palsy (fixed and dilated pupil) and medial occipital infarction (posterior cerebral artery compression) (Jefferson 1938), deterioration of consciousness (Cairns 1952), contralateral and sometimes ipsilateral weakness due to compression of the opposite cerebral penduncle by the edge of tentorium (Gurdjian and Thomas 1974). This pressure cone is also known as uncal or tentorial herniation.

Tonsillar herniation When supra-tentorial compression continues unchecked or the expanding mass is situated beneath the tentorium, tonsillar herniation follows, in which the cerebellar tonsils prolapse through the foramen magnum, obliterating the cisterna magna and compressing the medulla oblongata, with resultant apnoea. The characteristic finding of such herniation is depression of respiration which develops very early, perhaps before or commensurate with depression of consciousness.

Cerebral concussion

Cerebral concussion is deliberately described under a separate heading. This is purely a clinical term and is used to describe a transient loss of consciousness following a blow on the head of sufficient force. For practical purposes this is a clinically significant lesion. It signifies that the head injury was caused by a blow severe enough to produce further complications, particularly secondary expanding lesions, and is always associated with amnesia. Amnesia is the usual explanation in some patients who must have lost consciousness after an injury but cannot recall doing so.

Clinical management

Management concepts

Primary damage is predetermined; it occurs at the time of injury and before the patient is first seen. The best that can be offered is to maintain life and create favourable conditions for a recovery of reversibly damaged brain parenchyma. It is also important to prevent secondary changes that may occur from associated disorders such as hypotension or hypoxia. We are, however, entirely responsible for the early detection and treatment of secondary lesions. Delays in diagnosis and treatment will definitely lead to morbidity and mortality.

Plan of management

The plan of management depends on the patient's condition on admission. Patients may be allocated to one of two groups.

Group I Patients are conscious, able to converse, and give a good account of the medical history. This implies that primary damage was not all that serious and our goal is to ensure prompt recognition and treatment of any secondary expanding lesion.

All patients who have lost consciousness after a head injury, regardless of its duration, who have a neurological deficit, or who have a skull fracture, signs of skull fracture, or cerebrospinal fluid leakage ought to be admitted to hospital for observation.

Group II Patients who have impaired consciousness of any degree. They are unable to speak normally and cannot give a reliable history. If the patient has been brought to hospital immediately or soon after the injury, the condition is likely to be caused by primary damage. Alternatively if admission is delayed for some hours after the injury, especially if there is a history of deterioration of consciousness, it is probably caused by a secondary expanding lesion. In the case of the patient who has a history of momentary loss of consciousness after the injury, who has later regained consciousness and becomes unconscious again before hospitalization, the intervening clear period of full consciousness is called the *lucid interval* and is pathognomonic of a secondary expanding lesion. In these circumstances there is no phase for observation, and prompt action to investigate and treat the lesion concerned is immediately taken.

All patients in this group should be admitted to the intensive care unit. If a secondary expanding lesion is not suspected at the time of admission, the patient will require observation as for patients in the first group, in addition to other treatment designed to promote the best conditions for recovery.

Observation

In the management of head injury, observation implies constant surveillance of the patient to detect symptoms and signs of secondary expanding lesions. When there is any suggestion of the presence of a secondary lesion, prompt investigation must be undertaken and the lesion treated as soon as possible. Observation, therefore, requires constant evaluation of the patient's condition, based on possible symptoms, level of consciousness, vital and neurological signs.

Symptoms These may be voiced by patients in group I who are able to communicate. Headache is common after head injury of any severity, but progressively worsening headache is very suggestive of a secondary expanding lesion. Headache from a mass lesion in the skull is unlikely to be relieved by analgesics or bed rest. At a later stage it may be accompanied by vomiting, drowsiness, or restlessness.

Consciousness Coma has been defined as 'not obeying commands, not uttering words, and not opening the eyes' (Jennett and Teasdale 1981), and these three parameters have been utilized in the Glasgow coma scale and score. This method of recording levels of consciousness has been widely accepted and used all over the world. It offers an objective and simple assessment for all levels of medical personnel, while at the same time avoiding arbitrary staging or grading of patients and ambiguous terminology (Fig. 9.2). The total score of the Glasgow scale can also give easy and simple reference to the level of consciousness.

Vital signs Secondary expanding lesions at an early stage tend to slow the pulse rate and widen the pulse pressure. These are useful points of observation and must not be overlooked. Later decompensation of the brainstem, rapid rise in pulse rate, and lowering of blood pressure are ominous signs.

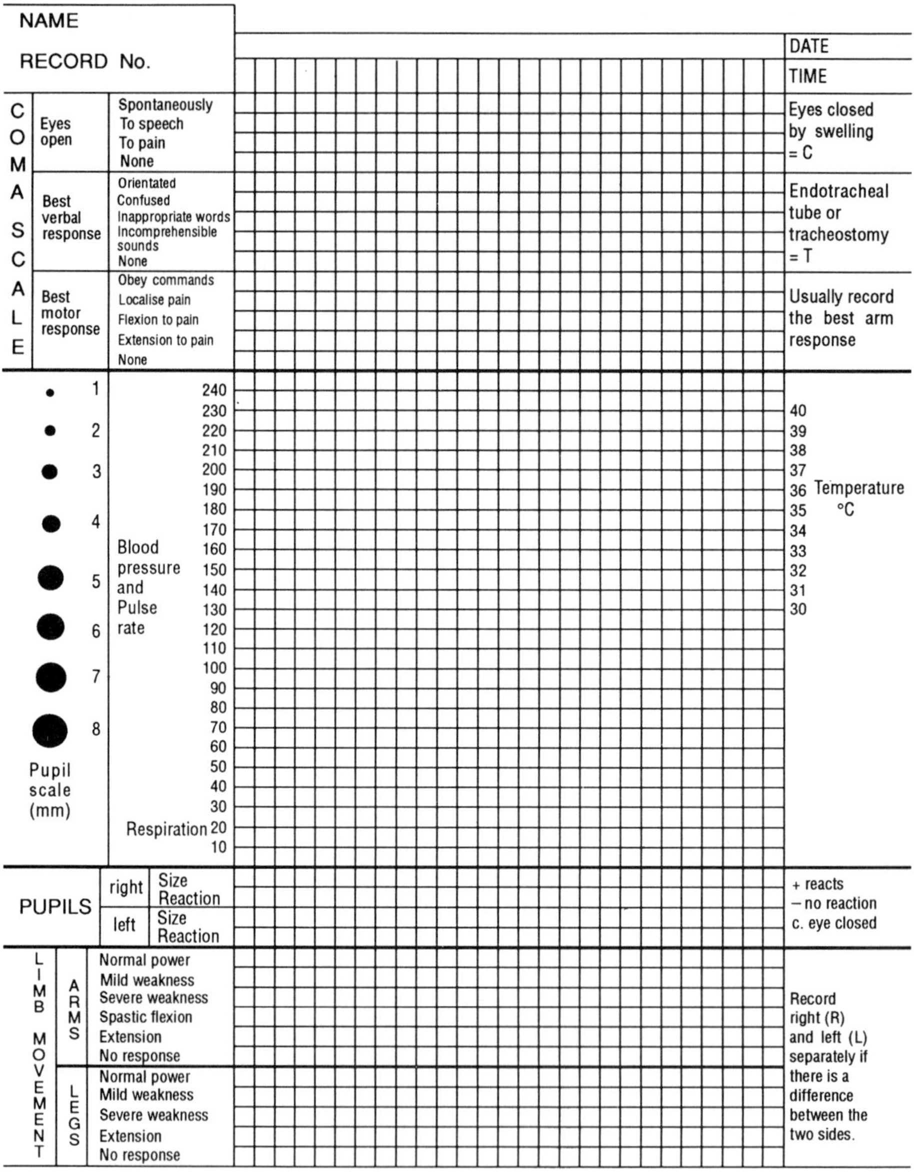

Fig. 9.2. Observation chart for the Glasgow coma scale.

Depression of respiration is highly suggestive of compression of the medulla by a clot in the posterior fossa and tonsillar herniation. Prompt removal of the clot is required to prevent the onset of apnoea. In contrast, supratentorial lesions produce irregular, ataxic, and rapid respiration.

Neurological signs Complete neurological examination must be repeated at intervals. Newly developed signs suggest a new pathological process which may be indicative of a secondary lesion. Monitoring for signs characteristic of secondary expanding lesions is mandatory. Of particular importance are pupillary sizes and reaction, plantar response, and weakness of the limbs. It should be noted that a patient who at one time has exhibited a unilateral extensor plantar response but who later develops bilateral extensor responses should be treated with extreme urgency, because the whole brainstem is now affected.

Observation should continue for at least 72 hours after injury because formation of most secondary lesions peaks within this period (Gade, Becker, Miller, and Dwan 1990). Patients in group I can be discharged after 3 days, provided that there are no symptoms or neurological deficit.

Diagnosis

A number of investigative procedures are employed in the management of head injury.

Skull films Skull films are definitely superfluous when a patient deteriorates and a secondary expanding lesion is suspected. These are performed when there is time to spare, such as when the patient is under observation and intervention is not required. Radiographs are useful, rapid, safe, and inexpensive and may be taken in the ward if necessary. The presence of a fracture indicates a relatively severe injury. Shift of the mid-line may be detected if there is calcification of the pineal gland. Skull films are also helpful for future reference. Conventionally three views — antero-posterior, lateral, and a Towne's view — should be taken.

Computed tomography Computed tomography is the most useful diagnostic tool in the management of head injury for the rapid detection and precise location of intracranial haematomas, brain contusion, and oedema. It is also of value for the detection of skull fractures, particularly of the skull base, which are often difficult to visualize in plain radiographic films. An assessment of the size of the haematoma, shift of the mid-line, and ventricular size facilitates appropriate clinical judgement. In order to expedite the examination in the acute situation, contrast enhancement may be omitted.

All patients in group II who are deeply unconscious should have computed tomography performed on admission. It must be remembered, however, that a new lesion may develop after an initial negative scan has been obtained and one must still be alert to this possibility even after a negative standing (Gudeman *et al.* 1979).

Angiography When computed tomography is not available, angiography can prove useful to detect mid-line shift, and is sometimes sufficient to warrant surgical intervention. Displacement of the angiographic triangle in the lateral view helps to localize a haematoma. Although computed tomographic scanning has replaced angiography for most conditions, the latter is still the investigation of choice in certain conditions such as thrombosis of blood vessels, traumatic aneurysm, and arterio-venous fistula.

Exploratory burr holes With the advent of computed tomography this operation has almost been completely abandoned by many neurosurgeons in the past decade. There are, however, surgeons who advocate that this procedure is reliable in the detection of a majority of traumatic haematomas and the most rapid method of doing so (Andrews, Pitts, Lovely, and Barkowski 1986). When the patient's condition dictates extreme urgency, and computed tomography is not available, or time for transportation of the patient to the scanning unit is likely to be prolonged, the author believes that this operation still has a very useful place. In a patient who exhibits clear-cut clinical features, such as a lucid interval, unilateral dilated pupil, and contralateral hemiparesis, and if scalp contusion and fracture strongly suggest the location of the haematoma, this operation may enable prompt removal of the clot, without the consequent delays to investigation.

Medical treatment

Patients in group I require little specific medical therapy and are primarily in the hospital for observation. Sedation must not be given as this will interfere with the patient's level of consciousness. Simple analgesics alone are permitted for treatment of headache.

Patients in group II require greater attention and should be admitted to an intensive care unit with more facilities and trained personnel. Aims are to provide an optimal milieu for recovery from the primary damage; to avoid adverse conditions such as hypoxia or hypovolaemia, which will not only hinder the recovery but may produce further damage; and to observe any suggestion of secondary expanding lesions.

Associated injuries Head injury is frequently associated with injuries to other parts of the body (Miller *et al.* 1981) and such injuries are easily overlooked in unconscious patients who cannot communicate. Low blood pressure, rapid thready pulse, and other signs of hypovolaemia are unusual in pure head injury, but may indicate a haemothorax, abdominal injury, or even a femoral fracture. Urinary retention is very rarely attributable to head injury, but is suggestive of spinal or pelvic injury. Fat embolism may lead to deterioration of consciousness and can be mistaken as a sign of a secondary expanding lesion.

Posture Unconscious patients who do not have a tracheostomy or an endotracheal tube should be put in the semi-prone position. This posture will keep the airway clear and provide good drainage of secretions from bronchi, trachea, and throat. This position is achieved by bending the under-leg to provide a base for support with the upper leg stretched over a pillow to protect pressure points. The under-arm should be positioned behind rather than in front or beneath the trunk. A pillow is used to support the front of the trunk to prevent the patient from turning into the prone position. If the patient is turned every 2 hours, the drainage from each side of the lung is alternately effective. Good nursing in this posture can keep the airway clear and make endotracheal tube or tracheostomy unnecessary (Miller 1987).

For the patient who requires a tracheostomy or an endotracheal tube, only supine and semi-supine positions can be used. These positions must also be alternated every 2 hours to prevent pressure sores.

Ventilation Most head-injured patients vomit, and most patients in group II aspirate gastic contents into the lungs before being brought to the hospital. Acidic gastric contents provoke a chemical pneumonitis which is most severe by 12–36 hours. If uncomplicated by bacterial pneumonia, this resolves over 72 hours. In some patients endotracheal intubation is needed in order to maintain the airway and to clear the excessive bronchial secretions. The endotracheal tube can be kept *in situ* for several weeks and a tracheostomy avoided in most patients.

Positive end-expiratory pressure, if required to maintain oxygenation, appears to be well tolerated from the standpoint of intracranial pressure up to pressures of 10 mmHg, provided the patient's head is elevated by 20° (Gildenberg and Frost 1985).

Cardiovascular function Cerebrovascular autoregulation is frequently deranged in association with head trauma, and any abnormality of systemic cardiovascular function may be harmful as regards cerebral blood flow (Muizelaar and Obrist 1985). Loss of autoregulation in the presence of hypertension may lead to cerebral hyperaemia and swelling (Miller, *et al.* 1975). It is advisable, therefore, that during the acute period when the autoregulation may be defective, blood pressure is maintained at normal or low normal levels at all times.

The importance of adequate plasma volume has been emphasized by experimental data which have indicated that cardiac output has a major influence on cerebral flow (Davis and Sundt 1980), and normal and even elevated plasma volume (using capillary wedge pressure) does not predispose to intracranial hypertension (Clifton, Robertson, and Grossman 1985). It is important, therefore, to administer normal daily requirements of fluid rather than to restrict fluid intake as previously advocated.

Electrolytes Most abnormalities of fluid and electrolytes associated with head trauma involve derangements of sodium and water balance. Since hyponatraemia promotes cerebral oedema and may provoke seizures, it is potentially the most serious abnormality. Inappropriate volume replacement with hypotonic fluids is a common cause, or an exacerbating factor, of hyponatraemia. In addition, intracranial disease, trauma, surgery, anaesthesia, and mechanical ventilation stimulate secretion of antidiuretic hormone (ADH) with free water retention that continues despite low serum sodium levels, decreased osmolarity, and expanded intravascular volume (Nelson 1987). This state is termed the syndrome of inappropriate ADH secretion. In this condition expansion of extracellular volume results in suppression of aldosterone secretion or increase in glomerular filtration, or both, causing urinary sodium loss despite hyponatraemia. Inappropriate secretion of ADH thus results in the characteristic laboratory picture of hyponatraemia and serum hypo-osmolality, increased urinary sodium concentration, and increased urine osmolarity.

The author has observed that the syndrome of inappropriate ADH secretion is not uncommon following severe head injury. Clinically the patient shows deterioration of consciousness, and quite often exhibits hyperkinesia in the form of fidgeting movements of the hands and fingers. In severe forms there may be convulsions. Blood and urine osmolarity, serum sodium, and urine sodium estimations will confirm the presence of the syndrome. Useful and easy parameters to determine the amount of water in the vascular compartment are levels of sodium and blood urea nitrogen (BUN). In the absence of kidney and adrenal disease, raised levels of BUN suggest dehydration. If the level is in the range of low normal this suggests overload of fluid, and if there is also a low serum sodium level, there is a very high possibility of the syndrome of inappropriate ADH secretion. If the patient's clinical condition also suggests the syndrome, further laboratory tests are required to confirm the diagnosis. Treatment of this condition is simply to limit fluid intake in most adults, to 500 ml per day. Once again the serum levels of sodium and BUN may be used as guides to the state of hydration.

Nutrition Metabolic responses to injury involve increased sympathetic tone and neuropeptide release mediated by the hypothalamus. Levels of adrenaline, glycogen, growth hormone, ADH, cortisol, and aldosterone levels are increased, whereas insulin secretion is inhibited. As a result, patients with severe injuries may have an elevated basal metabolic rate of 115–215 per cent of normal, consuming energy stores in the form of glycogen and lipid, and catabolizing up to 200–300 g protein per day (Epstein, Ward, and Becker 1987). During the first 2 weeks after injury, patients are in a catabolic phase, and attempts to match protein breakdown with increased intake simply result in urinary nitrogen excretion. The aim is to minimize losses rather than to achieve positive nitrogen balance. The daily caloric requirement consist of basal energy needs plus that required by the extent and severity of the injury, e.g. severe extensor rigidity which results in loss of large numbers of calories.

Nutritional support can be given on the second or third day after the injury, and is best given via a nasogastric tube. It is important to ensure that the patient can tolerate early feeding and, if not possible, other forms of feeding must be considered. It is also wise to start feeding slowly initially and subsequently increase this in amount and caloric content. Troublesome diarrhoea may result if the initial feeding volume is too great.

Temperature A high temperature tends to interfere with the patient's recovery in several ways including the dilatation of cerebral vessels with a rise in intracranial pressure. The rate of development of vasogenic oedema is also increased by pyrexia (Clasen, Pandolfi, Laing, and Casey 1974). Whether the cause of the fever is central, infective, or attributable to blood in the cerebrospinal fluid, reduction of temperature is necessary for recovery of brain cells. Aspirin suppositories are the best and safest medication. This, together with sponging and other means of cooling and the patient, is usually sufficient provided that shivering, which may produce more body heat, is controlled by medication, most commonly achieved with chlorpromazine hydrochloride.

Gastrointestinal complications Gastritis and ulceration are frequently associated with head injury and may be due to vagal stimulation due to diencephalic or brainstem injury. Another proposal is that an adrenergic surge resulting from brain injury may play a role by altering mucosal blood flow and physiology. Prophylaxis by cimetidine or antacids is useful in severe cases (French, Porter, von Amerongen, and Raney 1957, Epstein *et al.* 1987).

Seizures About 5 per cent of patients with head injury have seizures in the immediate post-injury period (Bricola 1976). During seizures, there are increases in cerebral metabolic demands and blood flow to the brain. The increase in blood flow may raise intracranial pressure, and the increase in metabolic demand may lead to anoxia, as blood flow may not keep pace with requirements. Any patient who appears to have moderate to severe brain contusion should receive prophylactic therapy. The most commonly employed and useful therapy is phenytoin, 300 mg per day. Acute seizures and status epilepticus may be controlled by diazepam or lorazepam.

Seizure that occurs in the first week after the injury carries important clinical implications. Twenty-eight per cent of patients with acute post-traumatic haematoma have one or more fits in the first week after the injury (Jennett 1974, 1975*a*). Early seizure also increases the risk of late epilepsy (Jennett 1975*b*).

Bladder and bowel care In the acute phase and in severely head-injured patients, the use of an indwelling catheter is necessary to ensure accurate measurement of urinary output. When fluid balance becomes less critical, and such measurements are not needed, the use of a condom strapped to the penis and connected to drainage tubing is commonly employed in male patients, and diapers in female patients. Bowel care of the head-injured patient is usually not difficult provided regular attention is given at the outset. Laxative suppositories suffice in most cases.

Physiotherapy It is important to ensure that a full range of passive movements of the limbs is performed early. This is essential to combat abnormal postures due to excessive spasm or paralysis. Quite often this aspect has been neglected until the patient recovers from the injury, and a longer period is required in hospital to correct deformities.

Monitoring of intracranial pressure Monitoring of intracranial pressure involves special training, equipment, and constant care. It can be very useful in patients who need artificial ventilation, since muscle relaxants and the administration of sedatives make it impossible to determine the patient's conscious level. It is also useful following surgery in a patient with brain swelling without any mass lesion or after removal of an haematoma. A pressure of 10–15 mmHg is regarded as normal whereas values of 25–30 mmHg require therapeatic intervention to reduce pressure.

Medical treatment for increased intracranial pressure Treatment is necessary when there is generalized brain swelling or before surgery for removal of an intracranial mass lesion, in order to limit the effects of the mass lesion until surgery can be performed. Osmotherapy, using mannitol, is the most common practice in head injury. A dosage of 1 g per kg body-weight, given intravenously over a period of 10 minutes, is commonly used in the acute period. The mechanism of action of osmotic agents in this situation is still controversial. In parts of the brain where vasogenic oedema exists, there is failure of the blood–brain barrier, such that osmotherapy is not, theoretically, efficacious. Overall reduction of the intracranial pressure is claimed to occur following the effects that these agents produce on normal portions of the brain.

The author has been using frusemide rather than mannitol for a number of years and believes the former to be advantageous. At a dosage of 1 mg per kg body-weight, given intravenously as a bolus dosage, it is cheaper and much easier to administer. It is equally effective in the reduction of pressure, without an initial period of rise in pressure as encountered with the use of mannitol. Electrolytic changes are also found less often than following mannitol administration (Pausawasdi and Bunyaratavej 1982).

The use of barbiturates to lower intracranial pressure in patients with head injury was advocated on the basis that barbiturates reduce brain metabolism, blood flow, and blood volume (Shapiro, Wyite, and Leosser 1974). A randomized prospective study, however, of the use of pentobarbitone in head-injured patients failed to show any beneficial effect on incidence, duration, or response to treatment of intracranial hypertension, or on overall outcome (Ward, *et al.* 1985). Therapy was also complicated by hypotensive episodes in 55 per cent of patients despite intensive cardiovascular monitoring and support. Another multi-centre trial has also been completed (Marshall and Marshall 1987), which showed a beneficial effect in terms of intracranial pressure control and survival with barbiturate use.

Steroid therapy Because steroids have proven to be very useful in the treatment of vasogenic oedema around a tumour, and because post-traumatic oedema is also vasogenic in experimental animals, steroids have been used liberally in the prevention and treatment of post-traumatic oedema. Nevertheless, all the current evident concerning the use of steroid therapy in normal or high-dose regimens in head injury has failed to influence morbidity and the incidence of raised intracranial pressure (Cooper, Moody, Clark, Kirkpatrick, Maravilla, Gould, and Dranne 1979).

Surgical treatment

Operative treatment of intracranial haematoma

When an intracranial clot is found at angiography or computed tomography, a judgement must be made as to whether the clot is the cause of clinical deterioration or whether it may delay patient recovery. Some clots are small and do not account for clinical deterioration. Efforts to remove such clots are unnecessary and often other causes for the patient's deterioration may be overlooked or recognized far too late. Degrees of cerebral displacement, particularly mid-line shift, usually indicate the severity of brain compression. An exception to this rule occurs when there are bilateral lesions, and the degree of mid-line shift may be less than expected due to counter-compression from the contralateral side.

The aim of surgery is to remove the clot, to bring intracranial pressure down to normal, and to eliminate cerebral displacement effects produced by the clot as soon as possible.

The operation is usually conducted under general anaesthesia, with the exception of chronic subdural haematoma which may require only a few burr holes over the haematoma and which can be performed under local anaesthesia. With computed tomography or angiography, the nature and exact location of the clot is known and an appropriate bone flap over the clot may be carefully planned and executed. It is wise to make a large bone flap covering the haematoma, if possible, in order to deal effectively with the sources of bleeding. Extradural haematoma usually arises from a bleeding middle meningeal artery and, although there may be only one bleeding point initially, the separation of the dura from the inner table of the skull by the clot will also tear several small branches of the artery running to the inner table of the skull. Acute subdural haematoma usually develops with haemorrhage from several bridging veins coursing to the superior sagittal sinus. Haemostatsis may only be possible by coagulating along the middle meningeal artery or ligating the stem of the artery itself. Occasionally a subdural haematoma extends into a brain laceration, and extension of the clot gives the impression of intracerebral haemorrhage. Not only must all surface and intracerebral clots be removed, but also the necrotic tissue surrounding the clot. Necrotic brain is removed by well-regulated suction which is able to aspirate necrotic tissue, but spare the normal brain. On removal of necrotic brain, more space is provided in the intracranial compartment for further brain expansion. This process is known as internal decompression.

When a diagnosis is made purely on a clinical basis and without confirmation by angiography or computed tomography, the exact location of the clot is not known. Burr-hole exploration may be required to determine the side of the lesion, but one has to rely on clinical findings. A fixed dilated pupil usually occurs on the side of the lesion, due to involvement of the third nerve following tentorial herniation. At a later stage, when both pupils are fixed and dilated, the side of the lesion is determined by the knowledge of which pupil was first to dilate. Hemiparesis can be also a useful guide to a clot on the contralateral side, particularly at an early stage. Subsequently, when full-blown tentorial herniation takes place, paresis can develop on the same side as the clot due to compression of the cerebral peduncle on the edge of the tentorium cerebelli (Kernohan's notch). As a rule, the first burr hole should be made just above the zygomatic process, about one inch in front of the external meatus. If a surface clot is not found, then parietal and frontal burr holes are made. In the absence of positive findings the same procedure is repeated on the opposite side.

Compound depressed fracture

All compound depressed fractures must receive operative treatment, the main risk of this condition being infection. To inexperienced eyes or exploring fingers there may not be any gap at the fracture site, which is usually tightly locked, to suggest that the dura underneath is torn and the brain is implanted by contaminated material, such as bone fragments, hair, or dirt. It is important, therefore, to enlarge widely the overlying wound and remove the bone fragments to expose the dura. Extreme care must be taken when removing the fragments overlying the dural venous sinuses, damage to which will cause alarming haemorrhage. The torn dura is then opened to allow further exploration of the lacerated brain and removal of all contaminated material. If the wound is badly soiled, it is preferable to remove all the bone fragments and undertake cranioplasty at a later date when the dangers of infection are eliminated.

Missile penetrating injury

Low velocity missiles, such as bullets from guns which are not war weapons, may penetrate the head and either traverse it completely or remain *in situ*. The entry wound should be treated in the same manner as a compound depressed fracture. There usually are foreign bodies in the bullet tract, together with necrotic brain material which should be removed after the skull hole is enlarged sufficiently by craniectomy to facilitate the procedure. The retained bullet should be removed together with other foreign body material unless it is in an area where removal might result in more damage to vital structures.

Operative brain swelling

The word brain swelling is here used in its descriptive sense to imply an increased volume of the brain due to any cause. This must not be confused with the term brain oedema, which we shall see later, forms a subset group of patients with brain swelling. When the skull and dura are opened, sometimes the brain herniates through the opening, indicating that it is under great pressure. This may take place during surgery, or immediately at the commencement of the operation. The cause of the swelling must be quickly diagnosed and remedied before the brain is damaged beyond repair (Bunyaratavej and Pausawasdi 1980). The following are the possible causes of post-traumatic brain swelling:

1. *Wrong location of craniotomy site* When the craniotomy is small and misses the clot, even by a few centimetres, or when there is also a clot on the other side, pressure of the clot will give rise to brain protrusion. This error is more likely when computed tomography is not performed.

2. *Increased blood volume in the intravascular compartment* When there is impairment of venous return from the brain, a rise of arterial carbon dioxide saturation, or when there is loss of autoregulation and hypertension, the volume of blood in the intravascular compartment increases and brain swelling occurs. Tension pneumothorax is the best example of impairment of venous return.

3. *Distension of ventricles or subarachnoid space* A posterior fossa clot may compress the fourth ventricle and thereby obstruct the ventricular system. Although uncommon, this is encountered from time to time. It is very difficult to diagnose without computed tomography, but tapping the ventricle with release of cerebrospinal fluid may improve the condition and lead to diagnosis. The problem is even more serious when bleeding arises from a large vessel in the subarachnoid space.

4. *Brain oedema* Following head injury, several kinds of brain oedema may occur, each requiring diagnosis and treatment. Vasogenic oedema is

said to follow head injury in experimental animals. Cytotoxic oedema can also be found when there is anoxia, which is a common occurrence after head injury. Hypo-osmotic oedema caused by hyponatraemia and the syndrome of inappropriate secretion of ADH are also common problems in the management of head injury. Treatment of these conditions then consists of prompt and correct diagnosis and appropriate therapy. In the patient in whose brain swelling cannot be reversed, removal of the skull flap is required and the wound is closed with the dura left open. This procedure is called external decompression.

Cerebrospinal fluid leakage

Leakage of cerebrospinal fluid from the nose implies a tear in the dura and arachnoid with cerebrospinal fluid leaking directly through the roof of the nose or indirectly through a paranasal sinus. In the case of aural leakage, there is usually a tear of the tympanic membrane and leakage is either directly into the middle ear or indirectly from the mastoid air cells. Usually leakage subsides spontaneously after a few days but if the fistula is very large, or if there is increased intracranial pressure, the leakage may be protracted, posing the threat of infection. Further investigation to identify the cause of its appropriate treatment are necessary.

Recommended initial treatment is to place the patient in a slightly head-elevated position, sufficient to maintain the intracranial pressure as low as possible, but not to induce negative pressure lest it encourage ascending infection. If rhinorrhoea is present, the patient is advised not to blow the nose for fear of intracerebral aerocele. Lumbar puncture is similarly not recommended in the initial treatment period. Acetazolamide is said to reduce cerebrospinal fluid production by half (Fishman 1975) and, if not contra-indicated, is worthy of a trial for a few days. Full antibiotic coverage of the normal flora in the paranasal sinus is essential. If the leakage does not stop within 7 days, surgical repair is probably advisable.

References

Adams, J.H. (1984). Head injury. In *Greenfield's neuropathology* (ed. J.H. Adams, J.A.N. Corsellis, and L.W. Duchen) (4th edn), pp. 85–124. Edward Arnold, London.

Adams, J.H., Graham, D.I., and Gennarelli, T.A. (1983). Head injury in man and experimental animals: neuropathology. *Acta Neurochir.* **S32**, 15–30.

Adams, J.H., Mitchell, D.E., Graham, D.I., and Doyle, D. (1977). Diffuse brain damage of immediate impact type. Its relationship to 'primary brain stem damage' in head injury. *Brain* **100**, 489–502.

Anderson, D.W. and McLaurin, R.L. (1980). Report on the national head and spinal cord injury survey: introduction *J. Neurosurg*. Supplement, S1.

Andrews, B.T., Pitts, L.H., Lovely, M.P., and Barkowski, H. (1986). Is computed tomographic scanning necessary in patients with tentorial herniation? *Neurosurgery* **19**, 408–14.

Bakay, L., and Glasauer, F.E. (1980). Mechanism of head injuries. In *Head injury* (ed. L. Bakey and F.E. Glassauer) pp. 3–10. Little, Brown and Co., Boston.

Becker, D.P., Gade, G.F., Young, H.F., and Feuerman, T.F. (1990). Diagnosis and treatment of head injury in adults. In *Neurological surgery* (ed. J.R. Youmans) (3rd edn), pp. 2018–19. Philadelphia.

Bollinger, O. (1891). Uber traumatische spat-apoplexie. Ein beitragzur lehre von der hirnerschutterung. Internationale beitrage zur wissenschaftlichen medicine Festschrift Rodolph Virchow. Berlin, Hirschwald. **2**, 457–70.

Bricola, A. (1976). Electroencephalography in neurotraumatology. *Clin. Electroencephalogr.* **7**, 184–97.

Bunyaratavej, S. and Pausawasdi, S. (1980). Brain swelling and brain edema. *Thai J. Surg.* **1**, 65–71.

Cairns, H. (1952). Disturbances of consciousness with lesions of the brain stem and diencephalon. *Brain* **75**, 109–46.

Cairns, H. and Holbourn, H. (1943). Head injuries in motor cyclists with special reference to crash helmets. *Br. Med. J.* **1**, 591–8.

Caveness, W.F. (1979). Incidence of craniocerebral trauma in the United States in 1976 with trend from 1970–1975. *Adv. Neurol.* **22**, 1–3.

Clasen, R.A. Pandolfi, S., Laing, I., and Casey, D. (1974). Experimental study of relation of fever to cerebral edema. *J. Neurosurg.* **41**, 576–81.

Clifton, G.L., Robertson, C.S., and Grossman, R.G. (1985). Management of the cardiovascular and metabolic response to severe head injury. In *Central nervous system trauma: status report* (ed. D.P. Becker and J.D. Povlishock) pp. 139–59. National Institute of Neurological and Communicative Disorders and Stroke, Bethesda, Maryland.

Cooper, P.R. (1982). Epidemiology of head injury. In *Head injury* (ed. P.R. Cooper) pp. 12–13. Williams & Wilkins, Baltimore.

Cooper, P.R., Moody, S., Clark, W.K., Kirkpatrick, J., Maravilla, K., Gould, A.L., and Dranne, W. (1979). Dexamethasone and severe head injury. *J. Neurosurg.* **51**, 307–16.

Davis, D.H. and Sundt, T.M. (1980). Relationship of cerebral blood flow to cardiac output, mean arterial pressure, blood volume, and alpha and beta blockade in cats. *J. Neurosurg.* **52**, 745–54.

Dott, N.M. (1960). Brain, movement and time. *Br. Med. J.* **5191**, 12–16.

Epstein, F.M., Ward, J.D., and Becker, D.P. (1987). Medical complications of head injury. In *Head injury* (ed. P.R. Cooper) (2nd edn), pp. 390–421. Williams & Wilkins, Baltimore.

Fishman, R.S. (1975). Brain edema. *N. Engl. J. Med.* **293**, 706–11.

French, J.D., Porter, R.W., von Amerongen, F.K., and Raney, R.B. (1957). Gastrointestinal hemorrhage and ulceration associated with intracranial lesions: a clinical and experimental study. *Surgery* **32**, 395–407.

Gade, G.F., Becker, D.P., Miller, J.D., and Dwan, P.S.: Pathology and pathophysiology of head injury. In *Neurological surgery* (ed. J.R. Youmans) pp. 1965–2016. W.B. Saunders, Philadelphia.

Gennarelli, T.A. (1964). Mechanisms of cerebral concussion, contusion, and other effects of head injury. In *Neurological surgery* (ed. J.R. Youmans) pp. 1953–64. W.B. Saunders, Philadelphia.

Gennarelli, T.A. (1983). Head injury in man and experimental animals, clinical aspects. *Acta Neurochir.* **S32**, 1–13.
Gildenberg, P.L. and Frost, E.A.M. (1985). Respiratory care in head trauma. In *Central nervous system trauma — status report* (ed. D.P. Becker and J.T. Povlishock) pp. 161–76. National Institute of Neurological and Communicative Disorders and Stroke, Bethesda, Maryland.
Goldsmith, W. and Ommaya, A.K. (1984). Head neck injury criteria and tolerance levels. In *The biomechanics of impact trauma* (ed. B. Aldman and A. Chapon) pp. 149–87. Elsevier, Amsterdam.
Graham, D.I., Adams, J.H., and Gennerelli, T.A. (1987). Pathology of brain damage in head injury. In *Head injury* (ed. T.R. Copper) (2nd edn), pp. 72–88. Williams & Wilkins, Baltimore.
Gudeman, S.K., Kishore, P.R.S., Miller, J.D., Girevendulis, A.K., Lipper, M.H., and Becker, D.P. (1979). The genesis and significance of delayed traumatic intracerebral hematoma. *Neurosurgery* **5**, 309–11.
Gurdjian, E.S. and Thomas, L.M. (1974). Traumatic intracranial hemorrhage. In *Brock's injuries of the brain and spinal cord and their coverings* (ed. E.H. Feiring) (5th edn), pp. 203–67. Springer Publishing, New York.
Holbourn, A.H.S. (1943). Mechanisms of brain injuries. *Lancet* **ii**, 438–41.
Jagger, J., Levine, J., Jane, J., *et al.* (1984). Epidemiologic features of head injury in a predominantly rural population. *J. Trauma* **24**, 40–4.
Jefferson, G. (1938). The tentorial pressure cone. *Arch. Neurol. Psychiatry* **40**, 857–76.
Jennett, B. (1974). Early traumatic epilapsy. Incidence and significance after non-missile injuries. *Arch. Neurol.* **30**, 394–8.
Jennett, B. (1975*a*). Epilepsy and acute traumatic intracranial hematoma. *J. Neurol. Neurosurg. Psychiatry* **38**, 378–81.
Jennett, B. (1975*b*). *Epilepsy after non-missile head injuries* (2nd edn). Heinemann, London.
Jennett, B. and McMillan, R. (1981). Epidemiology of head injury. *Br. Med. J.* **282**, 101–4.
Jennett, B. and Teasdale, G. (1981). *Management of head injuries*, p. 80. F.A. Davis, Philadelphia.
Kalsbeek, W.D., McLaurin, R.L., Harris, B.S.H., and Miller, J.D. (1980). The national head and spinal cord injury survey: major findings. *J. Neurosurg.* **53**, S19–S31.
Klauber, M.R., Barrett-Connor, E., and Marshall, L.F. (1984). A model for predicting intracranial hypertension following severe head injury. *J. Neurosurg.* **61**, 695–9.
Lewin, W. and Kennedy, W.F.C. (1950). Motorcyclists, crash helmets, and head injuries. *Br. Med. J.* **1**, 1253.
Liu, Y.K. (1979). Biomechanics and biophysics of CNS trauma. In *Central nervous system trauma research: status report* (ed. G.L. Odom) pp. 36–52. National Institute of Neurological and Communicative Disorders and Stroke, Bethesda, Maryland.
McLaurin, R.L. and King, L.R. (1975). Metabolic effects of head injury. In *Handbook of clinical neurology* (ed. P.J. Vinken and G.W. Bruyn) Vol. 23, pp. 109–31. Elsevier-North Holland, Amsterdam.
Marshall, L.F. and Marshall, S.B. (1987). Medical management of intracranial pressure. In *Head injury* (ed. P.R. Cooper) (2nd edn), Williams & Wilkins, Baltimore, pp. 177–96.

Miller, J.D. (1987). Head injury. In *Northfield's surgery of the central nervous system* (ed. J.D. Miller) pp. 797–8. Blackwell Scientific Publications, Oxford.
Miller, J.D., Butterworth, J.F., Gudman, S.K., Faulkner, J.E., Chot, S.C., Selhorst, J.B., Harrison, J.W., Lutz, H., Young, H.F., and Becker, D.P. (1981). *J. Neurosurg.* **54**, 289.
Miller, J.D., Garibi, J., North, J.B., *et al.* (1975). Effects of increased arterial pressure on blood flow in the damaged brain. *J. Neurol. Neurosurg. Psychiatry* **38**, 652–65.
Muizelaar, J.P. and Obrist, W.D. (1985). Cerebral blood flow and brain metabolism with brain injury. In *Central nervous system trauma: status report* (ed. D.P. Becker and J.T. Povlishock) pp. 123–38. National Institute of Communicative Disorders and Stroke, Bethesda, Maryland.
National Safety Council (1976). *Accident facts.* National Safety Council, Chicago.
Nelson, P.B. (1987). Fluid and electrolyte physiology, pathophysiology and management. In *Neurosurgical critical care* (ed. F.P. Wirth and R.A. Ratcheson) pp. 69–80. Williams & Wilkins, Baltimore.
Pausawasdi, S. and Bunyaratavej, S. (1982). Frusemide and mannitol induced changes intracranial pressure during the removal of intracranial tumours. *J. Med. Assoc. Thai.* **65**, 414–19.
Porter, R.J. and Miller, R.A. (1948). Diabetes insipidus following closed head injury. *J. Neurol. Neurosurg. Psychiatry* **11**, 259–62.
Rutherford, W.H., Greenfield, T., Hayes, H.R.M., and Nelson, J.K. (1985). *The medical effects of seatbelt legislation in the United Kingdom.* HMSO, London.
Shapiro, H.M., Wyite, S.R., and Leosser, J. (1974). Barbiturate augmented hypothermia for reduction of persistent intracranial hypertension. *J. Neurosurg.* **40**, 90–100.
Stritch, S.J. (1956). Diffuse degeneration of the cerebral white matter in severe dementia following head injury. *Neurol. Neurosurg. Psychiatry* **19**, 163–5.
Strich, S.J. (1961). Shearing of nerve fibres as a cause of brain damage due to head injury. A pathological study of 20 cases. *Lancet* **ii**, 443–8.
Thibault, L.E. and Gennarelli, T.A. (1985). Biomechanics and craniocerebral trauma. In *Central nervous system trauma research: status report* (ed. D.P. Becker and J.T. Povlishock) pp. 379–89. National Institute of Neurological and Communicative Disorder and Stroke, Bethesda, Maryland.
Ward, J.D., Becker, D.P., Miller, J.D., *et al.* Failure of prophylactic barbiturate coma in the treatment of severe head injury. *J. Neurosurg.* **62**, 383–8.
Whitman, S., Coonley-Hoganson, R., and Desai, B.T. (1984). Comparative head trauma experience in two socioeconominally different Chicago-area communities. A population study. *Am. J. Epidemiol.* **119**, 570–80.

10. Gastro-oesophageal reflux disease

David C. Gotley

The surgical management of gastro-oesophageal reflux (GOR) is currently in a state of flux. New knowledge about its pathophysiology and the development of modern potent antisecretory and pro-kinetic drugs are responsible for the changing trends in the treatment of this disease. This chapter outlines this new knowledge and highlights some controversial aspects of GOR and current guidelines in surgical management.

Definition

Since all individuals exhibit GOR (Kaye 1977), it is not surprising that the definition of pathological GOR has been a matter of controversy. The presence of oesophageal mucosal damage is not a reliable sole criterion for its diagnosis because half of patients with an abnormal amount of acid reflux (as determined by pH monitoring) do not have endoscopic oesophagitis (DeMeester, Johnson, Joseph, Toscano, Hall, and Skinner 1976). An abnormal duration of oesophageal acid exposure is also an unreliable sole criterion, since some patients with a normal amount of acid reflux are troubled with occasional severe heartburn (acid-sensitive oesophagus), while others with abnormal acid reflux are entirely asymptomatic. As a consequence, a definition of pathological GOR must take into account mucosal pathology (the presence of oesophagitis, stricture, Barrett's oesophagus) and/or troublesome symptoms (heartburn, regurgitation, dysphagia) which can be shown to be directly related to GOR. Based on this definition, a conservative estimate of the prevalence of the disease is 5 per cent (Tibbling 1985).

Pathophysiology

The pathogenesis of GOR and oesophagitis is multi-factorial (Dodds, Hogan, Helm, and Dent 1981). These factors are: defects in the antireflux mechanism, delayed oesophageal clearance, abnormal gastric emptying, composition of refluxed material, and mucosal resistance.

A resting tone exists in the lower oesophagus which prevents a natural tendency for reflux of gastric contents into the oesophagus. 'Physiological' reflux, present in all individuals, is usually post-prandial (almost never occurring at night), is rapidly cleared by primary oesophageal peristalsis, and is usually asymptomatic (Dent, Dodds, and Friedman 1980). The mechanism by which this occurs is known as transient lower oesophageal sphincter relaxation (TLOSR) (Dent, Holloway, Toouli, and Dodds 1988*b*). Possible precipitating factors include a failed primary peristaltic event (Kruse-Anderson, Wallin, and Madsen 1987*a*; Mittal and McCallum 1988) or a vagally mediated response to the activation of stretch receptors in the gastric fundus (Martin, Patrikios, and Dent 1986).

Excessive GOR, often nocturnal, is associated with oesophagitis (DeMeester *et al.* 1976; Kruse-Anderson, Wallin, and Madsen 1987*b*). It occurs through a hypotonic LOS, which may be permanently hypotensive or undergoing a TLOSR (Dent *et al.* 1988*b*). The LOS has considerable functional reserve, and a resting pressure of more than 4 mmHg is adequate to prevent GOR, even during straining (Dent, Dodds, Hogan, and Toouli 1988*a*).

Patients with a permanently low LOS pressure may have sphincter muscle damage (Biancini, Barwick, Selling, and McCallum 1984), since the sphincteric hypotension tends to remain after resolution of oesophagitis (Wesdorp, *et al.* 1978). In patients with oesophagitis, about two-thirds of reflux episodes occur in association with TLOSRs, and the remainder through a low resting LOS pressure; the preponderance of TLOSRs decreases and free reflux increases according to the increasing severity of the oesophagitis (Dent *et al.* 1988*b*). The discovery of TLOSR explains why some patients with abnormal GOR and oesophagitis have a resting LOS pressure within the normal range, and why short-term manometric assessment of sphincter competence and barium radiography are insensitive techniques for the diagnosis of GOR. Currently, the antireflux mechanism is thought to be due primarily to a resting LOS tone, bolstered by extrinsic compression effects of the diaphragmatic crura. The presence of a hiatal hernia, while associated with GOR on a population basis, 'permissive' at best of pathological GOR, is no longer an adequate sole criterion for its diagnosis.

Oesophageal acid clearance is an important protective mechanism after reflux has occurred. There are two main components: a motor response (primary and secondary peristalsis), which clears the fluid bolus into the stomach and which is aided by gravity, and the neutralizing effect of swallowed saliva (Helm, Dodds, Pelc, Palmer, Hogan, and Teeter 1984). The latter phenomenon accounts for the 'stepwise' restoration of normal oesophageal pH following a reflux episode. During standard oesophageal manometric testing, the majority of patients with oesophagitis have normal oesophageal peristalsis (Heddle, Dent, Toouli, and Lewis 1984; Kahrilas, Dodds, Hogan, Reece, and Arndorfer 1986). The remainder demonstrate abnormalities (often transient and non-specific) which may delay clearance. Unfortunately, detailed studies of peristalsis surrounding actual reflux event (especially in ambulant patients) is lacking. Identifying those with deficiencies in peristalsis may become important, since newly developed pro-kinetic agents (e.g. cisapride) are potentially valuable in improving acid clearance and, thereby, allowing healing of oesophagitis. Alternatively, treatment of patients with poor peristalsis with antireflux operations, which result in enhancement of the lower oesophageal high pressure zone, risks intractable dysphagia.

The amount of acid reflux is related to gastric volume (Ahtaridis, Snape, and Cohen 1981); GOR is increased after a meal, and is probably mediated by an increased rate of TLOSRs (Dent *et al.* 1980). Gastric volume is related to a variety of factors, but recent attention has been focused on delayed gastric emptying as a factor in the pathogenesis of GOR and oesophagitis. Early reports suggested that as many as 50 per cent of patients with GOR exhibit a delay in gastric emptying (McCallum, Berkowitz, and Lerner 1981), but a more recent detailed study refutes these findings (Schwizer, Hinder, and DeMeester 1989).

While there is little disagreement that (in patients who have not had gastric surgery) refluxed acid and pepsin cause oesophagitis (Goldberg, Dodds, Gee, and Montgomery 1969), the role of refluxed bile acids and trypsin from the duodenum is more contentious. Conjugated bile acids, which are injurious to the oesophageal epithelium in an acid medium, are infrequently found in oesophageal aspirates in concentrations which are known to be damaging (Gotley, Ball, Morgan, Owen, and Cooper, in press). Furthermore, bile acids inhibit peptic activity *in vitro* (Tompkins and Hayashi 1974), and there is evidence that, *in vivo*, oesophageal damage from pepsin is reduced by the addition of bile acid to the refluxate (Salo and Kivilaakso 1984). Trypsin is probably not important in acid reflux because it is active only at a neutral or alkaline pH and is rapidly destroyed by pepsin in the stomach (Heizer 1965).

Investigation

The majority of patients with typical symptoms of GOR do not need investigation. Those who fail medical therapy or whose symptoms recur, and those with atypical symptoms or with dysphagia, all require investigation. Several methods for the investigation of patients with GOR have been developed, of which endoscopy, histology, radiology, manometry, and 24-hour pH monitoring remain in common use. The fundamental difficulty in interpretation of the results is the somewhat arbitrary division between normal and abnormal physiological parameters.

Endoscopy is the recommended first investigation of choice, and the presence of ulcerative oesophagitis confirms the diagnosis of abnormal GOR. Interpretation of milder forms of inflammation (erythema granularity) suffers from marked inter-observer variation (DeMeester, *et al.* 1980). Histological examination does not improve the discrimination since it suffers from sampling error, and the diagnostic criteria of papillary elongation and epithelial hyperplasia, which are said to be induced by chronic GOR, have an unacceptable specificity. Histological appearances of gross ulceration are unmistakable, but this adds little additional information to the endoscopic diagnosis (except where exclusion of carcinoma is necessary). Histological examination is essential for the diagnosis of Barrett's oesophagus, however, as well as providing confirmation that a stricture is benign. Oesophagitis is usually graded endoscopically, which provides prognostic information about the potential for success with medical therapy (Koelz, *et al.* 1986).

Barium radiograms are no longer indicated for the routine investigation of symptomatic GOR for two reasons. First, the association of GOR with hiatal hernia is not predictive. Second, since GOR is intermittent and due predominantly to TLOSRs on the basis of a normal resting LOSP, short-term radiological screening is specific but does not have an acceptable sensitivity (Gotley and Cooper 1987). Although barium oesophagograms can demonstrate gross ulcerative oesophagitis, endoscopy is probably more sensitive and also permits biopsy of suspicious lesions.

Manometry alone cannot diagnose GOR. Whilst the absence of a resting LOSP is strongly predictive of GOR and oesophagitis, the majority of patients with reflux have a resting LOSP within the normal range (10–25 mmHg). Oesophageal manometry is the gold standard for the diagnosis of motor disorders, such as achalasia and diffuse oesophageal spasm, the symptoms of which can occasionally mimic those of GOR, and in these cases treatment with antireflux surgery is disastrous.

Twenty-four-hour pH monitoring remains the gold standard for the diagnosis of acid GOR disease (DeMeester *et al.* 1980). pH micro-electrodes, placed in the oesophagus 5 cm above the LOS and connected to portable digital recorders (worn at the waist), permit ambulatory out-patient studies in circumstances that are most likely to reproduce symptoms. The technique provides quantitative data about the frequency and duration and acid reflux (usually defined as a fall in pH to less than 4) and, perhaps most importantly in the clinical context, a correlation between symptoms (recorded in a diary) and acid reflux events. A suggested plan for the investigation of GOR is outlined in Table 10.1.

Results of medical therapy

The majority of patients with GOR are successfully treated with modern drug therapy (Heading 1989). H_2-receptor antagonists control symptomatic GOR in 63 per cent of patients and heal mild to moderate oesophagitis in 60–88 per cent (Stalnikowicz-Darvasi 1989). Omeprazole, a newly introduced proton pump inhibitor, heals mild oesophagitis (grades I–II — erythema, linear erosions) in 96 per cent cases by 8 weeks, but recurrence is the rule on cessation of therapy (Hetzel, *et al.* 1988) The healing rate of more

Table 10.1. Investigation of gastro-oesophageal reflux.

1. *Typical symptoms: unresponsive to or recurrent after medical therapy*	
Endoscopy	
Oesophagitis	Consider surgery
No oesophagitis	Progress to 24-hour pH monitoring
24-hour pH monitoring	
Normal	Retest if asymptomatic during study; investigate for heart disease/cholelithiasis or primary oesophageal motility disorder if symptoms unrelated to fall in pH
Abnormal	Consider surgery, especially if symptoms related to fall in pH
Manometry	If primary motility disorder suspected, or non-obstructive dysphagia, or prolonged clearance of acid from oesophagus on 24-hour pH monitoring
2. *Atypical symptoms*	No trial of medical therapy indicated — investigate
Endoscopy	
Oesophagitis	Trial of medical therapy
No oesophagitis	Progress to 24-hour pH monitoring
24-hour pH monitoring	
Normal	Investigate other conditions
Abnormal	Trial of medical therapy
3. *Dysphagia*	
Endoscopy/dilatation and biopsy	With or without barium swallow
4. *Suspected Barrett's oesophagus*	Must be confirmed by biopsy
Annual endoscopic surveillance whatever the treatment	

than 50 per cent for severe oesophagitis (grades III–IV — confluent ulceration, stricture) is much less satisfactory. Maintenance therapy with high-dose H_2-receptor antagonists is no better than with placebo (Koelz *et al.* 1986), with a 62 per cent relapse rate within 12 months, and intermittent ('weekend') therapy with omeprazole is even more disappointing, with an 85 per cent relapse rate (half of which recur within 6 weeks) (Bardhan, Daly, Singh, Morris, Thompson, and Hinchcliffe 1990). Omeprazole 20 mg daily has a 22 per cent recurrence rate at 12 months (Bardhan *et al.* 1990), but there is reluctance to use this drug in the long term until its safety has been established. Pro-kinetic agents (such as cisapride) are as effective in healing oesophagitis as the H_2-receptor antagonists (63 per cent) (Baldi, Bianchi

Table 10.2. Indications for operation in gastro-oesophageal reflux disease.

Failure of medical therapy to heal high-grade oesophagitis or control symptoms
Recurrence of symptoms or high-grade oesophagitis while on maintenance therapy
Fit patients with Barrett's oesophagus, especially complications of Barrett's oesophagus
Stricture patients who are young, male, or whose dysphagia recurs within months of dilatation and medical therapy
Recurrent aspiration while on medical therapy

Porro, Dobrilla, Iascone, Labello, Marzio, Sabbatini, Tittobello, and Verme 1988; Galmiche, Fraitag, Filoche, Evreux, Vitaux, Zeitoun, Fournet, and Soule 1990), and it is possible that combination therapy (pro-kinetic agent plus H_2-receptor antagonist) may give better results for maintenance therapy than either agent alone (Tytgat 1989).

Indications for operation

About 10 per cent of patients referred to hospital with GOR disease require operation (Heading 1989). The main indications for operation are failure to heal, high-grade oesophagitis, or the failure of maintenance therapy to control symptoms (particularly regurgitation) which can sometimes be disabling. Other indications are respiratory symptoms secondary to repeated aspiration, patients with a resistant stricture, and patients with a Barrett's oesophagus who are young or who have complications (Table 10.2). Pre-operative investigation with endoscopy is mandatory, as well as prolonged pH monitoring if the oesophageal mucosa is normal. Manometry is essential if there is non-obstructive dysphagia, excessively prolonged acid clearance, or a suspicion of a primary motility disorder.

Choice of operation

Most operations for reducing GOR employ some variant of fundoplication (Nissen 1961; Hill and Tobias 1967; Belsey 1985). The most popular operation in use today is probably the 'floppy' version of the Nissen fundoplication (Donohue, Samelson, Nyhus, and Bombeck 1985), which minimizes the post-operative incidence of 'gas-bloat' and dysphagia which are thought to be due to a tight fundoplication. The incidence of post-operative dysphagia may also be reduced by adopting a short (1.5–2 cm) wrap. Other fundoplication procedures which incorporate a partial wrap are designed to obviate post-operative problems of gas-bloat and dysphagia. Surprisingly, there is only one prospective randomized trial of the three most common anti-reflux procedures where the results have been evaluated by endoscopy, manometry, and pH monitoring (DeMeester, Johnson, and Kent 1974). Objective evaluation is necessary because symptoms alone are poor predictors of the degree of GOR, especially in the post-operative patient (Breumelhof, Smout, Schyns, Bronzwaer, Akkermans, and Jansen 1990). Only the Nissen fundoplication provided complete relief from all symptoms in every case, followed by the Belsey operation (80 per cent) and the Hill posterior gastropexy (47 per cent). The Nissen operation returned acid exposure to within normal limits in all patients, but acid reduction was less successful with the other operations (73 per cent for the Hill and 46 per cent for the Belsey procedures). A reduced ability to belch and vomit was experienced after each operation, least so following the Hill repair.

The ability to sustain these early findings after the Nissen fundoplication has been confirmed by the greater than 90 per cent satisfactory results after 10 years of follow-up (DeMeester, Bonavina, and Albertucci 1986).

Technical considerations

Exposure of the oesophageal hiatus (by the trans-abdominal route) is improved by the use of a sternal retractor and 15° head-up tilt of the operating table. Generous mobilization of the gastric fundus (with division of two or three short gastric vessels) ensures a loose fundoplication, and prevents the error of lateral invagination of the oesophagus into the gastric fundus which risks the possibility of post-operative dysphagia or recurrent reflux (Martin and Crookes 1990). A loose wrap is also aided by construction around a large-bore (54–60 Fr) intra-oesophageal tube or bougie. The risk of disruption of the fundoplication can be lessened by buttressing the sutures with Teflon® felt (DeMeester *et al.* 1986).

The Angelchik prosthesis

Introduced in 1979, this device consists of a silicone-filled silastic collar which is placed around the lower oesophagus and secured with tapes. An early design fault permitted separation of the collar from the tapes and subsequent migration, sometimes requiring reoperation. A design modification has eliminated this complication in the hands of the inventor, who achieves good to excellent results in 96 per cent of his cases (Angelchik and Cohen 1985). The results have been less satisfactory in other hands, where troublesome dysphagia (the prevalence of which increases with time) causes a reoperation rate of up to 10 per cent (Deakin, Mayer, and Temple 1989; Stuart, Dawson, Keeling, Bryne, and Hennessey 1989; Timoney, Kelly, and Welfare 1990). Oesophageal transit of food is slowed after insertion of the prosthesis, a phenomenon that does not appear to diminish with time

(Robertson, Smart, Amar, and Morris 1989). There is a higher incidence of post-operative dysphagia in those who complain of dysphagia before surgery (Timoney *et al.* 1990). Prosthesis migration (requiring reoperation) remains an occasional complication (Timoney *et al.* 1990; DeCaestaker, Ross, Heading, and Macleod 1989). In a prospective, randomized trial (mean follow-up 38 months), Visick grades I or II were achieved in 77 per cent of patients after insertion of the Angelchik device versus 94 per cent after Nissen fundoplication (Stuart *et al.* 1989). Both operations eliminated abnormal acid reflux, but almost a quarter of the Angelchik group developed late endoscopic ulcerative oesophagitis (versus none in the Nissen group). Ten per cent of prostheses required reoperation for removal.

The obvious advantage of the Angelchik prosthesis is its ease of insertion, which shortens operating time. Despite its disadvantages of high cost and complications (mainly intractable dysphagia) requiring a 10 per cent reoperation rate, the Angelchik prosthesis may still have a place in the treatment of the elderly or infirm with GOR, but who do not complain of dysphagia. The results from these recent studies suggest a cautionary approach toward its general use in younger, fit patients, especially in those who complain of dysphagia before operation.

Complicated gastro-oesophageal reflux

Peptic stricture

The management of peptic oesophageal stricture is controversial. The available options are dilatation followed by long-term medical therapy, or dilatation with antireflux surgery. The success rates with simple dilatation and medical therapy vary from 12.5 to 96 per cent (Ogilvie, Ferguson, and Atkinson 1980; Vantrappen and Hellemans 1981) and depend upon the definition and type of stricture (hard/fibrous or soft) and the criteria used to define success. More than half of these patients require more than one dilatation and no less than 40 per cent of male patients with a stricture will require dilatations beyond 2 years from diagnosis (Hands, Papavramidis, Bishop, Dennison, McIntyre, and Kettlewell 1989). Since these patients are often elderly and infirm (Hands *et al.* 1989), this choice of treatment may be appropriate. In younger patients (especially males) who have a rigid stricture with only short-term relief after dilatation, antireflux surgery should be considered.

Careful pre-operative biopsy is essential since unsuspected carcinoma may be lurking (Watson 1984). A preoperative barium swallow is prudent because it gives useful information about the length of the stricture and the possible presence of shortened oesophagus. Dilatation followed by a floppy Nissen fundoplication gives good to excellent results in 92–100 per cent of cases (Herrington, Wright, Edwards, and Sawyers 1975; Bremner 1982;

Zaninotto, DeMeester, Bremner, Smyrk, and Cheng 1989). A full fundoplication seems to give better results than a partial fundoplication in patients with a stricture (Siewert 1981). For the shortened oesophagus, a 'lengthening' procedure such as the Collis gastroplasty followed by a loose fundoplication returns a length of abdominal oesophagus to the abdomen, and is probably the operation of choice; the best exposure is afforded by a left thoracotomy (Orringer and Sloan 1978). In 261 patients with stricture treated by this technique and followed for a mean of 44 months, good reflux control (when assessed by objective testing) was achieved in 91 per cent of patients, and 86 per cent had none or only mild reflux symptoms (Stirling and Orringer 1989); 17 per cent continue to require periodic dilatation.

Patch oesophagoplasty (Maher, Hocking, and Woodward 1981; Hugh 1988), for resistant strictures, gives results which are similar to resection and replacement (with around 20 per cent requiring further dilatations), but with a lower mortality rate (0–4 per cent versus 4–10 per cent) (DeMeester 1981; Neville and Najem 1983; Negre and Markhula 1984; Zaninotto *et al.* 1989). Colonic interposition after resection is preferable to intrathoracic oesophagogastrostomy, after which continuing reflux is frequently troublesome and progresses to stricture formation in as many as 30 per cent of patients (Jackson, Cooper, Guvendik, and Reece-Smith 1979; King, Pairolero, Trastek, Payne, and Bernatz 1987). There is potential for severe gastritis to develop in the gastric tube. The colon is not completely immune from noxious attack, however, since peptic ulceration proximal to the cologastric anastomosis can occur (Bremner 1988). Orringer (1985) prefers a trans-hiatal subtotal oesophageal resection (which reduces cardiorespiratory complications) followed by anastomosis in the neck (which eliminates reflux (McKeown 1979). This procedure can be accomplished relatively atraumatically by the 'eversion/extraction' technique employing a vein stripper.

Barrett's oesophagus

Barrett's oesophagus is defined as at least 3 cm of columnar metaplastic epithelium lining the tubular oesophagus, which must be confirmed histologically (Skinner, Walther, Riddell, Schmidt, Iascone, and DeMeester 1983). Ascending 'tongues' of metaplastic epithelium or islands of squamous epithelium are commonly seen in conjunction with a developing columnar-lined oesophagus. Barrett's oesophagus is seen in 8–9.1 per cent of patients with symptomatic oesophagitis (Starnes, Adkins, Ballinger, and Sawyers 1984; Sarr, Hamilton, Marrone, and Cameron 1985; Ribet, Mensier, and Pruvot 1987), and there is little doubt that the condition is aquired (in most cases), and is associated with severe GOR (Iascone, DeMeester, Little, and Skinner 1983; Gillen, Keeling, Byrne, Healy, O'Moore, and Hennessey 1987; Gillen, Keeling, Byrne, West, and Hennessey 1988). Columnar-lined oesophagus may present with a complication, such as stricture (Lackey, Raukin, and Welsh 1984), peptic ulceration (in the Barrett's epithelium) or carcinoma. The carcinoma risk has excited considerable interest. Although the prevalence of adenocarcinoma in Barrett's oesophagus is as high as 15 per cent, the risk of developing carcinoma in a known Barrett's oesophagus is extremely low: two cases per 882 patient follow-up years in the Mayo Clinic experience (Cameron, Ott, and Payne 1985).

In patients who are fit, operation is the treatment of choice for columnar-lined oesophagus. Control of reflux heals oesophagitis, reverses stricture (Little, Naunheim, Ferguson, and Skinner 1988), heals Barrett's ulcer (Pearson, Cooper, Patterson, and Prakash 1987) and halts progress of the metaplastic epithelium (Naef and Savary 1972; Skinner *et al.* 1983). There is no evidence that antireflux surgery reduces the malignant potential of Barrett's oesophagus (Dent 1989); indeed it is possible to develop an adenocarcinoma long after surgical correction of GOR (Haggitt, Tryzelaar, Ellis, and Colcher 1978; Pearson *et al.* 1987). Despite sporadic case reports to the contrary, there is no convincing evidence that antireflux surgery causes regression of columnar metaplastic epithelium (Perniceni, Leymarios, Molas, and Fekete 1988). Whether medical therapy with omeprazole causes regression is not known. Although the occurrence of carcinoma in a known Barrett's oesophagus is low, annual endoscopic surveillance is worthwhile because dysplasia is a reliable indicator for impending malignancy (Kalish, Clancy, Orringer, and Appelman 1984). If a patient develops severe dysplasia, oesophagectomy is indicated (Skinner *et al.* 1983; Dent 1989). The place of cell kinetic studies in the follow-up of these patients is uncertain.

Failed antireflux surgery

Recurrent symptomatic reflux occurs in 9–20 per cent of patients after antireflux surgery (Belsey 1977; DeMeester *et al.* 1986; Low, Anderson, Ilves, Ricciardelli, and Hill 1989), and pre-operative physiological studies cannot predict the cases in which it is likely to occur (Mughal, Bancewicz, and Marples 1990). The commonest causes are slippage of the fundoplication (resulting in dysphagia and reflux) (Olsen, Lasser, and Ansell 1976) and wrap disruption. Wrap slippage can be difficult to distinguish from improper (distal) location of the wrap, even at reoperation, and sometimes there may be little evidence of a primary procedure. Few would disagree that patients with recurrent heartburn or regurgitation should be treated medically in the first instance. When dysphagia occurs in the early post-operative period it tends to improve over subsequent months, and is thus best treated expectantly. The decision to operate requires careful deliberation, and pre-operative objective evaluation is essential, since reoperation for failed antireflux surgery is technically demanding, and has a considerably higher mortality rate than primary antireflux surgery (4–18 per cent versus < 1 per cent) (Maher, Hocking, and Woodward 1985; Zucker, Peskin, and Saik 1982).

Recurrent reflux as a cause for the symptoms should be confirmed by 24-hour pH monitoring, and endoscopy is a worthwhile adjunct because the presence of high-grade oesophagitis has poor prognostic implications for medical therapy alone. The absence of the 'Nissen nipple' (a mucosal fold in the shape of an inverted cone at the cardia) at endoscopy suggests wrap disruption (O'Hanrahan, Marples, and Bancewicz 1990). Barium studies provide additional useful information (all antireflux operations have a characteristic radiological appearance); knowledge of the anatomy of the defect may reduce the incidence of damage to local structures (Martin and Crookes 1990). Finally, oesophageal manometry is indicated to rule out scleroderma, achalasia, diffuse oesophageal spasm, or a non-specific oesophageal motility disorder as possible causes of recurrent symptoms or the failure of conventional antireflux surgery.

Difficult reoperative surgery requires wide exposure. For recurrent reflux a left thoraco-abdominal incision may be appropriate, especially if the oesophagus is shortened and a Collis gastroplasty is necessary (Martin and Crookes 1990). Otherwise, as a general principle, the operative approach is via the cavity through which the original surgery took place. When possible, a short, floppy Nissen fundoplication returned to the positive pressure environment of the abdomen is the operation of choice. In cases where dense adhesions around the hiatus prevent safe dissection, a truncal vagotomy, antrectomy, and Roux-en-Y gastrojejunostomy via a left thoraco-abdominal approach is an effective alternative procedure.

Satisfactory results with reoperative antireflux surgery have been achieved in 80–92 per cent of cases (Leonardi, Crozier, and Ellis 1981; Maher *et al.* 1985; Martin and Crookes 1990). As stated above, a higher mortality rate can be expected with reoperation, and oesophageal leakage rates of up to 35 per cent have been encountered (Zucker *et al.* 1982). The results of reoperative surgery are worse with multiple attempts (Little, Ferguson, and Skinner 1986).

Conclusion

Modern medical management of GOR has undoubtedly improved the lot of patients with troublesome symptomatic reflux and oesophagitis. About a tenth of them will have complications of GOR or will fail medical therapy and require surgery. In view of the efficacy and safety of modern antireflux drugs, a reasonable expectation from surgery (for what is essentially a benign condition) is a mortality rate which is close to zero, a low morbidity, and a greater than 90 per cent long-term success rate in controlling the disease. The keys to achieving these aims are an accurate diagnosis of GOR, the correct choice of operation, and an operator experienced in antireflux surgery.

References

Ahtaridis, G., Snape, W.J., and Cohen, S. (1981). Lower esophageal sphincter pressure as an index of gastroesophageal acid reflux. *Dig. Dis. Sci.* **26**, 993–8.

Angelchik, J.P. and Cohen, R. (1985). A silicone prosthesis for gastroesophageal reflux: long-term results. *Contemp. Surg.* **26**, 29–54.

Baldi, F., Bianchi Porro, G., Dobrilla, G., Iascone, C., Labello, R., Marzio, L., Sabbatini, F., Tittobello, A., and Verme, G. (1988). Cisapride versus placebo in reflux esophagitis. A multicenter double-blind trial. *J. Clin. Gastroenterol.* **10**, 614–18.

Bardhan, K.D., Daly, M.J., Singh, S., Morris, P., Thompson, M., and Hinchcliffe, R.C. (1990). Refractory erosive oesophagitis: results of maintenance treatment with high dose H_2-receptor antagonists or omeprazole. *Gut* **31**, A602 (Abstract).

Belsey, R.H.R. (1977). Mark IV repair of hiatal hernia by the trans-thoracic approach. *World J. Surg.* **1**, 475–81.

Belsey, R. (1985). Hiatal herniorrhaphy. In *Surgical techniques illustrated: a comparative atlas* (ed. R.A. Malt) pp. 29–41. Ardmore Medical Books, W.B. Saunders, Philadelphia.

Biancini, P., Barwick, K., Selling, J., and McCallum, R. (1984). Effects of acute experimental esophagitis on mechanical properties of the lower esophageal sphincter. *Gastroenterology* **87**, 8–16.

Bremner, C.G. (1982). Benign strictures of the esophagus. *Curr. Probl. Surg.* **19**, 402–12.

Bremner, C.G. (1988). Peptic strictures — an overview. In *Surgery of the oesophagus* (ed. G.G. Jamieson). Churchill Livingstone, Edinburgh.

Breumelhof, R., Smout, A.J., Schyns, M.W., Bronzwaer, P.W., Akkermans, L.M., and Jansen, A. (1990). Prospective evaluation of the effects of Nissen fundoplication on gastroesophageal reflux. *Surg. Gynecol. Obstet.* **171**, 115–19.

Cameron, A.J., Ott, B.J., and Payne, W.S. (1985). The incidence of adenocarcinoma in columnar-lined (Barrett's) esophagus. *N. Engl. J. Med.* **313**, 857–9.

Deakin, M., Mayer, D., and Temple, J.G. (1989). Surgery for GOR: the Angelchik prosthesis compared to the Nissen fundoplication. Two year follow-up study and a five year evaluation of the Angelchik prosthesis. *Ann. R. Coll. Surg. Engl.* **71**, 249–52.

DeCaestaker, J.S., Ross, H.M., Heading, R.C., and Macleod, I.B. (1989). Appraisal of the Angelchik anti-reflux prosthesis based on clinical and manometric data and pH monitoring. *J. R. Coll. Surg. Edinb.* **34**, 9–12.

DeMeester, T.R. (1981). Management of benign esophageal strictures. In *Serono Symposium* (ed. S. Stipa, R.H.R. Belsey and A. Moraldi) Vol. 43, pp. 159–64. Academic Press. London.

DeMeester, T.R., Bonavina, L., and Albertucci, M. (1986). Nissen fundoplication for gastroesophageal reflux disease: evaluation of primary repair in 100 consecutive patients. *Ann. Surg.* **204**, 9–20.

DeMeester, T.R., Johnson, L.F., and Kent, A.H. (1974). Evaluation of current operations for the prevention of gastroesophageal reflux. *Ann. Surg.* **180**, 511–25.

DeMeester, T.R., Johnson, L.F., Joseph, G.J., Toscano, M.S., Hall, A.W., and Skinner, D. (1976). Patterns of gastroesophageal reflux in health and disease. *Ann. Surg.* **184**, 459–70.

DeMeester, T.R., Ching, I.W., Wernly, J.A., *et al.* (1980). Technique, indications and clinical use of 24-hour esophageal pH monitoring. *J. Thorac. Cardiovasc. Surg.* **79**, 656–70.

Dent, J. (1989). Approaches to oesophageal columnar metaplasia (Barrett's oesophagus). *Scand. J. Gastroenterol. Suppl.* **168**, 60–6.

Dent, J., Dodds, W.J., and Friedman, R.H. (1980). Mechanism of gastroesophageal reflux in recumbent asymptomatic human subjects. *J. Clin. Invest.* **65**, 256–67.

Dent, J., Dodds, W.J., Hogan, W.J., and Toouli, J. (1988*a*). Factors that influence induction of gastroesophageal reflux in normal human subjects. *Dig. Dis. Sci.* **33**, 270–5.

Dent, J., Holloway, R.H., Toouli, J., and Dodds, W.J. (1988*b*). Mechanisms of lower oesophageal sphincter incompetence in patients with symptomatic gastro-oesophageal reflux. *Gut* **29**, 1020–8.

Dodds, W.J., Hogan, W.J., Helm, J.F., and Dent, J. (1981). Pathogenesis of reflux esophagitis. *Gastroenterology*, **81**, 376–94.

Donohue, P.E., Samelson, S., Nyhus, L.M., and Bombeck, T. (1985). The floppy Nissen fundoplication: effective long-term control of pathologic reflux. *Arch. Surg.* **120**, 663–8.

Galmiche, J.P., Fraitag, B., Filoche, B., Evreux, M., Vitaux, J., Zeitoun, P., Fournet, J., and Soule, J.C. (1990). Double-blind comparison of cisapride and cimetidine in the treatment of reflux esophagitis. *Dig. Dis. Sci.* **35**, 649–55.

Gillen, P., Keeling, P., Byrne, P.J., West, A.B., and Hennessey, T.P.J. (1988). Experimental columnar metaplasia in the canine oesophagus. *Br. J. Surg.* **75**, 113–15.

Gillen, P., Keeling, P., Byrne, P.J. Healy, M., O'Moore, R.R. and Hennessey, T.P. (1987). Barrett's oesophagus: pH profile. *Br. J. Surg.* **74**, 774–6.

Goldberg, H.I., Dodds, W.J., Gee, S. and Montgomery, C. (1969). Role of acid and pepsin in acute experimental esophagitis. *Gastroenterology* **56**, 223–30.

Gotley, D.C. and Cooper, M.J. (1987). The investigation of gastro-oesophageal reflux. *Surg. Res. Commun.* **2**, 1–17.

Gotley, D.C., Ball, D., Morgan, A.P., Owen, R.W. and Cooper, M.J. Composition of gastro-oesophageal refluxate. *Gut* (in press).

Haggitt, R.C., Tryzelaar, J., Ellis, F.H. and Colcher, H. (1978). Adenocarcinoma complicating columnar epithelial-lined Barrett's oesophagus. *Am. J. Clin. Pathol.* **70**, 1–5.

Hands, L.J., Papavramidis, S., Bishop, H., Dennison, A.R., McIntyre, R.L., and Kettlewell, M.G. (1989). The natural history of peptic oesophageal strictures treated by dilatation and antireflux therapy alone. *Ann. R. Coll. Surg. Engl.* **71**, 306–9.

Heading, R.C. (1989). Epidemiology of oesophageal reflux disease. *Scand. J. Gastroenterol. Suppl.* **168**, 33–7.

Heddle, R., Dent, J., Toouli, J. and Lewis, I. (1984). Esophageal peristaltic dysfunction in peptic esophagitis. *Gastroenterology* **85**, 1109 (Abstract).

Heizer, W.D. (1965). Gastric inactivation of pancreatic supplement. *Bull. Johns Hopkins Med. J.* **116**, 261–70.

Helm, J.F., Dodds, W.J., Pelc, L.R., Palmer, D.W., Hogan, W.J., and Teeter, B.C. (1984). Effect of esophageal emptying and saliva on clearance of acid from the esophagus. *N. Engl. J. Med.* **310**, 284–8.

Herrington, J.L. Jr., Wright, R.S., Edwards, W.H., and Sawyers, J.L. (1975). Conservative surgical treatment of reflux esophagitis and esophageal stricture. *Ann. Surg.* **181**, 552–66.

Hetzel, D.J., Dent, J., Reed, W.D., *et al.* (1988). Healing and relapse of severe peptic esophagitis after treatment with omeprazole. *Gastroenterology* **95**, 903–12.

Hill, L.D. and Tobias, J.A. (1967). An effective operation for hiatal hernia: an eight year appraisal. *Ann. Surg.* **166**, 861–92.

Hugh, T.B. (1988). Antral patch oesophagoplasty for oesophageal stricture. In *Surgery of the oesophagus* (ed. G.G. Jamieson) pp. 355–60. Churchill Livingstone, Edinburgh.

Iascone, C., DeMeester, T.R., Little, A.G. and Skinner, D.B. (1983). Barrett's esophagus: functional assessment, proposed pathogenesis and surgical therapy. *Arch Surg.* **118**, 543–9.

Jackson, J.W., Cooper, D.K.C., Guvendik, L. and Reece-Smith, H. (1979). The surgical management of malignant tumours of the esophagus and cardia. *Br. J. Surg.* **66**, 98–104.

Kahrilas, P.J., Dodds, W.J., Hogan, W.J. Reece, A., and Arndorfer, R.C. (1986). Esophageal peristaltic dysfunction in peptic esophagitis. *Gastroenterology* **91**, 897–904.

Kalish, R.J., Clancy, P.E., Orringer, M.B., and Appelman, H.D. (1984). Clinical epidemiological and morphologic comparison between adenocarcinoma arising in Barrett's esophageal mucosa and in the gastric cardia. *Gastroenterology* **86**, 461–7.

Kaye, M.D. (1977). Postprandial gastroesophageal reflux in healthy people. *Gut* **18**, 709–12.

King, R.M., Pairolero, P.C., Trastek, V.F., Payne, W.S. and Bernatz, P.E. (1987). Ivor–Lewis esophagogastrectomy for carcinoma of the esophagus: early and late functional results. *Ann. Thorac. Surg.* **44**, 119–22.

Koelz, H.R., Birchler, R., Bretholz, A., *et al.* (1986). Healing and relapse of reflux esophagitis during treatment with ranitidine. *Gastroenterology* **91**, 1198–205.

Kruse-Anderson, S., Wallin, L. and Madsen, T. (1987*a*). Relationship between non-propagating peristaltic activity in the oesophagus and acid gastro-oesophageal reflux in pathological and non-pathological refluxers. *Gut* **28**, 1478–83.

Kruse-Anderson, S., Wallin, L., and Madsen, T. (1987*b*). Acid gastro-oesophageal reflux and oesophageal pressure activity during postprandial and nocturnal periods. *Scand. J. Gastroenterol.* **22**, 926–30.

Lackey, C., Rankin, R.A., and Welsh, J.D. (1984). Stricture location in Barrett's esophagus. *Gastrointest. Endosc.* **30**, 331–3.

Leonardi, H.K., Crozier, R.E. and Ellis, F.H. Jr. (1981). Reoperation for complications of the Nissen fundoplication. *J. Thorac. Cardiovasc. Surg.* **81**, 50–6.

Little, A.G., Ferguson, M.K., and Skinner, D.B. (1986). Reoperation for failed antireflux operations. *J. Thorac. Cardiovasc. Surg.* **91**, 511–17.

Little, A.G., Naunheim, K.S., Ferguson, M.K., and Skinner, D.B. (1988). Surgical management of esophageal strictures. *Ann. Thorac. Surg.* **45**, 144–7.

Low, D.E., Anderson, R.P., Ilves, R., Ricciardelli, E., and Hill, L.D. (1989). Fifteen to twenty-year results after the Hill antireflux operation. *J. Thorac. Cardiovasc. Surg.* **98**, 444–9.

Maher, J.W., Hocking, M.P., and Woodward, E.R. (1981). Long-term follow-up of the combined fundic patch fundoplication for treatment of longitudinal peptic strictures of the esophagus. *Ann. Surg.* **194**, 64–9.

Maher, J.W., Hocking, M.P., and Woodward, E.R. (1985). Reoperations for esophagitis following failed antireflux procedures. *Ann. Surg.* **201**, 723–7.

Martin, C.J. and Crookes, P.F. (1990). Reoperation for failed antireflux surgery. *Aust. N.Z. J. Surg.* **60**, 773–8.

Martin, C.J., Patrikios, J., and Dent, J. (1986). Abolition of gas reflex and transient lower esophageal sphincter relaxation by vagal blockade in the dog. *Gastroenterology* **91**, 890–6.
McCallum, R.W., Berkowitz, D.M., and Lerner, E. (1981). Gastric emptying in patients with gastroesophageal reflux. *Gastroenterology* **80**, 285–91.
McKeown, K.C. (1979). Carcinoma of the oesophagus. *J. R. Coll. Surg. Edinb.* **24**, 253–74.
Mittal, R.K. and McCallum, R.W. (1988). Characteristics and frequency of transient relaxations of the lower esophageal sphincter in patients with reflux esophagitis. *Gastroenterology* **95**, 593–9.
Mughal, M.M., Bancewicz, J., and Marples, M. (1990). Oesophageal manometry and pH recording does not predict the bad results of Nissen fundoplication. *Br. J. Surg.* **77**, 43–5.
Naef, A.P. and Savary, M. (1972). Conservative operations for peptic esophagitis with stenosis in columnar-lined lower esophagus. *Ann. Thorac. Surg.* **13**, 543–51.
Negre, J. and Markhula, H. (1984). Esophagectomy and colon interposition for benign esophageal stricture. *Acta Chir. Scand.* **150**, 639–42.
Neville, W.E. and Najem, A.Z. (1983). Colon replacement of the esophagus for congenital and benign disease. *Ann. Thorac. Surg.* **36**, 626–33.
Nissen, R. (1961). Gastropexy and fundoplication in surgical treatment of hiatus hernia. *Am. J. Dig. Dis.* **61**, 954–61.
Ogilvie, A.L., Ferguson, R., and Atkinson, M. (1980). Outlook with conservation treatment of peptic oesophageal stricture. *Gut* **21**, 23–5.
O'Hanrahan, T., Marples, M., and Bancewicz, J. (1990). Recurrent reflux and wrap disruption after Nissen fundoplication: detection, incidence and timing. *Br. J. Surg.* **77**, 545–7.
Olsen, R.C., Lasser, R.B., and Ansell, H. (1976). The 'slipped Nissen'. *Gastroenterology* **70**, 924 (Abstract).
Orringer, M.B. (1985). Transhiatal esophagectomy for benign disease. *J. Thorac. Cardiovasc. Surg.* **90**, 649–55.
Orringer, M.B. and Sloan, H. (1978). Combined Collis–Nissen reconstruction of the esophagogastric junction. *Ann. Thorac. Cardiovasc. Surg.* **25**, 16–21.
Pearson, F.G., Cooper, J.D., Patterson, G.A., and Prakash, D. (1987). Peptic ulcer in acquired columnar-lined esophagus: results of surgical treatment. *Ann. Thorac. Surg.* **43**, 241–4.
Perniceni, T., Leymarios, J., Molas, G., and Fekete, F. (1988). Does Barrett esophagus regress after total duodenal diversion? *Gastroenterol. Clin. Biol. et al.* **12**, 709–12.
Ribet, M., Mensier, E., and Pruvot, F.R. (1987). Barrett's esophagus and adenocarcinoma. *Eur. J. Cardiovasc. Surg.* **1**, 29–32.
Robertson, C.S., Smart, H., Amar, S.S., and Morris, D.L. (1989). Oesophageal transit of marshmallow after the Angelchik procedure. *Br. J. Surg.* **76**, 245–7.
Salo, J.A., and Kivilaakso, E. (1984). Contribution of trypsin and cholate to the pathogenesis of experimental alkaline esophagitis. *Scand. J. Gastroenterol.* **19**, 875–81.
Sarr, M.G., Hamilton, S.R.T., Marrone, G.C., and Cameron, J.L. (1985). Barrett's esophagus, its prevalence and association with adenocarcinoma in patients with symptoms of gastroesophageal reflux. *Am. J. Surg.* **149**, 187–93.
Schwizer, W., Hinder, R.A., and DeMeester, T.R. (1989). Does delayed gastric emptying contribute to gastroesophageal reflux disease? *Am. J. Surg.* **157**, 74–81.

Siewert, R. (1981). Surgical therapy of peptic stenoses. In *Medical and surgical problems of the esophagus. Serono Symposium* (ed. S. Stipa, R.H.R. Belsey, and A. Moraldi) Vol. 43, pp. 146–54. Academic Press. London.

Skinner, D.B., Walther, B.C., Riddell, R.H., Schmidt, H., Iascone, C., and DeMeester, T.R. (1983). Barrett's esophagus: comparison of benign and malignant cases. *Ann. Surg.* **198**, 554–66.

Stalnikowicz-Darvasi, R. (1989). H_2 antagonists in the treatment of reflux esophagitis: a critical analysis. *Am. J. Gastroenterol.* **84**, 245–8.

Starnes, V.A., Adkins, R.B., Ballinger, J.F., and Sawyers, J.L. (1984). Barrett's esophagus: a surgical entity. *Arch. Surg.*, **119**, 563–7.

Stirling, M.C. and Orringer, M.B. (1989). Continued assessment of the combined Collis–Nissen operation. *Ann. Thorac. Surg.* **47**, 224–30.

Stuart, R.C., Dawson, K., Keeling, P., Byrne, P.J., and Hennessey, T.P.J. (1989). A prospective, randomised trial of Angelchik prosthesis versus Nissen fundoplication. *Br. J. Surg.* **76**, 86–9.

Tibbling, L. (1985). Epidemiology of gastro-oesophageal reflux disease. In *Function and disease of the oesophagus* (ed. N. Sandberg and A. Walan) pp. 14–15. Smith Kline and French. UK.

Timoney, A.G., Kelly, J.M., and Welfare, M.R. (1990). The Angelchik antireflux device: a 5-year experience. *Ann. R. Coll. Surg. Engl.* **72**, 185–7.

Tompkins, R.K., and Hayashi, R.M. (1974). Investigations into the reduction of pepsin activity by bile. *Am. J. Surg.* **128**, 633–7.

Tytgat, G.N. (1989). Drug therapy of reflux oesophagitis: an update. *Scand. J. Gastroenterol. Suppl.* **168**, 38–49.

Vantrappen, G. and Hellemans, J. (1981). Dilatation of esophageal strictures. In *Medical and surgical problems of the esophagus. Serono Symposium* (ed. S. Stipa, R.H.R. Belsey and A. Moraldi) Vol. 43, pp. 138–40. Academic Press. London.

Watson, A. (1984). The role of antireflux surgery combined with fibreoptic endoscopic dilatation in peptic esophageal stricture. *Am. J. Surg.* **148**, 346–9.

Wesdorp, E., Bartelsman, J., Pape, K., *et al.* (1978) Oral cimetidine in reflux esophagitis: a double blind controlled trial. *Gastroenterology* **74**, 821–4.

Zaninotto, G., DeMeester, T.R., Bremner, C.G., Smyrk, T.C., and Cheng, S.C. (1989). Esophageal function in patients with reflux-induced strictures and its relevance to surgical treatment. *Ann. Thorac. Surg.* **47**, 362–70.

Zucker, K., Peskin, G.W., and Saik, R.P. (1982). Recurrent hiatal hernia repair: a potential surgical dilemma. *Arch. Surg.* **117**, 413–14.

11. Carcinoma of the oesophagus: epidemiology and surgical experience in China

Guo Jun Huang

Epidemiology

Carcinoma of the oesophagus in one of the most prevalent cancers in China and is perhaps more prevalent in China than in most countries of the world. The age-adjusted mortality rate for this disease is 31.7 per 100 000 population in males and 15.9 per 100 000 in females. It accounts for 26.5 per cent and 19.7 per cent of all cancer deaths in men and women respectively. Its cumulative mortality rate up to 74 years of age is 4.0 per cent for men and 2.0 per cent for women. The male:female ratio of this disease is about 2:1.

There is a great variation in the geographical distribution of oesophageal cancer in both males and females, with distinctly higher incidence areas in certain parts of China. One of these areas extends from the port of Lianyun in the east to Mianyang county of Sichuan province in the west. The northern boundary of this area extends to the suburbs of Beijing, and its southern boundary reaches Jiujiang city of Jiagxi province. Other high-incidence area include the coastline of Guangdong (Canton) and Fujian provinces, in Inner Mongolia, and parts of Xinjiang autonomous regions mostly inhabited by Kazakh minorities.

At a county level, the difference between high and low mortality rates of oesophageal cancer can be as high as 645-fold in men and 791-fold in women. Linxian of Henan province is well known for its extremely high incidence of oesophageal cancer, where the age-adjusted mortality rates are 161 per 100 000 in males and 103 per 100 000 in females, being 5 and 6.5 times, respectively, higher than those of the whole country; the cumulative death rates, up to 74 years of age, are 32.5 per cent for males and 20.4 per cent for females.

Surgical experience

Modern surgical treatment for carcinoma of the oesophagus dates back to 1938 when Marshall (1938) and Adams and Phemister (1938) independently reported their success in single-stage resection of the tumour with intrathoracic oesophagogastrostomy. Sweet (1945), Garlock (1944), and others further developed the procedure during the next decade. In China the first successful resection of oesophageal carcinoma with intrathoracic oesophagogastrostomy was performed by Wu and associates (Wu and Loucks 1941, 1942).

To date, it is well accepted that surgery is the treatment of choice for carcinoma of the oesophagus. Experience in high-incidence areas of oesophageal carcinoma, such as Linxian County of Henan Province where mass screening by means of balloon cytology led to the discovery of numerous early cases (stage I), showed that the results of surgery for early cases is excellent. For example, in a series of 253 resections of stage I oesophageal carcinoma reported by Shao, *et al.* (1981), the resectability rate was 100 per cent, the 30-day operative mortality rate was 2.4 per cent, the 5-year survival rate was 89.9 per cent, and the 10-year survival rate was 60.0 per cent. Pathology showed carcinoma *in situ* in 99 cases (39.1 per cent) and early infiltrative (submucosal) carcinoma in 154 (60.9 per cent).

Nevertheless, early oesophageal carcinoma is seen only infrequently in non-prevalent areas of this disease and, as is the experience world-wide, most patients coming to hospital have advanced disease. This may be exemplified by a series of 1874 surgically selected cases of oesophageal carcinoma reported by Huang, *et al.* (1985), in which stage I carcinoma was seen in only 3 per cent stage II in 16.8 per cent stage III in 70.4 per cent, and stage IV in 9.7 per cent of cases.

Operability

Obviously, patients selected for surgery (operability) represent only the minority of cases seen with the disease. It is disheartening to see that the majority of patients with oesophageal carcinoma seeking medical care are denied surgery, either because of far-advanced disease or poor general condition. The high expenses, risks, and fear of an oesophageal operation undeniably further decrease the number of patients accepting surgery. Operability rates differ in different medical centres. At the author's clinic where approximately 1700 new patients with carcinoma of the oesophagus or gastric cardia are seen annually, only 350 undergo surgery, an operability rate of about 21 per cent.

Patient selection

In general the selection of patients for surgery depends on three major factors: the predicted resectability of the tumour, the stage of the disease, and the general condition of the patient. Surgery is strongly indicated in patients predicted to be resectable with a localized disease process and in otherwise good health. It is generally contra-indicated, however, under the following circumstances:

1. Non-resectability as evidenced by gross invasion of the tumour into adjacent vital organs such as the trachea, bronchus, or aorta.
2. Distant lymph node metastases, or metastases in the liver, lung, bone, or brain, for example, or recurrent nerve paralysis. It is our experience that under cover of radiotherapy, given either before or after operation, or both, supra-clavicular lymph node metastasis, although a sign of poor prognosis, may not be a contra-indication to surgery if the primary tumour is likely to be resectable, as reasonably good palliation may still be obtained by this combined modality therapy.
3. Poor general condition, severe impairment of cardiopulmonary reserves, bloody ascites, cachexia.

The role of surgery

As carcinoma of the oesophagus is primarily an obstructive malignancy of the food conduit, patients usually suffer even more from the obstruction than from the malignancy. The role of surgery is to resect the primary tumour whenever technically feasible. Efforts are made to obtain a curative resection by completely eradicating all cancer-bearing tissues. This is mandatory and can usually be accomplished in relatively early cases where the disease has certain anatomical confinements. In relatively advanced cases, however, where disease is widespread with micrometastases and extra-oesophageal invasion to adjacent vital organs, surgery alone is of limited avail in complete eradication of cancerous involvement. The role of surgery is then to provide optimal palliative resection of the tumour, in order to promote the quality of life of the patient and to pave the way for multi-modality therapy. It is often unwise, in such circumstances, to over-extend the scope of operation, with the inevitable increase in surgical morbidity and mortality rates.

In patients with severe dysphagia, but in whom at operation the tumour is found to be unresectable, it may be advisable to perform a bypass procedure, such as a side-to-side oesophagogastrostomy proximal to the obstruction, in order to relieve dysphagia. It is to be noted that a high intrathoracic bypass procedure is of no less magnitude and risk than a regular oesophagectomy and oesophagogastrostomy, and so should be decided with caution. Our experience has shown that a bypass operation usually affords good relief of dysphagia but not significant prolongation of life.

Pre-operative determination of resectability

Experienced surgeons may comprehend fairly accurately the status of resectability of carcinoma of the oesophagus by reviewing the patient's contrast oesophagram and chest films and after careful physical examination of the patient. Today, computed tomography, magnetic resonance imaging, and endoscopic ultrasonography may further help to assess the degree of tumour invasion to surrounding vital organs. None the less, in borderline cases, the final determination of tumour resectability can be made only at the time of operative exploration.

Resectability of oesophageal cancer, upon which indications for surgery are dependent, can be estimated before operation by a correlated study of the following factors, discussed below in the order of decreasing importance.

Tumour location

This is by far the most important factor that determines resectability. Tumours located below the pulmonary hilum or in the distal segment of the oesophagus are less likely to involve surrounding vital organs and have the highest resectability rates for tumours of all sites of the oesophagus. Lesions located behind the tracheal bifurcation and the arch of aorta have the lowest resectability rates because of their close contiguity to these organs, which are easily involved by any extra-oesophageal extension of the disease.

Gross size of tumour

The length of tumour as shown by contrast roentgenograms, approximately reflects the stage of the disease. Resectability is high when the lesion in under 5 cm in length and is almost 100 per cent when located in the lower segment of the oesophagus. Resectability rates of tumours at the same location decrease with increasing tumour length, with perhaps the exception of the comparatively infrequent intraluminal type of oesophageal cancer, to be described. Resectability rates are much lower for lesions of more than 7 cm in length.

Clinicopathological type

In China, five clinicopathological types of oesophageal carcinoma are distinguished. Of the five types, the intraluminal and the fungating types are less likely to have penetrated the wall and have the highest resectability rates. The medullary, scirrhous, and ulcerative types offer less favourable prospects.

Roentgenological manifestations

A factor of some importance in the pre-operative assessment of resectability are the roentgenological manifestations of the tumour such as the general configuration of the filling defect, wall and luminal changes, soft tissue shadows of the cancer mass when evident, and fistulous extension of the growth. These are all significant parameters of extra-oesophageal invasion. Oesophageal axis abnormalities such as tortuosity, angulation, and deviation of the barium stream are also indications of extra-oesophageal infiltration of tumour (Akiyama, Kogure, and Itai 1972). These and other signs, such as irregularity of the filling defect, large and deep niches, and the presence of a soft tissue shadow, usually shown on oblique projections, are common signs of low or non-resectability. They are also signs of poor radiation sensitivity and in some cases may even be contra-indications to radiotherapy. In such circumstances pre-operative irradiation will not improve resectability.

Effect of pre-operative therapy

In patients who receive planned pre-operative irradiation, with a total dose of about 4000 cGy divided in 20 fractions and a rest period of less than a month after the completion of radiation as currently practised at the author's institution (Huang 1988), a good radiotherapeutic response of the tumour (as shown roentgenographically) usually indicates good resectability. In such cases it is not infrequent to find at operation that the tumour has softened and become smaller in size, with inconspicuous margins, and that tissue planes between the tumour and the surrounding structures are readily developed on dissection. In cases where prospects for tumour resection are borderline, such a planned pre-operative irradiation may be recommended as a means of promoting resectability.

In patients treated primarily with a full dose (6000 cGy or more) of radiation who come to surgery (because of poor control of the lesion, recurrence, or stenosis), resection of the lesion is usually very difficult. In such cases post-irradiation fibrosis, which usually reaches a peak at about 1 year after irradiation, may be so dense that no tissue plane can be developed at operation.

Pre-operative chemotherapy, with good roentgenographic response of the tumour, likewise improves resectability.

Clinical manifestations

Sex and age do not seem to influence overall resectability rates. However, in elderly patients with moderate to marked tortuosity and elongation of the arch and descending part of the aorta, higher resectability rates of oesophageal carcinoma can be expected because of increased interstitial spaces between the tumour and surrounding vital organs. Deep-seated pain in the chest, the back, or the epigastrum, may indicate tumour infiltration of regional nerves or organs and is often an indication that resection is unlikely to be feasible.

Surgical approaches

Today, while the abdominal and right chest approach, as advocated by Lewis in 1946 and Tanner in 1947, for resection of intrathoracic oesophageal carcinoma is most frequently used, the benefits of a left thoracotomy approach may not be fully appreciated and practised. It is sometimes hard to explain why the left approach is not used for carcinoma of the distal oesophagus or the gastric cardia (Payne, Trastek, Piehler, Pairolero, and Bernatz 1986). In China, while the Lewis–Tanner approach is used for carcinoma of the oesophagus cephalad to the tracheal bifurcation, the left thoracotomy approach is used almost exclusively for carcinoma of the oesophagus distal to this level and for that of the gastric cardia, with general satisfaction.

The advantages of a left thoracotomy approach may be summarized as follows:

1. There is only one incision needed and excellent access to the oesophago-gastric junction and the left upper abdomen can be obtained through an incision of the left hemi-diaphragm. Mobilization of the stomach, dissection of draining perigastric lymph nodes, and splenectomy, if necessary, can be performed most conveniently through the left approach.
2. There is no need to change the position of the patient at operation even when a supra-aortic or a cervical anastomosis is to be fashioned, thus saving intra-operative time.
3. Resectability of oesophageal cancer, often determined by the degree of tumour involvement of the aorta or the left main bronchus, is more clearly and quickly assessed from the left than from the right thoracotomy approach. Cancer involvement of these vital organs is more easily dissected, and repair of these organs, in case of injury, is more readily accomplished with a left rather than a right thoracotomy approach.
4. Post-operative pain, which restrains coughing and airway clearance, is more severe with an added abdominal incision as in the Lewis–Tanner approach than without, as in the left thoracotomy approach.

The major disadvantages of the left thoracotomy approach are that the dissection of the subcarinal lymph nodes is difficult and that exposure of the oesophagus behind and above the arch of aorta is less satisfactory. Injury of the arch of azygos vein, which may occur during dissection of tumour at this site, is sometimes not noticed promptly with a left approach if the right mediastinal pleura has been opened. Ligation of this vein, of course, is much more difficult from the left than from the right chest.

Resection

Surgery for carcinoma of the oesophagus entails resection of carcinoma and reconstruction of the alimentary tract. For detailed technical descriptions readers are referred to the reports of Akiyama, Tsurumaru, Kawamura, and Ono (1981), Huang and Wu (1984), and Wong and Siu (1988).

Controversies exist, however, in various concepts and hence methods of resection, such as conventional versus extended lymph node dissections, partial versus complete oesophagectomies, *en bloc* (Skinner 1988) versus standard resections, and thoracotomy versus non-thoracotomy trans-hiatal approaches for oesophagectomy (Orringer 1988; Peracchia 1988). The author and his associates and most other surgeons, in China particularly, are in favour of a standard oesophagectomy performed through a thoracotomy.

Table 11.1. Tumour node metastasis (TNM) staging of 1874 surgical patients with oesophageal carcinoma.

Stage	No. of patients	Percentage
I	57	3.0
II	314	16.8
III	1320	70.5
IV	181	9.7
No record	1	0.1
Total	1873	100.0

Our concept is that carcinoma of the oesophagus is a surgically curable disease at its relatively early stage, when the malignant process is limited to the oesophagus itself or with only regional lymph node metastasis. In such cases meticulous extirpation of all tumour-bearing tissues is possible and mandatory. Our usual practice of resection is to eradicate, as completely as possible, all the connective and tumour-bearing tissues around the oesophagus and the draining lymph nodes of the peri-gastric group up to the root of the left gastric artery. This includes the para-cardiac, para-oesophageal, and the subcarinal groups, which are resected during the dissection and mobilization of the oesophagus and the stomach. The stomach is used in the vast majority of cases as a substitute for the resected oesophagus (Huang 1989). No attempt is made to undertake an extended lymph node dissection, but the oesophagus is resected not less than 5 cm above the upper gross margin of the tumour. Total oesophagectomy, however, is not a routine practice except in cases with high thoracic or cervical lesions.

In more advanced cases of oesophageal carcinoma with extra-oesophageal invasion of adjacent vital organs and more extensive lymph node involvement, it is very likely that the cancer has already permeated through lymphatic and vascular networks into a wide area and become systemic. At this stage of the disease, surgery is palliative, although long-term survival may still be possible in a small number of patients. Further improvement in therapeutic results will depend on more effective use of multi-modality therapy rather than on further extending the scope of resection.

Results of surgery

Of 1874 patients with squamous cell carcinoma of the oesophagus treated surgically at the author's institute (Huang *et al.* 1985), 1501 (80.1 per cent) had stage III and IV disease with either extra-oesophageal tumour invasion and/or distant lymph node metastases, or organ metastasis (Table 11.1). In this series there was an overall resectability of 1572 out of 1874 (83.9 per cent) patients. The resectability rate was 87.0 per cent for lesions of the lower segment of the oesophagus and 82.5 per cent each for the middle and the upper segments. It is to be noted that of the 1874 cases in this series, 690 (36.8 per cent) received various modes of pre-operative irradiation.

Of the 1159 resections for non-irradiated oesophageal carcinoma under study, lymph node metastasis was found in 593 (51.2 per cent). It is obvious that the true frequency would be higher and that practically all unresectable cases, which accounted for about 16 per cent of the cases operated on, had lymph node metastasis, although fixation and severe infiltration of the tumour to the adjacent vital organs usually constituted the major cause of unresectability. Consequently, the actual occurrence of lymph node metastasis in our patients who came to surgery was no less than 67 per cent.

Operative mortality

There were 66 deaths in 1572 patients within 30 days of resection, a resection mortality rate of 4.2 per cent. The major causes of death were pulmonary complications in 20 (30.3 per cent) patients, anastomotic leaks in 17 (25.8 per cent), cardiocascular complications in 11 (16.7 per cent), empyema without leakage and internal haemorrhage each occurred in four (6.1 per cent) patients and miscellaneous causes occurred in 10 (15.2 per cent) patients.

Of the 66 deaths, nine were recorded in 41 (22.0 per cent) resections for a special group of patients who had a 'curative' radiotherapy (usually for doses of more than 6500 cGy) over 3 months before surgery, chiefly because of uncontrolled primary tumour, local recurrence, or severe stricture. The resection mortality rate of this group of patients was much higher than that of patients without pre-operative 'curative' radiotherapy. If this special group of patients were excluded, the resection mortality rate of the remaining patients was 57 of 1531 patients (3.7 per cent).

Long-term survival

Long-term survival rates for surgical treatment for oesophageal carcinoma have been discouraging in the past and around the world, but recent statistics from a number of clinics in China have been more encouraging (Table 11.2).

In the present series of 1572 resections, the 5-, 10-, 15-, and 20-year survivals after resection were 29.6 per cent (390 of 1317), 22.5 per cent (210 of 922), 19.7 per cent (122 of 620) and 11.0 per cent (20 of 181) respectively.

Causes of remote death

Analysis of the present series showed that recurrence and/or metastasis of the primary cancer were the main causes of death within 5 years of resection. These also constituted the cause of death in as many as 40.0 per cent of patients who died more than 5 years after resection, 24.2 per cent of those

Table 11.2. Results of surgical treatment for carcinoma of the oesophagus by various authors in China

Authors	Year	No. of resections	Resectability (per cent)	Operative mortality (per cent)	5-year survival (per cent)
Zhang Y.D., *et al.*	1982	2070	80.6	6.5	23.5
Li E.L., *et al.*	1985	679	95.4	3.8	36.2
Shao L.F., *et al.*	1985	3869	93.7	3.0	36.8
Huang G.J., *et al.*	1985	1572	83.9	3.7	29.6
Liu G.S., *et al.*	1986	309	83.5	6.1	32.5

who died more than 10 years after resection, and in 85.1 per cent of these patients the initial resection was classified as curative (Huang, Wang, Zhang, and Zhang 1988).

It is interesting to note from this analysis that many of the resections initially classified as being curative were in reality palliative in nature, as patients eventually developed and died from recurrence and/or metastasis of the original cancer, and that some of these patients who had, in reality, palliative resections, could be long-term survivors.

Prognostic factors

In a study of 474 consecutive resections of non-irradiated squamous cell carcinoma of the thoracic oesophagus carried out in a period of 4 years ending in 1984 at the author's department, it was documented that surgical radicality, either curative or palliative resection, and lymph node metastases (which to a certain extent reflects stages of the disease) were two important prognostic factors that influenced long-term survival, and that these were closely interrelated.

The overall 5-year survival rate of the 474 resections was 30.6 per cent (Table 11.3). It is of interest that in the group of 145 patients with lymph node metastasis, when the metastatic lymph nodes were fewer than five in number, the 5-year survival rate was 14.7 per cent (Table 11.4).

These findings serve to indicate that surgical radicality is of great prognostic importance when the cancer process is relatively early and localized, but is of much less importance when the disease process is relatively advanced.

Summary

Carcinoma of the oesophagus is unfortunately very prevalent in China. To date, surgery remains the treatment of choice for this disease. The results

Table 11.3. Prognostic factors influencing 5-year survivals in 474 resections for non-irradiated squamous carcinoma of the oesophagus

Factors	% 5-year survival (cases)		*P*
Overall	30.6	(145/474)	
with LNM*	12.8	(27/211)	
without LNM	44.9	(118/263)	0.0001
Curative resections	37.8	(132/349)	
with LNM	17.4	(25/144)	
without LNM	52.2	(107/205)	0.0001
Palliative resections	10.4	(13/125)	
with LNM	3.0	(2/67)	
without LNM	19.0	(11/58)	0.0035

* LNM = lymph node metastasis

Table 11.4. 5-year survivals in relation to number of metastatic lymph nodes (LNM)

No. of LNM	% 5-year survival (cases)		*P*
Less than 5	14.7	(27/184)	
Curative resections	19.4	(25/129)	
Palliative resections	3.6	(2/55)	0.0057
More than 5	0	(0/27)	
Curative resections	0	(0/15)	
Palliative resections	0	(0/12)	

of surgery for early or stage I oesophageal cancer are excellent. However, except in high-incidence areas of this disease where early detection may be practised by means of balloon cytology screening, most patients are seen at relatively advanced stages of the disease. Although large numbers of new patients are seen annually at the author's institution, the operability rate is only about 21 per cent. In a series of 1874 patients with oesophageal squamous cell carcinoma treated surgically, there was a resectability rate of 83.9 per cent, a 30-day resection mortality rate of 4.2 per cent, and a 5-, 10-, 15-, and 20-year survival rate of 29.6, 22.5, 19.7 and 11.0 per cent, respectively. Similar results have been reported by many authors in China.

It is evident that recurrence and/or metastasis are the main obstacles to long-term survival. They were the cause of death in 40.0 per cent of patients who died more than 5 years after resection, and in 24.2 per cent of those who died more than 10 years after resection of oesophageal carcinoma; in 85 per cent of these patients the initial resection was classified as curative.

Analysis of 474 consecutive resections of carcinoma of the oesophagus showed that surgical radicality and the status of lymph node metastasis were two important factors of prognostic significance. In the absence of lymph node metastasis, and with a curative resection, the 5-year survival rate was at best 52.2 per cent, whereas in the presence of lymph node metastasis and with a palliative resection it was only 3.0 per cent. With metastatic lymph nodes fewer than five- in number per patient, the 5-year survival rate was 19.4 per cent with a curative resection, and only 3.6 per cent with a palliative resection. When the metastatic lymph nodes were more than five in number per patient, there were no 5-year survivors irrespective of surgical radicality, whether curative or palliative.

It is postulated that carcinoma of the oesophagus is a surgically curable disease when the cancer process is localized or at a relatively early stage. However, surgery alone is of only palliative value in relatively advanced cases in which the cancer process has dispersed to a wide extent with gross and microscopic metastases, and extra-oesophageal invasion to adjacent vital organs, although long-term survival may still be possible in a small number of patients. In these circumstances it is often unwise to over-extend the scope of surgery, with an inevitable increase in operative morbidity and mortality rates.

References

Adams, W.E. and Phemister, D.B. (1938). Carcinoma of the lower thoracic esophagus: report of a successful resection and esophagogastrostomy. *J. Thorac. Surg.* **7**, 621–32.

Akiyama, H., Kogure, T., and Itai, Y. (1972). The esophageal axis and its relationship to the resectability of carcinoma of the esophagus. *Ann. Surg.* **176**, 30–6.

Akiyama, H., Tsurumaru, M., Kawamura, T., and Ono, Y. (1981). Principles of surgical treatment for carcinoma of the esophagus: analysis of lymph node involvement. *Ann. Surg.* **194**, 438–45.

Garlock, J.H. (1944). Re-establishment of esophagogastric continuity following resection of esophagus for carcinoma of middle third. *Surg. Gynecol. Obstet.* **78**, 23–8.

Huang, G.J. and Wu, Y.K. (1984). Operative technique for carcinoma of the esophagus. In *Carcinoma of the esophagus and gastric cardia* (ed. G.J. Huang, and Y.K. Wu) pp. 314–48. Springer-Verlag, Berlin.

Huang, G.J., Wang, L.J., Liu, J.S., *et al.* (1985). Surgery of esophageal carcinoma. *Semin. Surg. Oncol.* **1**, 74.

Huang, G.J. (1988). Preoperative radiotherapy and surgery for carcinoma of the esophagus. In *Thoracic surgery series. Vol. 4, Esophageal cancer* (ed. N.C. de la Rue, E.W. Wilkins Jr., and J. Wong) pp. 315–18. C.V. Mosby, St. Louis.

Huang, G.J., Wang, L.J., Zhang, D.W., and Zhang, R.G. (1988). Late results of surgical treatment for carcinoma of the esophagus. In *Diseases of the esophagus* (ed. J.R. Siewert and A.H. Hoelscher) Springer, New York.

Huang, G.J. (1989). Replacement of the esophagus with the stomach. In *General thoracic surgery* (ed. T.W. Shields) (3rd edn) pp. 433–42. Lea & Febiger, Philadelphia.

Lewis, I. (1946). The surgical treatment of carcinoma of the oesophagus with special reference to a new operation for growths of the middle third. *Br. J. Surg.* **34**, 18–31.

Marshall, S.R. (1938). Carcinoma of the esophagus. *Surg. Clin. North. Am.* **18**, 643–8.

Orringer, M.B. (1988). Transhiatal esophagectomy without thoracotomy for esophageal carcinoma. In *Thoracic surgery series. Vol. 4, Esophageal cancer* (ed. N.C. de la Rue, E.W. Wilkins Jr., and J. Wong) pp. 200–9. C.V. Mosby, St. Louis.

Payne, W.S., Trastek, V.F., Piehler, J.M., Pairolero, P.C., and Bernatz, P.E. (1986). Current techniques for the surgical management of malignant lesions of the thoracic esophagus and cardia. *Mayo Clin. Proc.* **61**, 564–72.

Peracchia, A. (1988). Discussion on Orringer's and Skinner's reports. In Thoracic surgery series. *Vol. 4, Esophageal cancer* (ed. N.C. de la Rue, E.W. Wilkins Jr., and J. Wong) pp. 210–12. C.V. Mosby, St. Louis.

Shao, L.F., Huang, G.J., Zhang, D.W., *et al.* (1981). Detection and surgical treatment of early esophageal carcinoma. In *Proceedings of the Beijing Symposium on Cardiothoracic Surgery*, pp. 168–71. China Academic Publishers and John Wiley & Sons Incorporated., Beijing.

Skinner, D.B. (1988). *En bloc* resection for esophageal carcinoma. In *Thoracic surgery series. Vol. 4, Esophageal cancer* (ed. N.C. de la Rue, E.W. Wilkins Jr., and J. Wong) pp. 193–9. C.V. Mosby, St. Louis.

Sweet, R.H. (1945). Transthoracic resection of the esophagus and stomach for carcinoma. *Ann. Surg.* **121**, 272–84.

Tanner, N.C. (1947). The present position of carcinoma of the esophagus. *Postgrad. Med. J.* **23**, 109.

Wong, J. and Siu, K.F. (1988). Squamous cell carcinoma of the esophagus. In *Thoracic surgery series. Vol. 4, Esophageal cancer* (ed. N.C. de la Rue, E.W. Wilkins Jr., and J. Wong) pp. 164–80. C.V. Mosby, St. Louis.

Wu, Y.K. and Loucks, H.H. (1941). Carcinoma of the oesophagus or cardia of stomach: analysis of 172 cases with 81 resections. *Ann. Surg.* **134**, 946–56.

Wu, Y.K. and Loucks, H.H. (1942). Resection of the esophagus for carcinoma: an analysis of experience in eleven cases. *J. Thorac. Surg.* **11**, 516–28.

12. Gastric cancer

Jin-Pok Kim

Pathophysiology of gastric cancer

Incidence

In the past 40 years the incidence of gastric cancer has continuously and markedly decreased in most western countries but remains high in Korea, Japan, China, Russia, Finland, and Chile. The Korean Registry (based on teaching hospitals throughout the country) reported that the frequency of gastric cancer among all patients admitted with malignant disease was 24 per cent (30 per cent in males and 17 per cent in females). According to 1988 statistics issued by the Korean government, cancer is the most common cause of death (41 764 cancer fatalities of 229 336 total deaths), and of all fatalities due to malignant disease, cancer death was the highest in both males and females in 1988 (32 gastric cancer deaths per 100 000 population).

Aetiological factors

Environmental and host factors have been implicated in the aetiology of gastric cancer. Dietary carcinogens are perhaps responsible for about 80 per cent of cases and natural and socio-economic factors play the major roles in the environment, whereas race, age, sex, and hereditary factors are important considerations in the host. A high salt diet, red pepper, and pyrolytic fish and meat cause gastric carcinogenesis in both experimental rats and humans, and the high incidence of gastric cancer in Korea is probably related to these factors. In contrast, milk, yellow or green vegetables, soybean paste or soup, and ginseng suppress gastric carcinogenesis in experimental animals. There is some evidence of an hereditary familial tendency. Epidemiological studies of the incidence of gastric cancer among Japanese immigrants in Hawaii and California showed that the incidence of gastric cancer in first-generation Japanese is significantly higher than that of American Caucasians, whereas no such difference is observed in second and third generations of Japanese immigrants.

Symptoms and signs

Symptoms and signs are infrequent early in the course of the disease and this makes diagnosis difficult at this stage. Symptoms include gastrointestinal bleeding, epigastric discomfort, fullness, and pain, and unexplained indigestion. Signs observed include an epigastric mass, weight loss, and a palpable liver. A palpable left supra-clavicular lymph node (Virchow's node), palpable rectal shelf (Blumer's shelf), and ascites are generally considered to be absolute contra-indications for surgery.

Diagnosis

Double-contrast upper gastrointestinal fluoroscopic series, gastroscopy with endoscopic biopsy and cytology, ultrasonography of peri-gastric lymph nodes and liver, and computed tomography (CT) scanning of pancreas, liver, and peri-gastric lymph nodes are used for the diagnosis of gastric cancer. Resectability of the tumour can often be determined by stomach movability in the upper gastrointestinal series. If the stomach moves more than one vertebral space on moving the patient from the upright to the supine position, the tumour is usually resectable. If gastric movement is less than half a vertebral space, then the tumour is considered to be unresectable. Ultrasonography or CT scanning can be used to determine the advisability of exploration for resection of the tumour, particularly when liver metastasis or pancreatic invasion is suspected.

Differential diagnosis between benign and malignant ulcer

This differentiation can be made using radiological and endoscopic features, which are shown in Table 12.1.

Pathological features

UICC clinical stage

By the Union International Contra le Cancrum tumour node metastasis (UICC TNM) staging method, any gastric cancer, even early gastric cancer, with lymph node metastasis should be classified as stage III. Alternatively, according to the Japanese concept of early gastric cancer, mucosal or submucosal cancers, even with lymph node metastasis, are classified as stage I disease early gastric cancer. By the new classification, proposed in 1985 by the Japanese and American Study Group, stage I and III disease is subgrouped into stage I_{a-b} and III_{a-b}. The problem was that a T_1 lesion with lymph node metastases was classified into stage I_b. In all staging systems of malignancy, any cancer with lymph node metastases can no longer be classified as stage I.

Good correlation was found between post-operative survival rate and the number of lymph node metastases in 214 patients undergoing surgery at Seoul National University Hospital (1974–7). The 5-year survival rate was 75.7 per cent in the group without lymph node involvement, 44.9 per cent with one to three lymph node metastases, and 24.1 per cent when metastases occurred in more than three lymph nodes. According to my own modification of the UICC classification, patients classified as $T_1N_{1(3)}M_0$ should be

Table 12.1. Radiological and endoscopic findings in benign and malignant ulcers.

	Benign	Malignant
Ulcer crater		
Shape	Round or ovoid	Irregular
Edge	Punched out	Irregular
Size	Usually small to medium	Variable
Location	Lesser curvature	Greater curvature
Number	May be multiple	Single
Base	Clear	Shallow
Mucosal fold		
Convergence	+	–
Interrupted	–	+
Clubbing	–	+
Fusion	–	+
Mucosal surface around ulcer	Oedematous but smooth	Heaped-up crater
Peristalsis in ulcer area	+	–
Healing with drugs	Rapid	Slow
Duodenal ulcer	May be present	Almost never present

classified as stage II_a and $T_2N_{1(3)}$ as stage II_b. The post-operative survival rate of these 214 gastric cancer patients showed a good positive correlation with the modification. It is proposed, therefore, that his modification of UICC classification would be more useful, on the premise that a T_1 lesion with lymph node metastasis can not be classified into stage I but is better classified into stage II_a.

Clinicopathological features

The overall male: female ration in Seoul patients was 1.9:1, but it was 1:1.5 in the third decade. The most frequent location of the tumour was the pyloric antrum (61.6 per cent). Advanced gastric carcinoma was present in 83.3 per cent, the remainder of the group having early carcinoma; Borrmann type III and early gastric carcinoma type II_c were the most common gross types, respectively. The most common histological type was poorly differentiated adenocarcinoma (39.9 per cent). The serosa was already invaded in 64 per cent of all patients at diagnosis. The mean number of regional lymph nodes for each patient was 28, and 61.9 per cent of all patients had regional lymph node metastasis. Polypoid tumours metastasized to regional lymph nodes less often than did infiltrative tumours. The poorly

Table 12.2. Results of multi-variate analysis of prognostic factors in stomach cancer (1981–6, Seoul National University Hospital).

Variable	Degrees of freedom	χ^2	p
Lymph node	2	73.59	0.001*
Depth of invasion	5	16.82	0.004*
Gross type	4	9.41	0.051
Age	5	10.93	0.054
Location	2	4.08	$p > 0.10$
Resection	2	3.86	$p > 0.10$
Histology	5	8.11	$p > 0.10$
Sex	1	0.31	$p > 0.10$

* Statistically significant difference.

differentiated lesions invaded the gastric wall more deeply and metastasized to regional lymph nodes more frequently than well-differentiated tumours. Tumours of the cardia invaded the gastric wall more deeply and more frequently metastasized to the regional lymph nodes than tumours of the body. There was no relationship between tumour location and cell differentiation. Regional lymph node metastasis was related to the depth of the tumour invasion into the gastric wall.

Several clinical and pathological features such as age, tumour location, gross appearance, histological type, depth of tumour invasion, and regional lymph node metastasis may be of prognostic value for ultimate survival by uni-variate analysis. Only two factors, regional lymph node metastasis and depth of gastric wall invasion, are significant on multi-variate analysis (Table 12.2).

Treatment

The principal goal of treatment of gastric cancer is radical curative surgery including subtotal, total, or extended total gastrectomy with systemic regional lymph node dissection. The best therapy is adequate curative surgery followed by early post-operative immunochemotherapy to control any remaining cancer cells or micrometastases.

Operability and resectability

In 5949 cases of gastric cancer, the overall operability rate was 93 per cent, which improved from 87 per cent in early 1979 to 94 per cent in 1987. Eighty per cent of patients with resected gastric cancer underwent subtotal gastrectomy and 20 per cent underwent total or extended total gastrectomy. Total gastrectomy is preferred for Borrmann type IV, cardia, or fundus cancer, and for signet ring cell or poorly differentiated tumours.

Extent of gastric resection

Due to the distal location of most primary gastric cancers, 80 per cent distal curative subtotal gastrectomy is the most common type of gastrectomy performed, but proximal subtotal gastrectomy is occasionally undertaken for early cancers which involve the cardia, fundus, or upper body. Because proximal subtotal gastrectomy is less likely to be curative, most surgeons prefer to undertake total gastrectomy for advanced cancers in the cardia, fundus, or upper body. On all occasions the proximal resection margin should be more than 2 cm in early gastric cancer and 6 cm in advanced gastric cancer, and the distal margin should extend more than 2 cm from the pylorus. For cancers in the fundus or along the greater curvature with direct infiltration into the distal pancreas, splenic hilum, mesocolon, or transverse colon, or with solitary direct extension into the left hepatic lobe, extended total gastrectomy including distal pancreas, spleen, transverse colon, or the left lobe of the liver is recommended.

Extent of lymph node dissection

Systematic regional lymph node dissection along the perigastric vessels, including the coeliac axis, common hepatic artery, hepatic artery, splenic artery, and portal vein (so-called skeletonization), with retropancreatic lymph node dissection, is the most important surgical procedure (R_2 + Nos. 12 and 13 lymph node dissection).

Reconstruction after subtotal gastrectomy

Billroth I gastroduodenostomy is rarely advocated for pre-pyloric or antral early gastric cancer and Billroth II retrocolic gastrojejunostomy is always performed whenever feasible because there are unlikely to be cancer cells in the mesocolon, the blind loop syndrome is less frequent with a short afferent loop, retrostomal internal herniation is less likely, and iron and nutritional absorption improve.

Reconstruction after total gastrectomy

Reconstruction after total gastrectomy is a controversial problem of the various reconstruction methods; loop oesophagojejunostomy and Roux-en-Y oesophagojejunostomy are the two most commonly practised basic reconstructive procedures. Post-operative oesophageal reflux following loop oesophagojejunostomy and a higher anastomotic leakage rate after Roux-en-Y oesophagojejunostomy have, however, been troublesome problems. We have found that simple loop oesophagojejunostomy, with closure of the afferent loop and a long jejunojejunostomy, is satisfactory and without significant oesophageal reflux and leakage, and with less post-operative immune depression.

Table 12.3. TNM Stages of 5949 patients with gastric cancer at the Department of Surgery, Seoul National University Hospital (1970–89).

Period	No. of patients	Stage I	II	III	IV
1970–9	1209	42 (3.5)	140 (11.6)	547 (45.2)	480 (39.7)
1980–4	1858	158 (8.5)	175 (9.4)	957 (51.5)	568 (30.6)
1985	454	67 (14.8)	81 (17.8)	181 (39.9)	125 (27.5)
1986	535	85 (15.9)	65 (12.1)	256 (47.9)	129 (24.1)
1987	523	72 (13.8)	66 (12.6)	291 (55.6)	94 (18.0)
1988	710	94 (13.2)	91 (12.8)	364 (51.3)	161 (22.7)
1989	660	106 (16.1)	99 (15.0)	304 (46.1)	151 (22.9)
Total	5949	624 (10.5)	717 (12.1)	2900 (48.7)	1708 (28.7)

Values in parentheses are percentages.

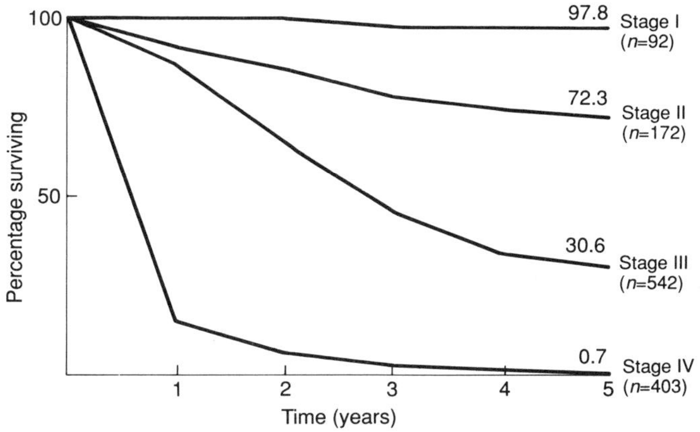

Fig. 12.1. Survival curves of patients with gastric cancer according to TNM stage (Seoul National University Hospital, 1975–81). Number of follow-up cases was 1209 of a total 1387 (87 per cent).

Immunochemosurgery as a reasonable treatment of advanced gastric carcinoma

Despite the development of diagnostic techniques, the majority of patients with gastric cancer have stage III or IV disease at first diagnosis (Table 12.3). The 5-year survival rate for stage III gastric cancer is only 30.6 per cent, which is disappointing (Fig. 12.1). The question therefore arises: 'Can surgery alone cure gastric cancer patients?' Whilst the answer may be yes, in stage I and II patients surgery alone can not cure patients with gastric cancer at an advanced stage. Stage III disease must be considered to be already systemic in nature. In order to improve the prognosis of advanced stomach cancer, systemic treatment such as immunotherapy or chemotherapy is required in the early post-operative period to eradicate micrometastases or remaining cancer cells even after 'curative' resection.

There are many reports concerning the beneficial effects of adjuvant immunotherapy and chemotherapy (Morton, Eiber, Malmgren, and Wood 1970; Okudaira, Sugimachi, Inokuchi, Kari, Kuwano, and Matsuura 1982; Rosenberg 1985). Immunotherapy itself does not interfere with the effects of surgery, radiation therapy, and chemotherapy, and is best considered as complementary. Pre-operative cell-mediated immunity tests such as the T-cell count, T-cell percentage, and delayed cutaneous sensitivity test to dinitrochlorobenzene (DNCB) were markedly decreased in patients with advanced gastric cancer compared with normal controls (Kim and Yoo 1978). Natural killer cell activity and antibody-dependent cellular cytotoxicity were also decreased. In contrast, serum immunosuppressive acidic protein level was increased as the stage of disease advanced. Immunotherapy is necessary to improve competence of the immune system of patients with gastric cancer, and is also helpful in overcoming the depressive effects of chemotherapy on the immune system.

The purpose of our own study in Korea was to evaluate the therapeutic efficacy of early post-operative immunochemotherapy (so-called immunochemosurgery) and conventional adjuvant chemotherapy in advanced, but resectable, adenocarcinoma of stomach. Survival rates and the immune status of patients with stage III gastric carcinoma were compared in the treatment and surgery-alone groups.

Patients and methods in immunochemosurgery study

Before surgery all patients with stomach cancer underwent complete history-taking and physical examination, with measurements of disease and immune parameters as described below, performance status, routine laboratory tests, and a liver scan. If the history or physical examination suggested distant metastasis, special studies such as bone or brain scans were performed.

After operation, patients with histologically confirmed lymph node-positive stage III adenocarcinoma of the stomach, were randomized into one of three groups: immunochemosurgery, conventional adjuvant chemotherapy, or surgery alone provided routine examinations (including haemoglobin estimation, liver and renal function tests) were normal. Patients were ineligible for study if they has a previous history of chemotherapy or radiation therapy, or were over 70 years of age. Initial performance status was within the range of the Eastern Co-operative Oncology, Group, 0–2 in all patients.

Three hundred and seventy patients with histologically proven stage III gastric cancer, aged between 30 and 70 years, and with performance status 0–2, without systemic disease, were thus randomly assigned to the three

Table 12.4. Randomization of patients with gastric cancer.

Treatment	No. entered	No. evaluated
Immunochemosurgery	170	159*
Post-operative chemotherapy	100	77*
Surgery alone	100	94*
Total	370	330 (89%)

Criteria: age > 30 years; < 70 stage III, performance status 0–2; subtotal gastrectomy with lymph node dissection; Billroth II gastrojejunostomy.
* Discontinued or altered treatment cases were excluded for evaluation.

groups after curative subtotal gastrectomy; 170 were allocated to immunochemosurgery group, 100 to post-operative chemotherapy, and 100 to surgery alone (Table 12.4). Forty patients were excluded because their treatment was altered or discontinued.

Curative surgery for gastric cancer performed in our centre includes subtotal gastric resection, complete dissection, skeletonization of regional lymph nodes along the coeliac axis, hepatic artery, splenic artery, portal vein, and retropancreatic lymph nodes as well as peri-gastric lymph nodes and removal of omentum with adjacent tissues. All tissues were removed in *en-bloc* fashion. Frozen section biopsy of both resection margins was performed in all cases.

Post-operative immunochemotherapy

Patients randomized to post-operative immunochemotherapy or chemotherapy received the following therapy:

1. *Immunotherapy Streptococcus pyogenes* preparation (Picibanil) was given intramuscularly at a dosage of 1.0 KE (Klinische Einheit = clinical unit) every week from the fourth or fifth day after operation.

2. *Chemotherapy* The MF (mitomycin C, 5-fluorouracil) regimen was started on the eighth to tenth post-operative day in the immunochemosurgery group and after 3–6 weeks in the chemotherapy group. The dosage administration schedules for each regimen were as follows: 4 mg/50 kg mitomycin C, 500 mg/50 kg 5-fluorouracil, given intravenously twice a week for the first 2 weeks and then every week for next 6 weeks. Subsequently oral 5-fluorouracil was given daily at a dosage of 600 mg/50 kg. Immunochemotherapy was continued for 24 months following operation, if well tolerated. Immediately before each chemotherapy cycle, white blood cell and platelet counts were obtained and liver function tests were repeated, if considered necessary. Drug dosage was controlled based upon the parameters of haematological toxicity and other adverse reactions.

Immunological studies

The following immunological tests were performed before operation and at the third to fourth post-operative months:

1. *DNCB cutaneous hypersensitivity test* 0.1 ml of 2 per cent DNCB (J.T. Baker Chemical Co., Phillipsburg, New Jersey, USA) solution in acetone (sensitizing dose) and 0.05 per cent DNCB solution in acetone (challenging dose) were smeared over a skin area of the inner surface of a forearm respectively. The flare reaction was measured between 7 and 14 days after application and was evaluated as follows: (1) erythema on both sides of the sensitizing and challenge dose areas, ++++; (2) erythema on sensitizing dose area only, +++ (if there was no reaction until 14 days, 0.1 ml of 0.05 per cent DNCB solution was smeared again and the reaction evaluated 48 hours later); (3) extent of erythema and induration exceeding that of challenge dose area smeared, ++; (4) erythema and induration not exceeding half of challenge dose area smeared, +; and (5) no response, 0.

2. *T-lymphocyte count* Lymphocytes were isolated using the Ficollhypaque method from the heparinized peripheral blood of patients. Isolated lymphocytes were washed with saline and Hank's solution and then mixed with washed sheep erythrocytes and incubated for 18 hours at 37°C. After incubation, the number of rosette-forming cells with at least three sheep erythrocytes was counted among 200 lymphocytes and was represented as the percentage of T lymphocytes.

3. *Lymphoblastogenesis by phytohaemagglutinin (PHA) and concanavalin A stimulation* Lymphocytes were prepared by the Ficoll–Hypaque method from the peripheral blood of patients. The prepared lymphocytes were made up to 1.5 × 10/0.2 ml with tissue culture-199 media. PHA (0.1 ml) and 50 μg concanavalin A were added to the mixture of 0.2 ml cell suspension and 3 ml media, respectively, and incubated for 72 hours in the presence of 5 per cent carbon monoxide. Four hours before harvest, 0.5 μCi of tritiated thymidine was added to each culture tube. After culture, tubes were centrifuged at 4°C and washed with cold saline. Five millilitres 5 per cent trichloroacetic acid solution was added to the precipitates and centrifuged at 4°C and 0.5 ml 90 per cent formic acid solution was added and retained overnight. Radioactivity was determined using a scintillation counter.

4. *Antibody-dependent cellular cytotoxicity* Lymphomononuclear cells isolated from peripheral blood of patients, ^{51}Cr-labelled chicken red blood cells, anti-chicken red blood cell antibody from rabbit and 10 per cent fetal calf serum-RPMI (Roswell Park Memorial Institute, New York, USA) media were mixed and incubated for 18 hours at 37°C. After culture, radioactivity of the supernatant was determined. The lymphomononuclear

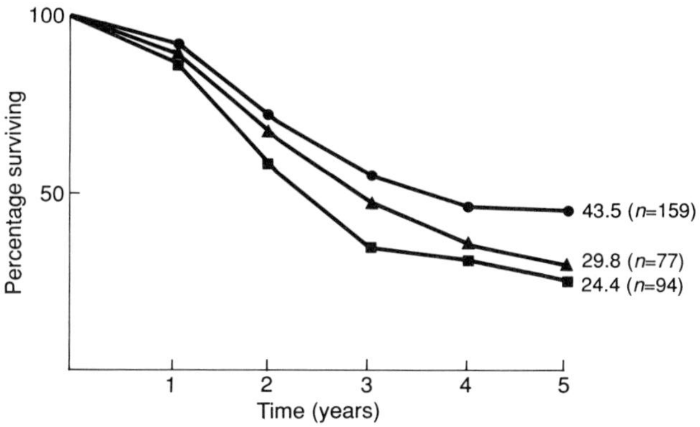

Fig. 12.2. Survival curves of immunochemosurgery group (●), surgery plus post-operative chemotherapy group (▲), and surgery-alone group (■) in patients with stage III stomach cancer (330 cases, 1975–82).

cells (effector cell) to ^{51}Cr-labelled chicken red blood cells (target cell) ratio was 10:1. Cytotoxicity was calculated as follows:

$$^{51}\text{Cr release (\%)} = \frac{\text{experimental release} - \text{spontaneous release}}{\text{maximum release} - \text{spontaneous release}} \times 100$$

Survival rate, calculated from the day of operation, and immune statue were compared in the three groups. Statistical comparison of patient characteristics and immune parameters was performed utilizing the χ^2 test or Student's t test. Differences were considered significant when p was less than 0.05. Differences in survival rate between groups were determined using the Cox–Mantel test.

Results

Three hundred and thirty patients were randomly divided into the three groups and followed for at least 5 years. Of these, 159 patients received post-operative immunochemotherapy, 77 received conventional adjuvant chemotherapy after operation, and 94 patients received no further therapy. Patient characteristics, pre-operative value of immune parameters, and the proportion of histological types and extent of lymph node involvement of the three groups of patients were similar.

Survival curves of three groups of patient are shown in Figure 12.2. The 5-year survival rate in the post-operative immunochemotherapy group was 45.3 per cent and that of the chemotherapy and surgery alone groups was 29.8 and 24.4 per cent, respectively. The difference in survival rate determined by Cox–Mantel test was statistically significant between the immunochemosurgery and the other two groups.

Post-operative T-cell percentage was increased in the immunochemosurgery group after immunochemotherapy, but was decreased in both the post-operative chemotherapy group and surgery-alone groups. A positive conversion rate of DNCB-negative patients after treatment was 85.9 per cent in the immunochemosurgery group, 72.5 per cent in the post-operative chemotherapy group, and 75 per cent in the surgery-alone group. Lymphoblastogenesis and antibody-dependent cellular cytotoxicity activity was also favourable in the immunochemosurgery group (Table 12.5).

Discussion

Certainly depth of invasion, presence or absence of lymph node metastases, particularly multiple involvement, and distant metastasis are the most important prognostic factors in gastric carcinoma. Lauren's histological type of stomach cancer, according to histotopographical investigation, is another important prognostic indicator (Lauren 1965). The author of this chapter analysed 448 cases of stomach cancer to evaluate the prognostic value of Lauren's histological types (Kim and Choi 1986) and documented that the 5-year survival rate of the intestinal type (43.7 per cent in 190 patients) was higher than that of the diffuse type (30.4 per cent in 138 patients, $p < 0.05$). The distribution of these histological types was similar among the three groups in this study.

The long-term survival rate of patients who underwent total gastrectomy is lower than that of patients who underwent subtotal gastrectomy, although patients were content to have the same stage of disease (Kim and Park 1983). This is probably not because mortality or serious morbidity rates following operation are high, but primarily because total gastrectomy is practical more often in advanced disease. Patients undergoing total gastrectomy were excluded in our study of immunochemosurgery. The presence or absence of metastatic lymph nodes and the extent of involved nodes are a significant prognostic indicator. It has been demonstrated previously that the 5-year survival rate of patients with one to three metastatic lymph nodes is significantly higher than that of patients with more than three metastatic lymph nodes (Kim and Jung 1986). The proportion of patients with between one and three lymph node metastases to those with more than three lymph node metastases was similar in each group in the immunochemosurgery study.

Although adjuvant therapy after radical gastric resection has been expected to be the most promising treatment for stomach cancer, there is no long-term follow-up report to demonstrate improvement of survival rate with use of adjuvant therapy, and many pessimistic results have been documented (Blake, Hardcastle, and Wilson 1981; Serlin, Keehn, Higgins, Harrower, and Mendeloff 1977). Several regimens for adjuvant chemotherapy have been suggested and evaluated clinically. The mitomycin C, 5-fluorouracil, and cytosine arabinoside (MFC) regimen (Ota, Kurita, Nishimura, Ogawa, Kunei, Imai, Ariyoshi, Kataoka, Murakami, Oyana, Hoshi-

Table 12.5. Values of immunoparameters before and after operation.

	Immunochemosurgery		Post-operative chemotherapy		Surgery alone	
Immune parameter	Before	After	Before	After	Before	After
DNCB positivity (%)	52.5 (41/78)	85.9 (67/78)	48.3 (14/29)	72.5 (21/29)	46.8 (15/32)	75.0 (24/32)
T-cell percentage	56.4 (6.1)	59.7 (5.8)	59.2 (7.4)	57.3 (6.8)	58.7 (7.9)	56.1 (6.8)
T-cell count/mm^3	1135 (507)	1182 (541)	1146 (352)	974 (496)	1154 (440)	1152 (364)
Blastogenesis (c.p.m.)						
PHA stimulated	5279 (759)	4638 (602)	5567 (1872)	2302 (290)	5536 (1321)	3654 (411)
Con-A stimulated	8879 (1301)	5327 (494)	8624 (1312)	2872 (340)	8502 (1321)	4409 (472)
ADCC activity (%)	37.8 (11.9)	40.2 (11.2)	36.7 (11.0)	37.8 (11.3)	36.8 (11.4)	37.9 (12.8)

DNCB, dinitrochlorobenzeve; PHA, phytohaemagglutinin; Con-A, concanavalin A; ADCC, antibody-dependent cellular cytotoxicity.

no, Ano, and Kato 1972) 5-fluorouracil and methyl CCNU® (FME) regimen (Moertel, Mittelman, Bakemeier, Engstrom, and Hanley 1976; Livstone and Stablein 1981) were reported to give good response rates in advanced gastric cancer. The Gastrointestinal Tumor Study Group (GITSG) reported a long-term follow-up result of adjuvant chemotherapy with the FME regimen following curative resection of gastric cancer (GITSG 1982*a*). Improvement in survival rate appeared to be associated with adjuvant treatment and an increase in survival rate began to be observed 12 months after surgery. The percentage survival rate difference between the control and adjuvant therapy groups was nearly 20 per cent at 4 years of follow-up. Survival in the author's study reported in this chapter is similar to that of the GITSG.

Since MacDonald, Schein, Woolley, Smythe, Veno, Hoth, Smith, Boiron, Gisselbrecht, Brunet, and Lagarde (1980) reported a response rate of 42 per cent with FAM (5-fluorouracil, Adriamycin®, mitomycin C) for advanced gastric cancer, there have been many reports that combination chemotherapy incorporating Adriamycin is more effective than other regimens (Bitran, Desser, Kozloff, Billings, and Shapero 1979; GITSG 1979, 1982*a*, 1982*b*; Kim and Park 1983). The author believes, however, that Adriamycin is too toxic to be used as an adjuvant chemotherapeutic agent. Many clinical studies using FAM are being investigated and their effects can be interpreted when long-term results become available.

There have been numerous reports of the efficacy of immunotherapy for certain malignancies, such as acute myeloblastic leukaemia, breast cancer, malignant melanoma, squamous cell carcinoma of head and neck, ovarian cancer, childhood neuroblastoma, stomach cancer, and oesophageal cancer (Morton, Malmgren, Holmes, and Ketcham 1968; Mathe, Amiel, Schwarzenberg, Schneidor, Cattan, Schlumberger, Hayat, and de Vassal 1969; Morton *et al.* 1970; Hattori *et al.* 1972; McElwain, Russell, Lister, Whitehouse, Wrigley, Pike, Alexander, Hamilton, and Fairly 1973; Gutterman, Mavligit, Blumenshein, Burgess, McBride, and Hersh 1976*a*; Gutlerman, Cardenas, Blumenschein, Hortobagyi, Burgess, Livingston, Mavligit, Freireich, Gottlieb, and Hersh 1976*b*; Necheles 1976; Richman, Livingston, Gutterman, Suen, and Hersh 1976; Alberts 1977; Hoerni, Chauvergne, and Hoerni, 1977; Wanebo, Hilal, Pinsky, Strong, Mike, Hirshaut, and Oettgen 1978; Okudaira *et al.* 1982; Kim and Park 1983). Theoretically specific immunotherapy could be more beneficial than non-specific immunotherapy, but it is not yet a practical reality. Non-specific immunotherapy using various immune potentiators or biological response modifiers (BRM) is now being commonly practised.

I believe that immunotherapy should be advocated in all the patients with advanced disease after curative operation. The immune status of patients with cancer is depressed by some tumour-related factors, host factors enhanced by tumour, and poor nutritional state. Immunotherapy is therefore not as effective as expected, because some patients have a poor response to active immunotherapy, and endogenous mechanisms to potentiate passive immunotherapy using antibody and cytotoxic lymphocyte are blocked in those patients. Surgery itself, however, is a kind of immunotherapy, removing many factors that act to depress the immune status as well as the tumour itself. Patients may then have better prospects for not only active immunotherapy, but also passive or adoptive immunotherapy using antibody and lymphokine-activated killer cells.

Advantages of post-operative immunochemotherapy have been documented as prolonged remission and survival (McElwain *et al.* 1973; Kim and Park 1983), decreased incidence of fatal infection (Holland, Bekesi, Cuttner, and Glidewell 1977; Rodriquez, Bodey, Freireich, McCredie, Gutterman, Keating, Smith, and Gehan 1978), improved bone marrow tolerance (Pouillart, Palangie, Schwarzenburg, Brugerie, Lheritier, and Mathe 1975), and delayed recurrence (Kim and Park 1983). The efficacy, however, of post-operative immunochemotherapy for gastric cancer remains the subject of considerable debate. Makowka, Falk, Ambus, Bugala, and Landi (1980) reported that adjuvant immunochemotherapy with 5-fluorouracil and BCG for gastric cancer was ineffective, but Suga, Tsunekawa, and Washino (1977) have shown longer survival times in patients treated with MFC and picibanil, compared with patients treated with MFC alone for advanced gastric cancer.

Treatment procedures consisted of two components in our study. First, radical gastrectomy was performed as thoroughly as possible and regional lymph nodes including adjacent tissues were removed in an *en-bloc* fashion. It is true that stage III gastric cancer is already a systemic disease and cannot be cured with local therapy alone, even though locoregional therapy is performed thoroughly and aggressively. Moreover, there are technical limitations for complete removal of tumour cells owing to anatomical complexity of lymphatic channels draining the stomach.

Immunochemotherapy, as a second treatment modality, was considered to eradicate microscopic residual tumour. In general, conventional adjuvant chemotherapy is commenced between 3 and 8 weeks after operation to avoid the post-operative immune depressive period similar to the chemotherapy group of the study. For the immunochemosurgery group we began immunotherapy on the fourth or fifth post-operative day when vital signs of the patients were stable, and started chemotherapy on the eight to tenth post-operative day, when sutures in the main wound were removed and the patient was able to tolerate an oral intake. The purpose of early adjuvant therapy is to achieve a cure by destroying residual tumour cells including micrometastases, when the burden of tumour cells is at a minimum. Post-operative adjuvant therapy should be started early to be effective, because from 24–48 hours up to several weeks after cancer resection the remaining or micrometastatic cancer cells are proliferating rapidly. These are sensitive to chemotherapy and because the immune defence ability of cancer patients is temporarily depressed in the immediate post-operative period until 2–3 weeks thereafter.

Gunduz, Fisher, and Staffer (1979) elaborated on the important rationale of early post-surgical use of adjuvant chemotherapy. These authors reported that the increase in growth fraction of residual foci was observed within 24 hours after primary tumour removal and that this increase was no longer evident after 7 days in the experimental mouse tumour mode. Nissen-Meyer, Kjellgren, Malmio, Mansson, and Norin (1978) reported a decreased recurrence and death rate with adjuvant chemotherapy when this was started in the early post-operative period for breast cancer, but no improvement when commenced 3 weeks after mastectomy.

Several reasons have been proposed to explain why Japanese reports have shown a better survival rate than those from western countries. Many surgeons recognized that extensive lymph node dissection might contribute to improved survival rates. Another important contributing factor may be differences in the mode of chemotherapy, especially the timing of therapy. As in our trial, adjuvant therapy was commenced immediately after operation in Japan.

The results have shown that the 5-year survival rate of patients receiving surgery with early immunochemotherapy is better than that of the chemotherapy group or control groups. Immune status data in this study also show better results in the immunochemotherapy group. Surgery with complete removal of visible tumour cells is of prime importance in multimodality therapy. Nevertheless, surgery is not considered adequate primary treatment in advanced disease and immunochemotherapy is no longer regarded as adjuvant, according to the concept that both types of therapy should be practised almost simultaneously to prolong the survival of gastric cancer patients. Immunochemotherapy is an important systemic therapeutic means to cure cancer patients. I have therefore proposed the use of the new terminology 'immunochemosurgery' rather than surgery and adjuvant chemotherapy.

Gastric carcinoma can, I believe, be cured with active immunochemosurgery in the near future. To reach that goal, further prospective, randomized, controlled, clinical studies of immunochemosurgery should be continued. Measures for local control such as intra-operative radiation therapy and intraperitoneal chemotherapy should be considered because local failure and intraperitoneal seedlings are the major causes of treatment failure.

Conclusions

1. Immunochemosurgery is the best multi-modality treatment for advanced gastric cancer. For success, surgery must encompass curative radical surgery including skeletonization of regional lymph nodes.

2. In order to kill micrometastasis and small numbers of remaining cancer cells, post-operative immunochemotherapy should be commenced in the early post-operative period. It is preferable to start immunotherapy from the fourth or fifth and chemotherapy from the eight to tenth post-operative day.

3. Post-operative immunotherapy may revive the depressed immunity of the patient with advanced cancer and may alleviate the adverse effects of post-operative chemotherapy.

References

Alberts, D.S. (1977). Adjuvant immunotherapy with BCG of advanced ovarian cancer: a preliminary report. In *Proceedings of the International Conference on the Adjuvant Therapy of Cancer* (ed. S.E. Jones), pp. 327–34. Amsterdam.

Bitran, J.D., Desser, R.K., Kozloff, J.F., Billings, A.A., and Shapero, C.M. (1979). Treatment of metastatic pancreatic and gastric adenocarcinoma with fluorouracil, adriamycin, and mitomycin-C (FAM). *Cancer Treat. Rep.* **63**, 2049.

Blake, J.R.S., Hardcastle, J.D., and Wilson, R.G. (1981). Gastric cancer: a controlled trial and adjuvant chemotherapy following gastrectomy. *Clin. Oncol.* **71**, 13.

Gastrointestinal Tumor Study Group (1979). Phase II–III chemotherapy study in advanced gastric cancer. *Cancer Treat. Rep.* **63**, 1871.

Gastrointestinal Tumor Study Group (1982*a*). Controlled trial of adjuvant chemotherapy following curative resection of gastric cancer. *Cancer* **49**, 1116.

Gastrointestinal Tumor Study Group (1982*b*). A comparative clinical assessment of combination chemotherapy in the management of advanced gastric carcinoma. *Cancer* **49**, 1362.

Gunduz, N., Fisher, B., and Staffer, E.A. (1979). Effect of surgical removal on the growth and kinetics of residual tumors. *Cancer Res.* **39**, 3861.

Gutterman, J.U., Mavligit, G.M., Blumenshein, G., Burgess, M.A., McBride, C.M., and Hersh, Z.M. (1976*a*). Immunotherapy of human solid tumors with BCG: prolongation of disease free interval and survival in malignant melanoma, breast and colorectal cancer. *Ann. N.Y. Acad. Sci.* **277**, 135.

Gutterman, J.U., Cardenas, J.O., Blumenschein, G.R., Hortobagyi, G., Burgess, M.A., Livingston, R.B., Mavligit, G.H., Freireich, E.J., Gottlieb, J.A., and Hersh, E.M. (1976*b*). Chemoimmunotherapy of advanced breast cancer: prolongation of remission and survival with BCG. *Br. Med. J.* **2**, 1222.

Hoerni, B., Chauvergne, J., and Hoerni, S.G. (1977). BCG in the immunotherapy of malignant lymphomas. Current results of a controlled trial. *Cancer Immunol. Immunother.* **3**, 57.

Holland, J.F., Bekesi, J.G., Cuttner, J., and Glidewell, O. (1977). Chemoimmunotherapy in acute myelocytic leukemia. *Isr. J. Med. Sci.* **13**, 694.

Kim, J.P. and Choi, W.J. (1986). A study on histologic type of gastric carcinoma: analysis of clinico pathologic characterization and its implication as a prognostic factor. *Journal of the Korean Cancer Research Association* **18**, 194.

Kim, J.P. and Jung, S.E. (1986). Staging patients with gastric cancer and their prognosis. *Journal of the Korean Cancer Research Association* **18**, 9.

Kim, J.P. and Park, J.G. (1983). The end-results of surgical treatment of gastric cancer. *Journal of the Korean Medical Association* **26**, 637.

Kim, J.P. and Yoo, I.H. (1978). Relationship between the advance of stomach cancer and the change in immunity. *Journal of the Korean Surgical Society* **20**, 195.

Lauren, P. (1965). The two histological main types of gastric carcinoma; diffuse and so-called intestinal type carcinoma. An attempt at a histoclinical classification. *Acta Pathol. Microbiol. Scand.* **64**, 31.

Livstone, E.M. and Stablein, D.M. (1981). Adjuvant chemotherapy with 5-FU and methyl CCNU prolongs recurrence free interval and survival following curative resection for gastric adenocarcinoma. *Gastroenterology* **80**, 1215.

MacDonald, J.S., Schein, P.S., Woolley, P.V., Smythe, T., Ueno, W., Hoth, D., Smith F., Boiron, M., Gisselbrecht, C., Brunet, R., and Lagarde, D. (1980). 5-Fluorouracil, doxorubicin, and mitomycin (FAM) combination chemotherapy for advanced gastric cancer. *Ann. Intern. Med.* **93**, 533.

Makowka, J., Falk, R.E., Ambus, U., Bugala, R., and Landi, S. (1980). Adjuvant chemoimmunotherapy for gastric carcinoma. *Can. J. Surg.* **23**, 429.

Mathe, G., Amiel, J.L., Schwarzenberg, L., Schneidor, M., Cattan, A., Schlumberger, J.R., Hayat, M., and de Vassal, F. (1969). Active immunotherapy for acute lymphoblastic leukemia. *Lancet* **i**, 697.

McElwain, T.J., Russell, J., Lister, T.A., Whitehouse, J.M.A., Wrigley, P.F.M., Pike, M., Alexander, P., and Hamilton Fairly, G. (1973). Immunotherapy for acute myelogenous leukemia. *Br. J. Cancer* **28**, 365.

Moertel, C.G., Mittelman, J.A., Bakemeier, R.F., Engstrom, P., and Hanley, J. (1976). Sequential and combination chemotherapy of advanced gastric cancer. *Cancer* **38**, 678.

Morton, D.L., Eilber, F.R., Malmgren, R.A., and Wood, W.C. (1970). Immunological factors which influence the response to immunotherapy in malignant melanoma. *Surgery* **68**, 158.

Morton, D.L., Malmgren, R.A., Holmes, E.C., and Ketcham, A.S. (1968). Demonstration of antibodies against malignant melanoma by immunofluorescence. *Surgery* **64**, 233.

Necheles, T.F. (1976). MER/BCG in the treatment of disseminated neuroblastoma. *Proc. Am. Soc. Clin. Oncol.* **17(c-86)**, 258.

Nissen-Meyer, R., Kjellgren, K., Malmio, K., Mansson, B., and Norin, T. (1978). Surgical adjuvant chemotherapy: results with one short course with cyclophosphamide after mastectomy for breast cancer. *Cancer* **41**, 2088.

Okudaira, Y., Sugimachi, K., Inokuchi, K., Kari, H., Kuwano, H., and Matsuura, H. (1982). Postoperative long-term immunochemotherapy for esophageal carcinoma. *Jpn. J. Surg.* **12**, 249.

Ota, K., Kurita, S., Nishimura, M., Ogawa, N., Kanei, Y., Imai, K., Ariyoshi, Y., Kataoka, K., Murakami, N., Oyana, A., Hoshino, A., Ano, H., and Kato, T. (1972). Combination therapy with mitomycin-C, 5-fluorouracil and cytosine arabinoside for advanced cancer in man. *Cancer Chemother. Rep.* **56**, 373.

Pouillart, P., Palangie, T., Schwarzenburg, L., Brugerie, H., Lheritier, J., and Mathe, G. (1975). Effect of BCG on hematopoietic stem cells. *Biomedicine* **23**, 469.

Richman, S.P., Livingston, R.B., Gutterman, J.U., Suen, J.Y., and Hersh, E.M. (1976). Chemotherapy versus chemoimmunotherapy of head and neck cancer: report of a randomized study. *Cancer Treat. Rep.* **60**, 353.

Rodriguez, V., Bodey, G.P., Freireich, E.J., McCredie, K.B., Gutterman, J.U., Keating, M.J., Smith T.L., and Gehan, E.A. (1978). Randomized trial of protected environment prophylactic antibodies in 145 adults with acute leukemia. *Medicine* **57**, 253.

Rosenberg, S.A. (1985). Lymphokine-activated killer cells: a new approach to immunotherapy of cancer. *J. Nat. Cancer Inst.* **7**, 595.

Serlin, O., Keehn, R.J., Higgins, G.A., Jr., Harrower, H.W., and Mendeloff, G.L. (1977). Factors related to survival following resection for gastric carcinoma. Analysis of 903 cases. *Cancer* **40**, 1318.

Suga, S., Tsunekawa, H., and Washino, M. (1977). Treatment of gastric cancer, with special reference to the survivals of the cancer patients treated with multiple combination MFC therapy or immunochemotherapy MFC plus OK-432(NSC B116209). *Gastroenterol. Jpn.* **12**, 20.

Wanebo, H.J., Hilal, E.Y., Pinsky, C.M., Strong, E.W., Mike, V., Hirshaut, Y., and Oettgen, H.F. (1978). Randomized trial of levamisole in patients with squamous cancer of the head and neck: a preliminary report. *Cancer Treat. Rep.* **62**, 1663.

13. Portal hypertension and oesophageal varices

Naofumi Nagasue

Following the introduction of a portacaval shunt in 1945 for the treatment of bleeding oesophageal varices (Blakemore and Lod 1945, Whipple 1945), this fatal complication of portal hypertension has become a potentially curable condition. Since then the pathophysiology of portal hypertension has been gradually elucidated and various further types of operation proposed. Pharmacological prophylaxis against variceal haemorrhage has also been advocated by some investigators. Studies of portal hypertension were initiated in the West, with Asian countries subsequently following this lead. Different approaches to management and concepts of the disease have appeared in western and Asian countries, particularly Japan, largely because the aetiological background of the condition differs between East and West. In this chapter Asian perspectives are reviewed, focusing on the treatment of oesophageal varices in particular.

Aetiological background

Around the world the most common cause of portal hypertension is cirrhosis of the liver. However, the aetiology of cirrhosis is mainly alcoholic in western countries, whereas post-hepatitis or cryptogenic cirrhosis is common in Asia. The incidence of alcoholic cirrhosis was between 10 and 20 per cent in the past (Sugiura and Futagawa 1984*a* and *b*.) but it is apparently increasing in Japan (Ohnishi, *et al.* 1982) and also in India (Sarin, Malhotra, Nayyar, Sundaram, and Broor 1988). Idiopathic portal hypertension is the second commonest cause of portal hypertension but the incidence of this disease is decreasing year by year in Japan (Okuda 1983). Idiopathic portal hypertension in Japan is probably identical to non-cirrhotic portal fibrosis in India, which is relatively prevalent in that area (Sama, *et al.* 1971). The frequency of this disorder may be related to standards of hygiene although its precise natural history is still unknown (Okuda, *et al.* 1984). Recently, Sugita, Ohnishi, Iida, Nomura, and Okuda (1988) succeeded in producing very similar lesions to those of idiopathic portal hypertension in dogs by repeated intraportal injections of killed *Escherichia coli*. Pre-hepatic portal obstruction, which is the main cause of portal hypertension in children, is probably due to peri-natal omphalitis in most cases. The relationship of idiopathic portal hypertension to extra-hepatic portal obstruction, however, remains to be elucidated.

The Budd–Chiari syndrome in western countries is largely due to thrombotic occlusion of the hepatic veins. In contrast, most patients with this syndrome in Japan (Yamamoto, Yokoyama, Takeshige, and Iwatsuki, 1968; Kimura, Matsuda, Koie, and Hirooka 1972; Ono, Sakoda, and Kawada 1983) and India (Khuroo and Datta 1980; Victor, Jayanthi, Kandasamy, Ratnasabathy, and Madanagopalan 1986) have occlusion of the inferior vena cava at the diaphragmatic level, with or without obstruction of the hepatic veins. This discrepancy between findings in patients in the West and East can be attributed of differing aetiologies. Most cases in the West are attributable to oral contraceptive ingestion, abdominal trauma, or coagulation disorders such as polycythaemia, myeloproliferative disease, paroxysmal nocturnal haemoglobinuria, and so forth. Hepatic veno-occlusive disease due to ingestion of toxic alkaloids has been reported from India (Datta, Khuroo, Mattocks, Aikat, and Chhuttani 1978) and Hong Kong (Kumana, Lin, Ko, Wu, and Todd 1985). The cause of membranous obstruction of the supra-hepatic inferior vena cava, which is common in Japan, India, and Africa, may be of congenital or acquired thrombotic origin. Because primary biliary cirrhosis is rather rare in Asian countries, it was rarely documented as the cause of portal hypertension in our series (Nagasue, *et al.* 1989).

Natural history

The natural history and prognosis of patients with portal hypertension is dependent upon the aetiology and complications. The prognosis of cirrhotic patients is apparently poorer than that of the patients with idiopathic portal hypertension or pre-hepatic portal obstruction, in whom liver function is normal or only slightly disturbed. In those with the acute type of the Budd–Chiari syndrome, hepatic function rapidly deteriorates and many patients die within 1 or 2 years. Marked ascites, overt jaundice, and variceal bleeding are usually ominous signs for those with portal hypertension.

Tanaka, Itoshima, and Nagashima (1987) have followed 582 Japanese patients with liver cirrhosis for 26 years and documented that 59 per cent had died. The causes of death were hepatocellular carcinoma (44 per cent), liver failure (30 per cent), bleeding from oesophageal varices (14 per cent), and non-hepatic causes (8 per cent). Inokuchi, *et al.* (1984*b*) followed up 52 cirrhotic patients with demonstrated oesophageal varices and observed cumulative bleeding rates of 16.8 per cent at 1 year and 31.6 per cent at 2 years. These observations are almost identical to those recorded in the West (Garceau, Chalmers, and the Bile Study Group 1963; Jackson, *et al.* 1968; Conn, Lindenmuth, May, and Ramsby 1972).

The long-term prognosis for patients who have bled from varices is dismal without treatment (Garceau *et al.* 1963; Powell and Klatskin 1968). According to Graham and Smith (1981) the mortality rate of medically treated patients was 42 per cent at 6 weeks, one-third of patients with haemorrhage rebled within 6 weeks, and only one-third of the patients survived 1 year after their first bleed. This sort of study has been rarely reported from Eastern countries.

Diagnosis and pathophysiology

Many clinical studies of the aetiology of upper gastrointestinal bleeding in patients with cirrhosis of portal hypertension have been reported in the West, particularly in the US (Dagradi, Mehler, Tan, and Stempieu 1970; Buset, Des Marez, Baize, Bourgeois, and Cremer 1987). Most reports stress the frequency of erosive lesions in the upper gastrointestinal tract of patients with varices which bleed. Dagradi and colleagues (1970), in a series of 121 patients, reported a variceal source in 27 per cent, erosive gastritis in 31 per cent, Mallory–Weiss syndrome in 11 per cent, and chronic peptic ulceration in 8 per cent. Hislop, Hall, and Grant (1976) also emphasized the significance of erosive lesions in Australian patients. Such erosive lesions in the stomach, recently described as 'congestive gastropathy', are most effectively treated by shunt surgery (Hosking, Kennedy, Seddon, and Triger 1987). The most accurate diagnostic procedure for the identification of oesophageal varices is an endoscopic examination, using fibre-optic instruments. Endoscopy also identifies other common sources of bleeding such as oesophagitis, peptic ulcer, erosive lesions, and the Mallory–Weiss syndrome.

In 1980, the Japanese Research Society for Portal Hypertension proposed a new endoscopic record system for oesophageal varices. Using this classification, Beppu, *et al.* (1981) found that the risk of bleeding was related to the size and extent of varices and the presence of red colour signs such as red wale markings, cherry-red spot, haematocystic spot, or diffuse redness. They also showed that blue varices are more likely to bleed when compared with white varices. The society have recently modified these criteria and proposed that expanded glossy blue varices are more related to bleeding (Koyanagi and the Co-operative Study Group 1988). The validity of the Japanese criteria was confirmed in 1987 by the Italian Liver Cirrhosis Project.

A systemic hyperkinetic state in cirrhosis is well known although its cause is not clearly elucidated. Several humoral factors such as glucagon, bile acids, endotoxin, or prostaglandins may be involved in the phenomenon. One explanation for the hyperdynamic circulation is that arterio-venous shunts open in various organs, the extent of which may increase according to the extent of hepatic dysfunction (Murray, Dawson, and Sherlock 1958;

Siegel, *et al.* 1974). Harada, Nonami, Kasai, Nakao and Takagi (1988) recently reported, however, that patients with pre-hepatic portal obstruction and idiopathic portal hypertension, who had no or minimal liver impairment, had increased cardiac output and decreased peripheral resistance compared with controls. They attributed this to increased plasma volume which may be due to an expanded portal bed volume.

The major blood supply to oesophageal varices is the left gastric vein, with the short gastric veins being more dominant in patients with gastric varices. Spontaneous spleno- or gastro-renal shunts are not infrequently seen in those with gastric varices (Ohnishi, *et al.* 1986). Detailed haemodynamic studies of the oesophago-gastric region show that a significant hyperdynamic circulation exists in this area, which may be secondarily related to exacerbation and rupture of varices (Koyanagi, Inokuchi, Nakayama, Sakata, and Beppu 1981). The present author has found such a phenomenon in 30 per cent of variceal patients by means of intra-operative direct splenoportography (Fig. 13.1). The pathophysiology, particularly of haemodynamics in the oesophage-gastro-splenic area is variable, and appropriate therapy must be offered on an individual basis.

Emergency treatment of variceal bleeding

Conventional therapy with intravenous administration of Pitressin® (antidiuretic hormone) and the Sengstaken–Blakemore tube is widely used and probably the first choice for acute variceal bleeding. Trans-hepatic obliteration of the coronary and short gastric veins, first attempted by Lunderquist and Vang (1974), produces only a temporary effect and is dangerous when performed for patients in whom the flow of the coronary vein is hepatopetal. Many institutions have adopted the use of endoscopic sclerotherapy for acute variceal bleeding. Sarin, Nanda, Kumar, Vij, and Anand in India (1985) achieved successful haemostasis in 35 (92 per cent) of 38 such patients. In Japan, successful control of active variceal bleeding in 97 and 100 per cent of patients has been reported (Takase, Ozaki, Orii, Nagoshi, Okamura, and Iwasaki 1982; Kitano, Koyanagi, Iso, Higashi, and Sugimachi 1987*a*).

In all these studies, sclerotherapy was performed in the first instance. Many patients actually have haemostasis secured by medical means and are electively treated. In contrast, emergency surgery is usually performed for those in whom medical management has failed to stop bleeding. This implies that the security of bleeding and the risk of mortality are different between patients treated by sclerotherapy, as initial therapy, and those undergoing emergency operation. In Table 13.1 the results are shown of various emergency treatment methods in Asia. Very few reports of major portasystemic shunts are available in our region. Nine of thirty patients died

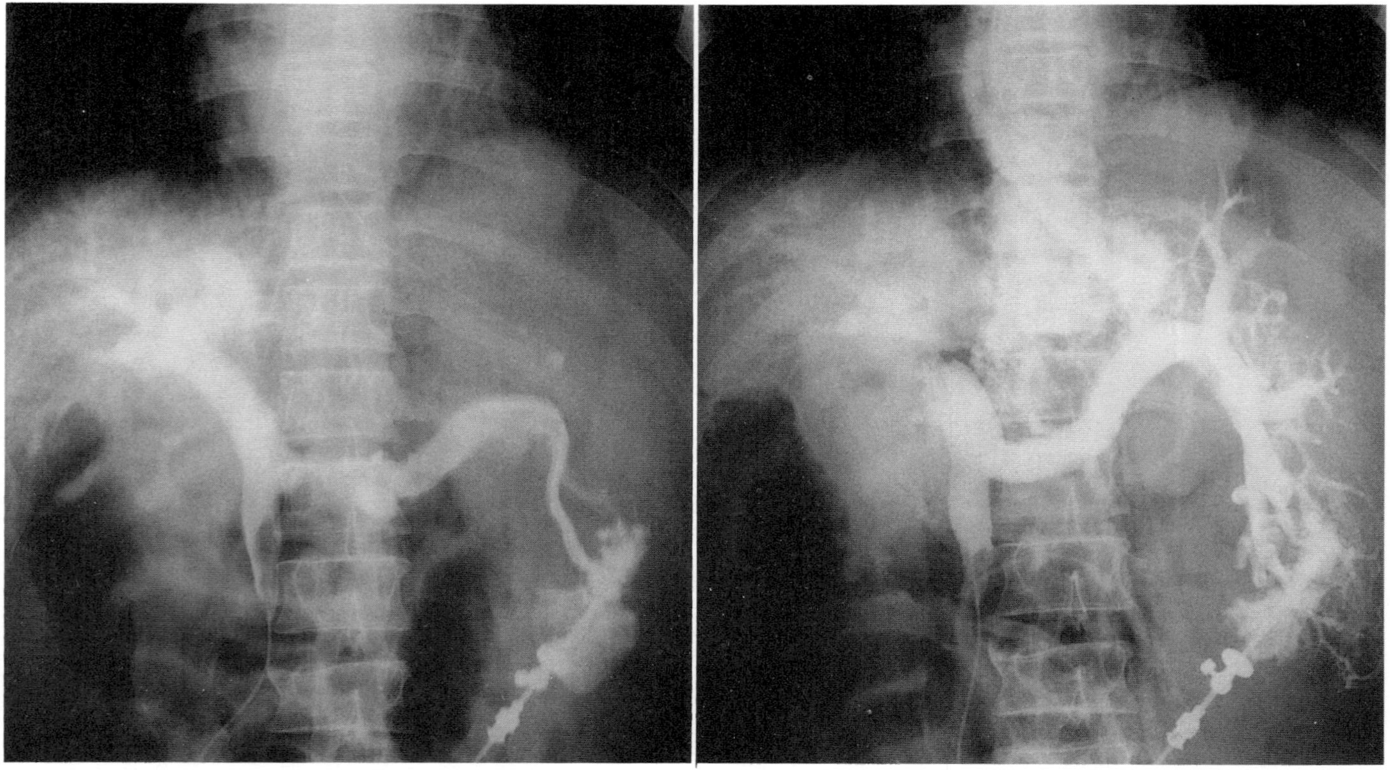

Fig. 13.1. Intra-operative direct splenoportography in a patient with large oesophageal varices. Collaterals towards the varices were visualized only with portal vein occlusion (right). This probably indicates that the blood flow of the coronary and short gastric veins is hepato-petal and a hyperdynamic state exists in the lower oesophagus and cardia.

Table 13.1. Results of emergency therapy for oesophageal variceal bleeding.

Reference	No. of patients	Child's class A	Child's class B	Child's class C	Method	Mortality rate (%)	Recurrent variceal bleeding (%)
Takase *et al*. (1982)	30				Sclerotherapy	10	8
Sarin *et al*. (1985)	38	8	9	21	Sclerotherapy	8	32
Kitano *et al*. (1987*a*)	40				Sclerotherapy	20	
Lam *et al*. (1977)	60	40	16	4	Trans-abdominal variceal ligation	40	74
Sugiura and Futagawa (1984*a*)	102	12	27	63	Sugiura's procedure	14	
Balasegaram and Damodaran (1970)	30				Portacaval shunt 27 Spleno-renal shunt 2 Mesocaval shunt 1	30	
Kuang *et al*. (1984)	7				Mesocaval shunt	0	0
Gibson *et al*. (1981)	9				Warren shunt	33	33
Nagasue *et al*. (1988*a*)	14	1	5	8	Warren shunt	21	0

post-operatively in the unselected series by Balasegaram and Damodaran (1970). Gibson, McInnes, Rosengarten, Jakobovits, Coventry, and Dudley (1981) reported three deaths after emergency distal spleno-renal shunt procedures; all had shunt thrombosis and subsequent variceal bleeding.

We have performed this operation on 14 patients, none of whom had recurrent variceal haemorrhage (Nagasue, Ogawa, Yukaya, Tamada, Chang, and Nakamura 1988*a*). Our limited experience has shown that variceal bleeding rarely occurs, as long as the shunt remains patent. Lam, Lam, Cheng, and Ong (1977) reported trans-abdominal trans-gastric variceal ligation with an operative mortality rate of 40 per cent. Thirty of sixty patients survived and 13 subsequently underwent elective spleno-renal shunt surgery. Five patients were lost to follow-up. Thus, of 16 patients followed up after variceal ligation, 14 had recurrent bleeding. The Sugiura procedure produced a very low mortality rate of 13.7 per cent in 102 emergency cases (Sugiura and Futagawa 1984*a*). Oesophageal transection using stapling instruments has the advantage that it is not technically demanding and can be accomplished expeditiously (Takasaki, Kobayashi, Muto, Suzuki, Harada, and Nakayama 1977). Immediate control of acute bleeding is usually satisfactory but the development of oesophageal strictures and later recurrent bleeding in 20–40 per cent of patients is problematic (Wexler 1980).

Elective management of oesophageal varices

Non-selective major shunts (Table 13.2)

The Tokyo University Group (Sugiura and Futagawa 1973) performed portacaval shunts in 78 elective cases between 1950 and 1964. Their operative mortality rate was 21 per cent and 44 per cent of surviving patients developed hepatic encephalopathy. Such poor results in Japan led us to abandon portacaval shunt, particularly in cirrhotic patients. Inokuchi, Kobayashi, and Ogawa (1971) proposed a controlled central spleno-renal shunt, in which the splenic vein was narrowed by sutures just above the anastomosis in the hope that too much portal blood would not be 'stolen' through the shunt. The results seemed to be superior to those with portacaval shunt, but selective shunts were later adopted.

Poor results with portacaval shunts in cirrhotic patients were published from India (Boyer, *et al.* 1967; Basu, *et al.* 1969). On the contrary, Chinese groups, including those in Taiwan, have had much better results (Hsu 1972; Chang 1981; Kuang, Chen, Jiang, Zhou, Sang, and Wu 1984; Sun, Zhang, and Wang 1984). Between 1960 and 1981, Sun and colleagues (1984) carried out a limited side-to-side portacaval shunt electively on 228 cirrhotic patients (163 Child's class A, 47 class B, and 18 class C). Their operative mortality rate was only 3.9 per cent. Rebleeding and encephalopathy rates were 11.4 and 19.8 per cent, respectively, and corresponding, 5- and 10-year survival

Table 13.2. Results of elective portosystemic shunts for oesophogeal varices.

Reference	No. of patients	Child's class or liver disease	Method of shunt	Operative mortality rate (%)	Recurrent bleeding (%)	Encephalopathy (%)	5-year survival rate (%)
Boyer *et al*. (1967)	72	LC 32	Portacaval	LC 25		LC 29	
		NCPF 21		NCPF 10		NCPF 13	
		PPO 19		PPO 16		PPO 42	
Basu *et al*. (1969)	84	LC 53	Portacaval	LC 25		LC 56	
		NCPF 31		NCPF 10		NCPF 29	
Inokuchi *et al*. (1971)	40	LC 23	Spleno-renal (controlled)	15	7	15	68
		IPH 11					
		PPO 6					
Hsu (1972)	48	A 30	Spleno-renal 24	10	7		63
		B 15	Portacaval 8				
		C 3	Mesocaval 17				
Sugiura and Futagawa (1973)	78		Portacaval	21		44	51
Chang (1981)	28		Mesocaval	0	0	4	
Sun *et al*. (1984)	228	A 163	Side-to-side portacaval	4	11	20	80
		B 47					
		C 18					
Kuang *et al*. (1984)	20	A 0	End-to-side mesocaval	0	15	0	
		B 17					
		C 3					

LC, liver cirrhosis; NCPF, non-cirrhotic portal fibrosis; PPO, pre-hepatic portal obstruction; IPH, idiopathic portal hypertension.

rates were 80 and 78 per cent. This survival rate is much higher than that expected from the natural history of cirrhosis. According to collective series in Japan, portacaval shunts gave an operative mortality rate of 21 per cent, variceal rebleeding rate of 7.6 per cent, and hepatic encephalopathy rate of 50 per cent (Inokuchi and the Japanese Research Society 1985).

When major portasystemic shunts were performed in idiopathic portal hypertension or non-cirrhotic portal fibrosis, the results were much better. The operative mortality rate was significantly lower than that in cirrhotics. Hepatic encephalopathy was less frequent and milder (Basu *et al.* 1969; Boyer *et al.* 1967) although subclinical encephalopathy was observed in one-third of the patients (Sarin and Nundy 1985). According to western experience, a side-to-side portacaval shunt may be indicated for patients with Budd–Chiari syndrome without caval obstruction (Orloff and Johansen 1978).

Selective shunts (Table 13.3)

Since the first report by Warren, Zeppa, and Fomon in 1967, distal spleno-renal shunt has been used in Asia. The original or modified Warren shunt produced operative death rates of 2.5–34.8 per cent (Gibson *et al.* 1981; Isomatsu 1983; Nagasue *et al.* 1989; Ashida, *et al.* in press). The shunt patency rate varied from 80 to 95.7 per cent. The incidence of recurrent variceal bleeding was usually less than 10 per cent. Hepatic encephalopathy occurred in 14.7 per cent in the author's series (Nagasue *et al.* 1989) and in 17.4 per cent in the report of Ashida and colleagues (in press). It has been well demonstrated that in western countries the result of distal spleno-renal shunt in alcoholic patients is significantly inferior to that in non-alcoholics. We have also confirmed this in Japanese patients (Nagasue *et al.* 1989). Guharay, Sain, Banerjee, Guha Majumdar, Sengupta, and Basu (1980) performed selective spleno-caval shunts in 10 children; eight with pre-hepatic portal obstruction and two with non-cirrhotic portal fibrosis. One child died from variceal bleeding secondary to shunt occlusion; encephalopathy was not seen in the nine surviving patients.

The problem of loss of selectively with time after the original Warren shunt (Isomatsu 1983; Gibson, McInnes, and Dudley 1986) has been challenged by several groups in Japan. Inokuchi and colleagues in 1984 (*a* and *b*), obtained better results in this context by avoiding pancreatic drainage. With a 4-year follow-up of the patients undergoing distal spleno-renal shunt with spleno-pancreatic disconnection, Henderson, Warren, Millikan, Galloway, Kawasaki, and Kutner (1989) recently reported that the disconnection could provide better portal perfusion and survival rates in alcoholic patients.

In Japan, two studies (Fig. 13.2) independently achieved similar results and have shown that spleno-pancreatic disconnection does not give rise to post-operative hepatic encephalopathy with higher long-term survival rates, compared with the original distal spleno-renal shunt procedure, although

Table 13.3. Results of elective selective shunts for oesophageal varices.

Reference	No. of patients	Child's class A	Child's class B	Child's class C	Method of shunt	Operative mortality rate (%)	Shunt patency (%)	Recurrent bleeding (%)	Encephalopathy (%)	5-year survival rate (%)
Gibson *et al.* (1981)	30*	10	11	9	DSRS	26.0	80.0	16.7		
Isomatsu (1983)	60				DSRS	6.7		8.9		54.4
Nagasue *et al.* (1989)	40	28	9	3	DSRS	2.5	94.1	0	14.7	55.2
Ashida *et al.* (in press)	69	12	25	32	DSRS	2.9	95.7	4.3	17.4	41.0
	43	10	15	18	DSRS + SPD	0	95.3	7.0	0	56.7
Katoh *et al.* (in press)	33	11	22	0	DSRS + SPD	0	100	3.0	0	88.0
Inokuchi *et al.* (1984*b*)	231				LGCS	2.2	86.8	7.4	0	69.8

* Nine emergency cases are included.

DSRS, distal spleno-renal shunt; SPD, spleno-pancreatic disconnection; LGCS, left gastric caval shunt.

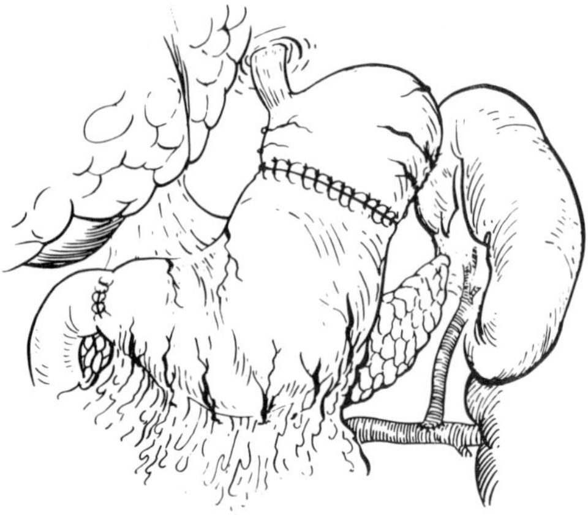

Fig. 13.2. Modification of distal spleno-renal shunt with spleno-pancreatic disconnection and gastric subserosal transection by Katoh, Shimozawa, Kojima, and Tanabe (1991).

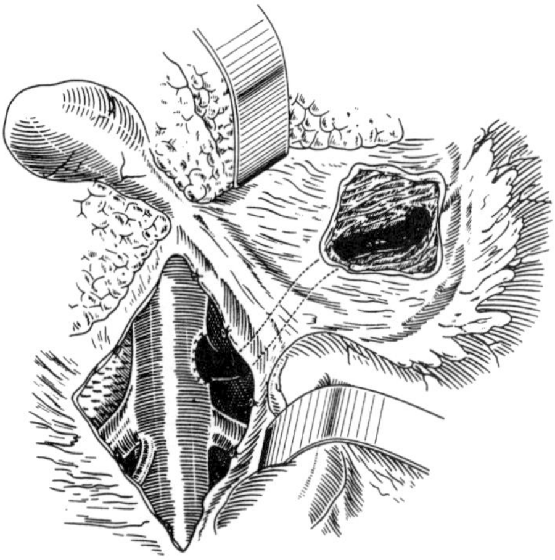

Fig. 13.3. Left gastric venous caval shunt by Inokuchi and his associates (1970).

neither study was randomized (Ashida *et al.* in press; Katoh, Shimozawa, Kojima, and Tanabe in press). Currently, it is believed that distal spleno-renal shunt with spleno-pancreatic disconnection will produce more satisfactory results when undertaken in selected patients.

The left gastric venous caval shunt devised by Inokuchi, Kobayashi, Kusaba, Ogawa, Saku, and Shiizaki (1970) is an alternative type of selective shunt procedure (Fig. 13.3), and they have subsequently performed this shunt operation in 231 patients, electively or prophylactically (Inokushi *et al.*

1984*b*). The operative mortality rate was 2.2 per cent, recurrent bleeding was seen in 7.4 per cent, and encephalopathy was not observed. The 5- and 10-year survival rates were 70 and 55 per cent, respectively. The Inokuchi shunt is the best operation theoretically but, unfortunately, it has not achieved wide popularity, probably because of technical difficulties encountered. The present author assumes that this operation does have a role and that it should be used for selected patients.

Devascularization procedures (Table 13.4)

Ligation of varices or oesophageal transection was first introduced by western surgeons to control acute bleeding (Boerema 1949; Crile 1950; Walker 1964). The high operative mortality rate and risk of recurrent bleeding led to gradual abandonment of this approach. In Japan the results of portacaval shunts were so poor that non-shunt operations became more popular and selective shunting was adopted by several groups. Oesophageal transection or oesophago-cardial resection, with or without splenectomy, is used in emergency and elective situations.

In 1973, Sugiura and Futagawa reported their experience with 87 patients treated by oesophageal transection with para-oesophago-gastric devascularization (Sugiura procedure) (Fig. 13.4). In 1984, they reported a large series of 671 patients; their operative mortality rate was 4.9 per cent and variceal bleeding occurred in only 1.5 per cent. The 5-year survival rate was 73 per cent for patients with cirrhosis and 97 per cent for those without (Sugiura and Futagawa 1984*b*). Hirashima, Sato, Takeuchi, Nakamuri, Hirota, and Hara (1981) obtained similar results with trans-abdominal oesophageal transection whereas poorer figures were presented by Koyama, Takagi, Ouchi, and Sato (1980), who performed almost the same operation as the Sugiura procedure.

Alternatively, Yamamoto, Hidemura, Sawada, Takeshige, and Iwatsuki (1976) had satisfactory results by trans-abdominal oesophago-cardial resection with splenectomy and extensive devascularization. It was reported from Hong Kong that trans-gastric suture of varices in emergency cases was undertaken with an operative mortality rate of 40 per cent, recurrent variceal bleeding being observed in 74 per cent of the survivors (Lam *et al.* 1977). Takasaki and his group (1977) used the EEA® stapler for oesophageal transection in 30 patients. Variceal bleeding recurred in 11.1 per cent during a relatively short follow-up period. Although this procedure is simple and easy to perform, it should probably be used only in an emergency or in poor-risk cases since recurrent bleeding occurs in 20–40 per cent.

Endoscopic sclerotherapy (Table 13.5)

The past decade has seen changes in basic concepts for treatment of oesophageal varices, largely brought about by a revival of interest in endoscopic sclerotherapy. Most endoscopists initially used a rigid oesophagoscope, as

Table 13.4. Results of devascularization operations for oesophageal varices.

Reference	No. of patients	Child's class or liver disease		Operative method	Operative mortality rate (%)	Recurrent bleeding (%)	5-year survival rate (%)	
Yamamoto *et al.* (1976)	112	Cirrhosis	79	Trans-abdominal cardiectomy with splenectomy	11.0	8.6	65	
		Non-cirrhosis	33					
Lam *et al.* (1977)	60*	A	40	Trans-abdominal suture of varices	40.0	74.0		
		B	16					
		C	4					
Takasaki *et al.* (1977)	30	Cirrhosis	26	Oesophageal transection with EEA stapler	10.0	11.1		
		IPH	3					
		PPO	1					
Koyama *et al.* (1980)	100	Cirrhosis	68	Trans-thoracic oesophageal transection	11.0	6.7	58	
		IPH	23					
		PPO	9					
Hirashima *et al.* (1981)	100	Cirrhosis	69	Trans-abdominal oesophageal transection	3.0	5.0	84	
		Non-cirrhosis	31					
Sugiura and Futagawa (1984*a* and *b*)	671	A	244	Sugiura's procedure	4.9	1.5	Cirrhosis	73
		B	251				Non-cirrhosis	97
		C	176					

IPH, idiopathic portal hypertension; PPO, pre-hepatic portal obstruction.
* Only emergency cases were included.

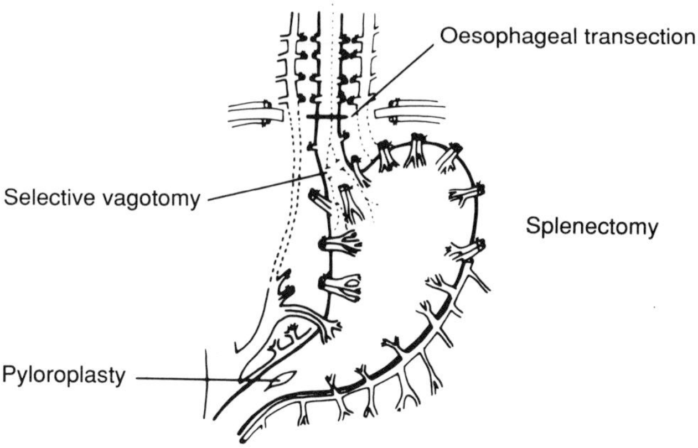

Fig. 13.4. The Sugiura procedure (Sugiura and Futagawa 1973).

originally described in 1939 by Crafoord and Frenckner. Recently, a fibre-optic endoscope seems to have been more widely used. Intravariceal injection of sclerosants is preferred by many groups. Para-variceal injection, predominantly advocated in Germany, is said to avoid interruption of portazygos collaterals, thereby preventing subsequent bleeding from gastric varices. As a sclerosant, 5 per cent ethanolamine oleate is the most popular agent in Japan (Takase *et al.* 1982; Kitano, Koyanagi, Iso, Higashi, and Sugimachi 1987*a*; Terabayashi, *et al.* 1987). According to the recent study by Kitano, *et al.* (1989) the addition of thrombin to 5 per cent ethanolamine oleate reduces the likelihood of immediate bleeding and helps expedite eradication of varices.

The same group devised a transparent over-tube through which a fibre-optic scope could be passed (Kitano and Sugimachi 1987) and which allows the oesophageal varix to protrude into the lumen through the slit of the tube. The protruded varix can be sclerosed easily and safely under direct vision. (Fig. 13.5). This technique is reported to be superior to usual methods (Kitano, Koyanagi, Iso, Iwanaga, Higushi, and Sugimachi 1987*b*). Terabayashi and colleagues (1987) recently conducted a randomized study of sclerotherapy and percutaneous transhepatic obliteration of oesophageal varices in elective patients only. In the sclerotherapy group, recurrent bleeding occurred in 9 per cent and their 3-year survival rate was 77 per cent. Sarin, Sachder, and Nanda of India, in 1986, followed up 101 patients after complete eradication of varices by intravariceal ethanol injections. Their early mortality rate was 10.9 per cent, oesophageal varices reappeared in 18.8 per cent and rebleeding was found in 2.9 per cent. The frequency of oesophageal stricture varied from 5.8 per cent (Kitano and Sugimachi 1987), to 14.9 per cent (Sarin *et al.* 1986) and 27 per cent (Terabayashi *et al.* 1987). These variations could be due to the differences in sclerosant, the volume

Table 13.5. Results of endoscopic sclerotherapy for oesophageal varices.

Reference	No. of patients	Mode of treatment		Method	Child's grade		Early mortality rate (%)	Recurrent bleeding (%)	Oesophageal structure (%)
Takase *et al.* (1982)	68	Emergency	30	Intravariceal				3.0	
		Elective	38	5 per cent ethanolamine oleate					
Sarin *et al.* (1986)	101	All elective*		Intravariceal	A	54	10.9	2.9	14.9
				Pure ethanol	B	16			
					C	31			
Kitano *et al.* (1987*a*)	155	Emergency	40						
		Elective	49	Intravariceal	A	17	5.2	4.9	5.8
		Prophylactic	66	5 per cent ethanolamine oleate	B	76			
					C	62			
Terabayashi *et al.* (1987)	33	All elective		5 per cent ethanolomine oleate	A	11	3.0	18.0	27.0
					B	15			
					C	7			

* Study was initiated after complete eradication of oesophageal varices.

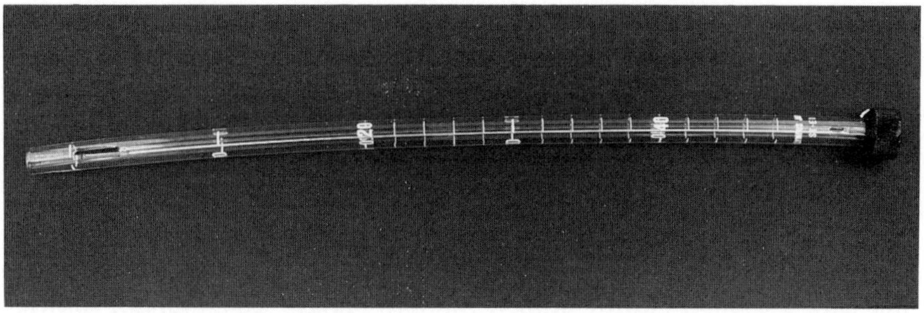

Fig. 13.5. Transparent over-tube for endoscopic injection sclerotherapy by Kitano and Sugimachi (1987).

injected, or the injection method and interval between injections. A schedule of weekly sclerosis is recommended (Dilawari, Raju, and Chawla 1989), or is routinely employed by many authors (Takase *et al.* 1982; Kitano *et al.* 1987*a*; Terabayashi *et al.* 1987). Sarin and associates (1986) observed an improvement of Child's grade, particularly in patients with cirrhosis, following sclerotherapy. In addition, the development of spontaneous portasystemic shunts has been reported to occur after the sclerotherapy (Dilawari *et al.* 1989). There is no single definitive treatment method for oesophageal varices and it is, perhaps, wise not to insist on a single approach. In 1989, Burroughs, Hamilton, Phillips, Mezzanotte, McIntyre, and Hobbs concluded from a well-conducted, randomized study that surgical treatment is recommended after two injection treatments have failed.

Budd–Chiari syndrome

The Budd–Chiari syndrome is a disorder caused by occlusion of the major hepatic veins and/or the inferior vena cava around the hepatic vein roots. This syndrome is a rare cause of portal hypertension in the western hemisphere but relatively common in Japan (Kimura *et al.* 1972; Ono *et al.* 1983; Yamamoto *et al.* 1986) and India (Datta *et al.* 1978; Khuroo and Datta 1980; Victor *et al.* 1986). The Budd–Chiari syndrome seen in our locality is mostly due to membranous obstruction of the inferior vena cava. Therapy for this condition varies whether or not the inferior cava is simultaneously obstructed.

When only the hepatic veins are occluded, side-to-side portacaval shunt is the most reliable operation, as shown by Orloff and Johansen (1978). For those with obstruction of both the hepatic veins and inferior vena cava, Cameron, *et al* (1983) recommended meso-atrial shunt with Dacron® grafts. This operation was carried out in three patients by Khanduri, *et al.* (1983) in India but only one patient survived. Late thrombosis of the graft seems to be a major problem in this operation. If the inferior vena cava is obstructed above the hepatic vein ostia and all or part of the hepatic veins are patent below the caval occlusion, retrohepatic cavo-atrial shunt can decompress both the portal system and inferior vena cava (Victor *et al.* 1986; Nagasue, Ogawa, Yukaya, Chang, and Kaneko 1987).

The present author used a stented Gortex® graft with excellent results (Nagasue *et al.* 1987) (Fig. 13.6). In the treatment of complete obstruction of both the hepatic veins and inferior vena cava, we believe that the combination of a side-to-side portacaval shunt and a retrohepatic cavo-atrial shunt with a stented Gortex graft is the best choice. Membranous obstruction of the inferior vena cava can be treated by transatrial membranotomy. In 1972, Kimura and his associates treated eight such patients by this method with a successful outcome in five patients. Akita and Sakoda (1980) treated 19 patients by splenoneumopexy, 10 of whom survived. Percutaneous transluminal angioplasty has been attempted by several Japanese groups (Eguchi, Takeuchi, and Asano 1974; Yamada, Sato, Kawadata, Nakatsuka, and Kobayashi 1983). The procedure was successful in most of their patients but the efficacy of this method is difficult to evaluate because of the short periods of follow-up.

Is prophylactic surgical treatment valid?

The ultimate aim of prophylactic therapy for oesophageal varices should be not only to improve survival by preventing the first variceal haemorrhage, but also to secure an acceptable quality of life. In this sense, portacaval shunt was shown to be beneficial (Jackson *et al.* 1968; Resnick, *et al.* 1969; Conn *et al.* 1972). Abrupt diversion of portal blood can, however, produce an unacceptably high incidence of hepatic encephalopathy and subsequent liver failure.

To date, there have been only a few randomized studies on prophylactic surgical treatment therapy other than the portacaval shunt. Inokuchi and colleagues (1984*a* and *b*) randomized Child's class A and B patients with oesophageal varices considered to be of risk, as judged by the Japanese endoscopic criteria (Japanese Research Society 1980), into two different groups; various surgical procedures which did not decompress portal pressure were compared with non-surgical therapy. The cumulative bleeding rate in the control group at 2 years was 31.6 per cent, whereas that in the surgical group was nil. Their interim results showed no difference in survival at 2 years and the final results of this study are awaited with interest. There are several prospective controlled studies of prophylactic endoscopic sclerotherapy (Paquet 1982; Witzel, Wolbergs, and Merki 1985; Koch, Henning, Grimm, and Soehendra 1987), all of which endorse the efficacy of this treatment modality when compared with medical therapy. Longer follow-up periods are, however, necessary. We have shown that distal spleno-renal

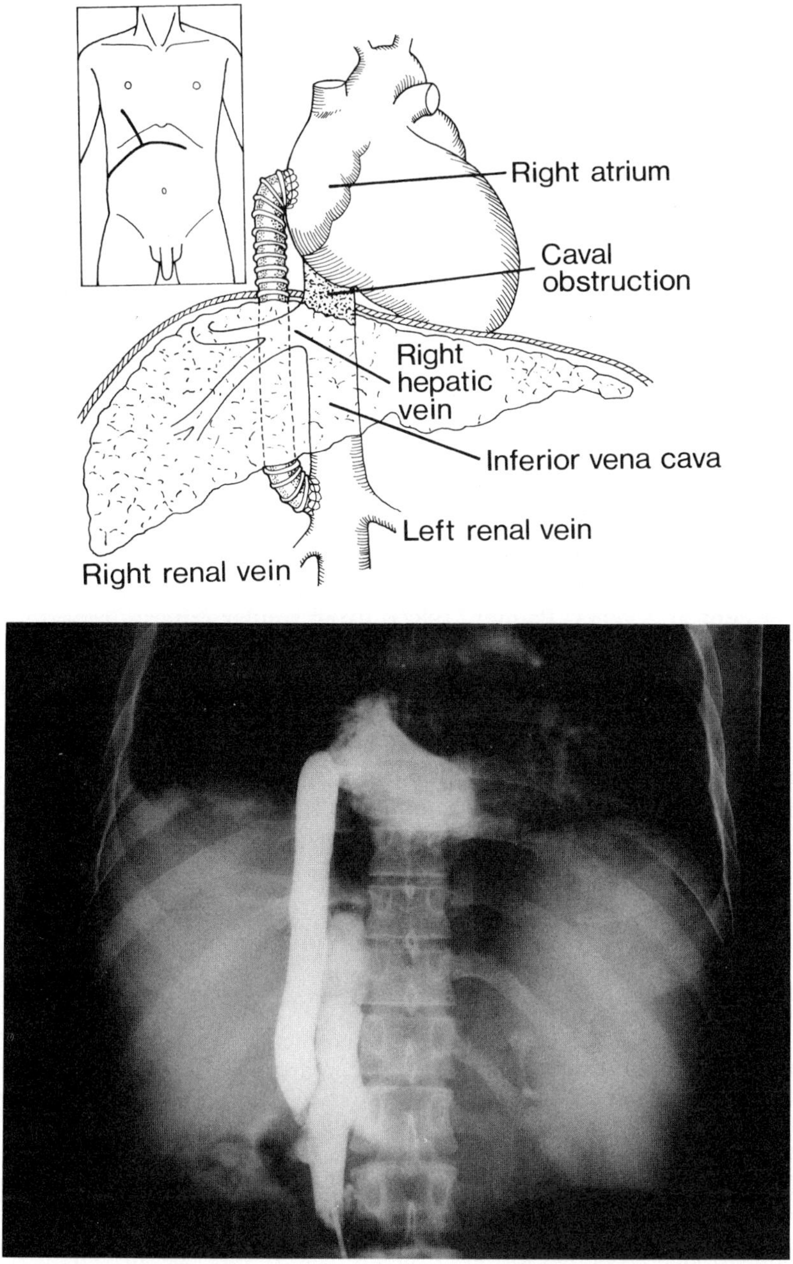

Fig. 13.6. Retrohepatic cavo-atrial shunt with externally stented Gortex graft in a patient with caval obstruction but with a patent right hepatic vein (Nagasue *et al.* 1987). The cavogram (bottom) was taken 3 weeks after operation.

shunt can produce a satisfactory result in selected patients (Nagasue, *et al.* 1988*b*).

In performing prophylactic therapy for oesophageal varices, several important questions remain unanswered. Which criteria should be used to select patients with oesophageal varices for prophylactic therapy? What findings or factors indicate the risk of haemorrhage? Burroughs, d'Heygere, and McIntyre (1986), in their excellent review, raise four items probably related to bleeding: portal and intravariceal pressure, endoscopic appearances of varices, alcohol abuse, and hepatic decompensation. Although the relationship between portal pressure and bleeding has been denied (Lebrec, de Fleury, Rueff, Nahum, and Benhamou 1980), we assume that portal pressure is one of the important factors since, in our series, the mean pressure was 34.7 cm H_2O in patients having prophylactic treatment in elective cases, and 39.9 cm H_2O in patients subjected to emergency intervention (Nagasue *et al.* 1989).

As to the size of varices, there seems to be general agreement that large varices are more liable to bleed. What of the endoscopic criteria we use in Japan? According to the study of Inokuchi and colleagues (1984*b*) the cumulative bleeding rate of the control patients with high-risk varices was 31.6 per cent at 2 years. Paquet (1982), using similar criteria, reported that 66.7 per cent of the control patients bled within 2 years. This difference can probably by explained by the fact that Japanese patients were predominantly non-alcoholics. At present, our own opinion is that the presence of 'red colour signs' may be related to variceal bleeding. As Child's class C usually implies terminal liver disease, major operations for such patients are best avoided. Thus, it is assumed that candidates for prophylactic operations are Child's class A or B patients with marked portal hypertension, large varices, and/or varices with 'red colour signs'. The most effective method for prophylaxis requires further elucidation.

References

Akita, H. and Sakoda, K. (1980). Portopulmonary shunt by splenopneumopexy as a surgical treatment of Budd–Chiari syndrome. *Surgery* **87**, 85–94.

Ashida, H., Utsunomiya, J., Kotoura, Y., *et al.* (1991). Results of distal splenorenal shunt with vs. without splenopancreatic disconnection. *J. Clin. Gastroenterol.* (in press).

Balasegaram, M. and Damodaran, A. (1970). Emergency shunt surgery for bleeding oesophagogastric varices. *Aust. N.Z. J. Surg.* **40**, 152–7.

Basu, A.K., Basu Mallik, K.C., Sengupta, K.P., *et al.* (1969). Long-term follow-up of 'non-cirrhotic portal fibrosis' after surgery. *Br. J. Surg.* **56**, 497–503.

Beppu, K., Inokuchi, K., Koyanagi, N., *et al.* Prediction of variceal hemorrhage by esophageal endoscopy. *Gastrointest. Endosc.* **27**, 213–18.

Blakemore, A.H. and Lod, J.W. Jr. (1945). The technique of using vitalium tubes in establishing portacaval shunts for portal hypertension. *Ann. Surg.* **122**, 476–89.

Boerema, I. (1949). Bleeding varices of the esophagus in cirrhosis of the liver and Banti's disease. *Arch. Chir. Neer-land* **1**, 253–60.

Boyer, J.L., Gupta, K.P.S., Biswas, S.K., *et al.* (1967). Idiopathic portal hypertension: comparison with the portal hypertension of cirrhosis and extrahepatic portal vein obstruction. *Ann. Intern. Med.* **66**, 41–68.

Burroughs, A.K., d'Heygere, F., and McIntyre, N. (1986). Pitfalls in studies of prophylactic therapy for variceal bleeding in cirrhotics. *Hepatology* **6**, 1407–13.

Burroughs, A.K., Hamilton, G., Phillips, A., Mezzanotte, G., McIntyre, N., and Hobbs, K.E.F. (1989). A comparison of sclerotherapy with staple transection of the esophagus for the emergency control of bleeding from esophageal varices. *N. Eng. J. Med.* **321**, 857–62.

Buset, M., des Marez, B., Baize, M., Bourgeois, N., and Cremer, M. (1987). Bleeding esophagogastric varices. An endoscopic study. *Am. J. Gastroenterol.* **82**, 241–4.

Cameron, J.L., Herlong, H.F., Sanfey, H., *et al.* (1983). The Budd–Chiari syndrome. Treatment by mesentric–systemic venous shunts. *Ann. Surg.* **198**, 335–46.

Chang, W.H. (1981). Side-to-side mesocaval anastomosis in portal hypertension. *Surg. Gynecol. Obstet.* **152**, 511–12.

Conn, H.O., Lindenmuth, W.W., May, C.J., and Ramsby, G.R. (1972). Prophylactic portacaval anastomosis. A tale of two studies. *Medicine (Baltimore)* **51**, 27–40.

Crafoord, C. and Frenckner, P. (1939). New surgical treatment of varicose veins of the oesophagus. *Acta. Otolaryngol.* **27**, 422–9.

Crile, G.S. (1950). Transesophageal ligation of bleeding oesophageal varices: a preliminary report of seven cases. *Arch. Surg.* **61**, 654–60.

Dagradi, A.E., Mehler, R., Tan, D.T., and Stempien, S.J. (1970). Sources of upper gastrointestinal bleeding in patients with liver cirrhosis and large esophagogastric varices. *Am. J. Gastroenterol.* **54**, 458–63.

Datta, D.V., Khuroo, M.S., Mattock, A.R., Aikat, B.K., and Chhuttani, P.N. (1978). Herbal medicines and veno-occlusive disease in India. *Postgrad. Med. J.* **54**, 511–15.

Dilawari, J.B., Raju, G.S., and Chawla, Y.K. (1989). Development of large splenoadreno-renal shunt after endoscopic sclerotherapy. *Gastroenterology* **97**, 421–6.

Eguchi, S., Takeuchi, Y., and Asano, K. (1974). Successful balloon membranotomy for obstruction of the hepatic portion of the inferior vena cava. *Surgery* **76**, 837–40.

Garceau, A.J., Chalmers, T.C., and the Bile Study Group (1963). The natural history of cirrhosis. I. Survival with esophageal varices. *N. Engl. J. Med.* **268**, 469–73.

Gibson, P.R., McInnes, I.E., and Dudley, F.J. (1986). The long-term effect of distal lienorenal shunt surgery on portal venous pressure. *Aust. N.Z. J. Surg.* **56**, 773–6.

Gibson, P.R., McInnes, I.E., Rosengarten, D.S., Jakobovits, A.W., Coventry, D.A., and Dudley, F.J. (1981). The distal lienorenal shunt: perioperative experience with 30 patients. *Aust. N.Z. J. Surg.* **51**, 336–40.

Graham, D.Y. and Smith, J.L. (1981). The course of patients after variceal hemorrhage. *Gastroenterology* **80**, 800–9.

Guharay, B.N., Sain, P., Banerjee, D., Guha Majumdar, D.N., Sengupta, K.P., and Basu, A.K. (1980). Direct splenocaval shunt for selective decompression of portal hypertension in children. *Surgery* **87**, 271–9.

Harada, A., Nonami, T., Kasai, Y., Nakao, A., and Takagi, H. (1988). Systemic hemodynamics in non-cirrhotic portal hypertension: a clinical study of 19 patients. *Jpn. J. Surg.* **18**, 620–5.

Henderson, J.M., Warren, W.D., Millikan, W.J., Galloway, J.R., Kawasaki, S., and Kutner, M.H. (1989). Distal splenorenal shunt with splenopancreatic disconnection: a 4-year assessment. *Ann. Surg.* **210**, 332–41.

Hirashima, J., Sato, H., Takeuchi, H., Nakamura, H., Hirota, K., and Hara, T. (1981). Evaluation of surgical treatment for esophageal varices. *World J. Surg.* **5**, 715–16.

Hislop, I.G., Hall, P., and Grant, A.K. (1976). Bleeding mucosal lesions in the upper gastrointestinal tracts of patients with oesophageal varices and hepatic cirrhosis. *Aust. N.Z. J. Surg.* **46**, 202–5.

Hosking, S.W., Kennedy, H.J., Seddon, I., and Triger, D.R. (1987). The role of propranolol in congestive gastropathy of portal hypertension. *Hepatology* **7**, 437–41.

Hsu, K.-Y. (1972). Portal systemic shunt for portal hypertension: importance of bromsulphalein retention for prediction of survival. *Ann. Surg.* **175**, 569–76.

Inokuchi, K. and the Japanese Research Society for Portal Hypertension (1985). Present status of surgical treatment of esophageal varices in Japan: a nationwide survery of 3588 patients. *World J. Surg.* **9**, 171–80.

Inokuchi, K., Kobayashi, M., and Ogawa, Y. (1971). Controlled splenorenal shunt for esophageal varices with the long term clinical observations. *Jpn. J. Surg.* **1**, 99–111.

Inokuchi, K., Beppu, K., Koyanagi, N., Nagamine, K., Hashizume, M., and Sugimachi, K. (1984*a*). Exclusion of nonisolated splenic vein in distal splenorenal shunt for prevention of portal malcirculation. *Ann. Surg.* **200**, 711–17.

Inokuchi, K., Kobayashi, M., Kusaba, A., Ogawa, Y., Saku, M., and Shiizaki, T. (1970). New selective decompression of esophageal varices by a left gastric venous–caval shunt. *Arch. Surg.* **100**, 157–62.

Inokuchi, K., Beppu, K., Koyanagi, N., *et al.* (1984*b*). Fifteen years' experience with left gastric venous caval shunt for esophageal varices. *World J. Surg.* **8**, 716–21.

Isomatsu, T. (1983). Loss of selectivity of Warren shunt in long-term observation. *Jpn. J. Surg.* **13**, 202–6.

Italian Liver Cirrhosis Project (1987). Reliability of endoscopy in the assessment of variceal features. *J. Hepatol.* **4**, 93–8.

Jackson, F.C., Perrin, E.B., Smith, A.G., *et al.* A clinical investigation of the portacaval shunt. II. Survival analysis of the prophylactic operation. *Am. J. Surg.* **115**, 22–42.

Japanese Research Society for Portal Hypertension (1980). The general rules for recording endoscopic findings on esophageal varices. *Jpn. J. Surg.* **10**, 84–7.

Katoh, H., Shimozawa, E., Kojima, T., and Tanabe, T. (1991). Modified splenorenal shunt with splenopancreatic disconnection. *Surgery* (in press).

Khanduri, P., Murlidharam, Nathaniel, P., *et al.* (1983). Meso-atrial shunt in the surgical treatment of Budd–Chiari syndrome. *Aust. N.Z. J. Surg.* **53**, 309–15.

Khuroo, M.S. and Datta, D.V. (1980). Budd–Chiari syndrome following pregnancy: report of 16 cases, with roentgenologic, hemodynamic and histologic studies of the hepatic outflow tract. *Am. J. Med.* **68**, 113–21.

Kimura, C., Matsuda, S., Koie, H., and Hirooka, M. (1972). Membranous obstruction of the hepatic portion of the inferior vena cava: clinical study of nine cases. *Surgery* **72**, 551–9.

Kitano, S. and Sugimachi, K. (1987). A rapid and relatively safer method of sclerosing esophageal varices utilizing a new transparent tube. *Am. J. Surg.* **153**, 317–19.

Kitano, S., Koyanagi, N., Iso, Y., Higashi, H., and Sugimachi, K. (1987*a*). Prevention of recurrence of esophageal varices after endoscopic injection sclerotherapy with ethanolamine oleate. *Hepatology* **7**, 810–15.

Kitano, S., Koyanagi, N., Iso, Y., Iwanaga, T., Higashi, H., and Sugimachi, K. (1987*b*). Prospective randomized trial comparing two injection techniques for sclerosing oesophageal varices: over-tube and free-hand. *Br. J. Surg.* **74**, 603–6.

Kitano, S., Hashizume, M., Yamada, H., *et al.* (1989). Human thrombin plus 5 per cent ethanolamine oleate injected to sclerose oesophageal varices: a prospective randomized trial. *Br. J. Surg.* **76**, 715–18.

Koch, H., Henning, H., Grimm, H., and Soehendra, N. (1987). Prophylactic sclerosing of esophageal varices. Results of a prospective controlled study. *Endoscopy* **18**, 40–3.

Koyama, K., Takagi, Y., Ouchi, K., and Sato, T. (1980). Results of esophageal transection for esophageal varices: experience in 100 cases. *Am. J. Surg.* **139**, 204–9.

Koyanagi, N. and the Co-operative Study Group of Portal Hypertension in Japan (1988). Prognostic blue varices as a discriminant factor of variceal hemorrhage: amendment of the criteria of endoscopic findings of esophageal varices. *Jpn. J. Surg.* **18**, 142–5.

Koyanagi, N., Inokuchi, K., Nakayama, S., Sakata, H., and Beppu, K. (1981). Decreased arteriovenous flow resistance in the left gastric venous area in cirrhotic patients. *Eur. J. Clin. Invest.* **11**, 355–9.

Kuang, Y.-L., Chen, Z.-P., Jiang, G.-J., Zhou, H.-G., Sang, J.-X., and Wu, X.-Y. (1984). Mesocaval shunt in treatment of rebleeding after splenectomy for portal hypertension. *Chin. Med. J.* **97**, 175–8.

Kumana, C.R., Lin, H.J., Ko, W., Wu, P.-C., and Todd, D. (1985). Herbal tea induced hepatic veno-occlusive disease: quantification of toxic alkaloid exposure in adults. *Gut* **26**, 101–4.

Lam, S.K., Lam, W.K., Cheng, F.C.Y., and Ong, G.B. (1977). Transabdominal suture of bleeding gastro-oesophageal varices in cryptogenic cirrhosis of the liver. *Br. J. Surg.* **64**, 428–32.

Lebrec, D., de Fleury, P., Rueff, B., Nahum, H., and Benhamou, J.P. (1980). Portal hypertension, size of esophageal varices, and risk of gastrointestinal bleeding in alcoholic cirrhosis. *Gastroenterology* **79**, 1139–44.

Lunderquist, A. and Vang, J. (1974). Transhepatic catheterization and obliteration of the coronary vein in patients with portal hypertension and oesophageal varices. *N. Engl. J. Med.* **291**, 646–9.

Murray, J.F., Dawson, A.M., and Sherlock, S. (1958). Circulatory changes in chronic liver disease. *Am. J. Med.* **24**, 358–67.

Nagasue, N., Ogawa, Y., Yukaya, H., Chang, Y.-C., and Kaneko, S. (1987). Cavo-atrial shunt with externally stented PTFE graft for Budd–Chiari syndrome with caval obstruction. *Br. J. Surg.* **74**, 1177–8.

Nagasue, N., Ogawa, Y., Yukaya, H., Tamada, R., Chang, Y., and Nakamura, T. (1988*a*). Emergency distal splenorenal shunt for medically uncontrollable variceal haemorrhage. *Zentralbl. Chir.* **113**, 446–54.

Nagasue, N., Ogawa, Y., Yukaya, H., *et al.* (1988*b*). Prophylactic distal splenorenal shunt for Child's class A and B patients at high risk of bleeding. *Zentralbl. Chir.* **113**, 1329–37.

Nagasue, N., Kohno, H., Ogawa, Y., *et al.* (1989). Appraisal of distal splenorenal shunt in the treatment of esophageal varices: an analysis of prophylactic, emergency, and elective shunts. *World J. Surg.* **13**, 92–9.

Ohnishi, K., Iida, S., Iwama, S., *et al.* (1982). The effect of chronic habitual alcohol intake on the development of liver cirrhosis and hepatocellular carcinoma. Relation to hepatitis B surface antigen carriage. *Cancer* **49**, 672–7.

Ohniski, K., Sato, S., Saito, M., *et al.* (1986). Clinical and portal hemodynamic features in cirrhotic patients having a large spontaneous splenorenal and/or gastrorenal shunt. *Am. J. Gastroenterol.* **81**, 450–5.

Okuda, K. (1983). Epidemiology of idiopathic portal hypertension. In *Idiopathic portal hypertension* University of Tokyo Press, Tokyo. (ed. K. Okuda and M. Omata pp. 3–12.

Okuda, K., Kono, K., Ohnishi, K., *et al.* (1984). Clinical study of eight-six cases of idiopathic portal hypertension and comparison with cirrhosis with splenomegaly. *Gastroenterology* **86**, 600–10.

Ono, J., Sakoda, K., and Kawada, T. (1983). Membranous obstruction of the inferior vena cava. *Ann. Surg.* **197**, 454–8.

Orloff, M.J. and Johansen, K.H. (1978). Treatment of Budd–Chiari syndrome by side-to-side portacaval shunt: experimental and clinical results. *Ann. Surg.* **188**, 494–512.

Paquet, K.J. (1982). Prophylactic endoscopic sclerosing treatment of the esophageal wall in varices. A prospective controlled randomized trial. *Endoscopy* **14**, 4–5.

Powell, W.J. and Klatskin, G. (1968). Duration of survival in patients with Laennec's cirrhosis: influence of alcohol withdrawal, and possible effects of recent changes in general management of the disease. *Am. J. Med.* **44**, 406–20.

Resnick, R.H., Chalmers, T.C., Ishihara, A.M., *et al.* (1969). A controlled study of the prophylactic portacaval shunt. A final report. *Ann. Intern. Med.* **70**, 675–88.

Sama, S.K., Bhargava, S., Gopi Nath, N., *et al.* (1971). Noncirrhotic portal fibrosis. *Am. J. Med.* **51**, 160–9.

Sarin, S.K. and Nundy, S. (1985). Subclinical encephalopathy after portosystemic shunts in patients with non-cirrhotic portal fibrosis. *Liver* **5**, 142–6.

Sarin, S.K., Sachdev, G., and Nanda, R. (1986). Follow-up of patients after variceal eradication: a comparison of patients with cirrhosis, noncirrhotic portal fibrosis, and extrahepatic obstruction. *Ann. Surg.* **204**, 78–82.

Sarin, S.K., Malhotra, V., Nayyar, A., Sundaram, K.R., and Broor, S.L. (1988). Profiles of alcoholic liver disease in an Indian hospital. A prospective analysis. *Liver* **8**, 132–7.

Sarin, S.K., Nanda, R., Kumar, N., Vij, J.C., and Anand, B.S. (1985). Repeated endoscopic sclerotherapy for active variceal bleeding. *Ann. Surg.* **202**, 708–11.

Siegel, J.H., Goldwin, R.M., Farrel, E.J., *et al.* (1974). Hemodynamic states and physiologic determinants of survival in patients with cirrhosis and portal hypertension. *Arch. Surg.* **108**, 282–92.

Sugita, S., Ohnishi, K., Iida, S., Nomura, F., and Okuda, K. (1988). Histological changes in the liver and portal hypertension subsequent to repeated intraportal injection of killed *E. coli* in the dog. *Liver* **8**, 1–9.

Sugiura, M. and Futagawa, S. (1973). A new technique for treating esophageal varices. *J. Thorac. Cardiovasc. Surg.* **66**, 677–85.

Sugiura, M. and Futagawa, S. (1984*a*). Esophageal transection with paraesophagogastric devascularizations (the Sugiura procedure) in the treatment of esophageal varices. *World J. Surg.* **8**, 673–82.

Sugiura, M. and Futagawa, S. (1984*b*). Results of six hundred thirty-six esophageal transections with paraesophagogastric devascularization in the treatment of esophageal varices. *J. Vasc. Surg.* **1**, 254–60.

Sun, Y.-Q., Zhang, J.-M., and Wang, Y. (1984). Limited side-to-side portacaval shunt: over 20 years' clinical experience. *Chin. Med. J.* **97**, 13–18.

Takasaki, T., Kobayashi, S., Muto, H., Suzuki, S., Harada, M., and Nakayama, K. (1977). Transabdominal esophageal transection by using a suture device in cases of esophageal varices. *Int. Surg.* **62**, 426–8.

Takase, Y., Ozaki, A., Orii, K., Nagoshi, K., Okamura, T., and Iwasaki, Y. (1982). Injection sclerotherapy of esophageal varices for patients undergoing emergency and elective surgery. *Surgery* **92**, 474–9.

Tanaka, R., Itoshima, T., and Nagashima, H. (1987). Follow-up study of 582 liver cirrhosis patients for 26 years in Japan. *Liver* 7, 316–24.

Terabayashi, H., Ohnishi, K., Tsunoda, T., *et al.* (1987). Prospective controlled trial of elective endoscopic sclerotherapy in comparison with percutaneous transhepatic obliteration of esophageal varices in patients with nonalcoholic cirrhosis. *Gastroenterology* **93**, 1205–9.

Victor, S., Jayanthi, V., Kandasamy, I., Ratnasabathy, A., and Madanagopalan, N. (1986). Retrohepatic cavoatrial bypass for coarctation of inferior vena cava with a polytetrafluoroethylene graft. *J. Thorac. Cardiovasc. Surg.* **91**, 99–105.

Walker, R.M. (1964). Esophageal transection for bleeding varices. *Surg. Gynecol. Obstet.* **118**, 323–9.

Warren, W.D., Zeppa, R., and Fomon, J.J. (1967). Selective trans-splenic decompression of gastroesophageal varices by distal splenorenal shunt. *Ann. Surg.* **166**, 437–54.

Wexler, M.J. (1980). Treatment of bleeding esophageal varices by transabdominal esophageal transection with the EEA stapling instrument. *Surgery* **88**, 406–16.

Whipple, A.O. (1945). The problem of portal hypertension in relation to the hepatosplenopathies. *Ann. Surg.* **122**, 449–75.

Witzel, L., Wolbergs, E., and Merki, H. (1985). Prophylactic endoscopic sclerotherapy of oesophageal varices. A prospective controlled study. *Lancet* **i**, 773–5.

Yamada, R., Sato, M., Kawabata, M., Nakatsuka, K., and Kobayashi, N. (1983). Segmental obstruction of the hepatic inferior vena cava treated by transluminal angioplasty. *Radiology* **149**, 91–6.

Yamamoto, S., Yokoyama, Y., Takeshige, K., and Iwatsuki, S. (1968). Budd–Chiari syndrome with obstruction of the inferior vena cava. *Gastroenterology* **54**, 1070–84.

Yamamoto, S., Hidemura, R., Sawada, M., Takeshige, K., and Iwatsuki, S. (1976). The late results of terminal esophagoproximal gastrectomy (TEPG) with extensive devascularization and splenectomy for bleeding esophageal varices in cirrhosis. *Surgery* **80**, 106–14.

14. Acalculous biliary disease

James Toouli

Increased understanding of the motility of the biliary tract in recent years has provided firm evidence for the existence of biliary tract motility disorders. These disorders, in common with other abnormalities of motility in the gastrointestinal tract, produce symptoms which often mimic other pathological conditions. In the biliary tract the major symptom produced by motility disorders is pain, the nature of which is often similar to that of calculous disease.

There are two separate areas of the biliary tract, the gallbladder and the sphincter of Oddi, which have been implicated in the production of acalculous biliary disease. The prevalence of motility disorders of the gallbladder and sphincter of Oddi is, however, unknown. Nevertheless, most investigators in this field would agree that patients with objective signs of motility disorders of the biliary tract are quite rare and constitute less than 1 per cent of patients with calculous biliary disease (Tondelli, Gyr, Stalder, and Allgower 1979).

Gallbladder motility abnormalities typically present with symptoms very similar to those in patients with gallbladder stones. Following extensive investigation for calculi, the patient is usually found to have no evidence of stones in either the gallbladder or the bile duct, raising the possibility of acalculous gallbladder disease. Similarly, in patients with a motility disorder of the sphincter of Oddi, initial symptoms at presentation suggest the presence of a stone in the bile duct. These patients usually present some years after cholecystectomy with features of recurrent biliary-type pain which may be associated with abnormal levels of liver enzymes.

Recent developments in endoscopic and radionuclide techniques have permitted a better understanding of the motility of the biliary tract. These advances have facilitated improvements in the definition of motility abnormalities and the development of objective investigations for the identification of patients with acalculous biliary disease.

Normal human biliary tract motility

Studies over the last decade have shown that the motility of the gallbladder and sphincter of Oddi are important in controlling the flow of bile from the liver into the duodenum. During fasting, approximately 50 per cent of secreted hepatic bile passes into the gallbladder where it is concentrated by absorption of water (Wood and Svanvik 1983). Resistance to flow through the sphincter of Oddi is produced by a basal pressure and phasic contractions which modulate the flow of bile either into the gallbladder or into the duodenum. During the inter-digestive period, expulsion of small volumes of concentrated bile from the gallbladder occurs just before the duodenal, migrating-motor complex (Toouli, Bushell, Stevenson, Dent, Wycherley, and Iannos 1986). This action of the gallbladder is associated with increased frequency of sphincter of Oddi contractions, which may promote the flow of small volumes of bile into the duodenum (Takahashi, Nakaya, Suzuki, and Itoh 1982). After a meal, the gallbladder contracts with slow sustained action so that most of its contents are expelled into the duodenum. Sphincter of Oddi contractions decrease in amplitude, thus allowing for an enhancement of passive flow of bile (Worthley, Baker, Iannos, Saccone, and Toouli 1989). The control of the motility of the gallbladder and sphincter of Oddi is achieved via both extrinsic and intrinsic nerves. In addition, a variety of hormones act on both the gallbladder and sphincter of Oddi, the primary hormone being cholecystokinin. The inter-play between neuronal and hormonal factors in controlling biliary motility has not, as yet, been totally elucidated.

Gallbladder motility disorders

Motility disorders of the gallbladder produce acalculous gallbladder disease. Both decreased contraction (hypokinesia) and excessive contraction (hyperkinesia) have been postulated to result in pain syndromes attributed to the gallbladder. A major difficulty in the diagnosis of these disorders has been the lack of an objective investigation to identify gallbladder dyskinesia.

The prevalence of gallbladder motility disorders in unknown. However, a recent prospective evaluation of its incidence in our own hospital population has shown it to be extremely rare and to constitute less than 1 per cent of the population of patients presenting with calculous disease. The patients are usually female and present with symptoms and signs typical of gallstone disease. Investigations such as ultrasonography of the gallbladder, oral cholecystography, and endoscopic retrograde cholangiopancreatography (ERCP) fail to determine the presence of gallstones in the biliary tract. These patients are either given the label of 'irritable bowel' or disease of a 'functional' disorder.

In the past a number of investigations aimed at reproducing symptoms have been used to identify patients with gallbladder motility disorders. Cholecystokinin provocation tests have been used to produce pain (Rhodes, Lennard, Farndon, and Taylor 1988). Prospective studies have, however, failed to show consistent results with respect to their usefulness in selecting patients with gallbladder dyskinesia for treatment. One of the difficulties with provocation tests is their dependence on the subjective response of the patient to pain. It is well known that cholecystokinin not only induces contraction of the gallbladder but also produces colonic spasm (Harvey and Read 1973). Thus, it is not surprising these investigations do not discriminate between patients with gallbladder symptoms and patients who may have pain as a result of an irritable bowel.

A recent study has used the radionuclide DIDA for gallbladder opacification and has defined a gallbladder ejection fraction to diagnose patients with acalculous gallbladder disease (Yap, McGee, McKenzie, Wycherley, and Toouli 1989). Following intravenous administration, the compound technetium-99m IDA (imino-diacetic acid) used for these studies is cleared through the liver into bile. Technetium-99m emits 140 keV gamma photons that are ideally suited for imaging and counting by gamma-camera. These properties have been used to image the gallbladder and the biliary tract and, by producing temporal profiles, monitor gallbladder emptying. The motor function of the gallbladder can be evaluated by determining the gallbladder ejection fraction. Following concentration of Technetium-99m DIDA in the gallbladder, cholecystokinin-octapeptide is infused intravenously for 45 minutes. Gallbladder emptying of the technetium-99m DIDA is monitored during the infusion period and for 15 minutes after cessation of infusion. The gallbladder ejection fraction is determined by the formula:

$$\frac{\text{Counts at specific time}}{\text{Maximal counts before infusion}} \times 100$$

The mean gallbladder ejection fraction at 15 minutes post-infusion is normally 70 per cent. Values lower than 40 per cent represent abnormalities in gallbladder ejection fraction which reflect disorders in gallbladder motility.

In a recent study, patients with abnormal gallbladder ejection fractions were randomized to either cholecystectomy or conservative management. At 3-year follow-up it was shown that the patients who underwent cholecystectomy remained asymptomatic, whereas the control group continued to have biliary-type symptoms (Yap *et al.* 1989). Gallbladders removed at cholecystectomy were evaluated histologically and showed thickening of the cystic duct, as well as gallbladder wall hypertrophy. None of the patients had stones in the gallbladder. It was concluded from this study that a motility disorder of the gallbladder produced biliary-type pain, probably due to relative resistance to outflow across the cystic duct. These patients were helped by cholecystectomy.

As a result of the above study, it is recommended that, in patients who are suspected of having a motility disorder of the gallbladder, a gallbladder ejection fraction be determined. Those patients with abnormal gallbladder ejection fractions qualify for the diagnosis of gallbladder dyskinesia and will benefit from cholecystectomy.

In addition to patients with a motility disorder of the gallbladder, there

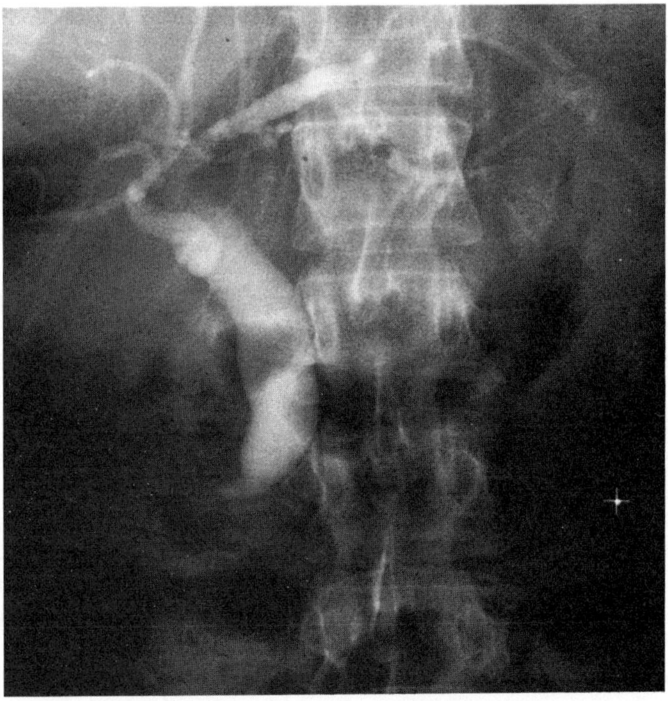

Fig. 14.1 Cholangiogram demonstrating a moderately dilated bile duct with delay in passage of contrast into the duodenum. The radiograph was taken 45 minutes after introduction of contrast medium into the bile duct via ERCP.

exists a small group of patients who present with biliary-type pain but in whom no gallstones are shown on standard investigations. In this group of patients microscopy of gallbladder bile, obtained from the duodenum, may reveal the presence of cholesterol crystals (Freeman, Cohen, and Den-Besten 1975). It is postulated that small calculi have been formed and are extruded through the biliary tract, producing symptoms. These patients do not have acalculous biliary disease but 'microcalculous' disease. Cholecystectomy is usually associated with resolution of symptoms.

Post-cholecystectomy sphincter of Oddi dysfunction

Following cholecystectomy for either calculous or acalculous gallbladder disease, a small percentage of patients present, usually 5–10 years later, with recurrent upper abdominal pain (Hess 1979). The pain may be associated with abnormal elevation of serum liver enzymes or a dilated bile duct, and patients show delayed emptying of contrast medium introduced into the bile duct at endoscopic cholangiography (Fig. 14.1). A separate group of patients may present with pain consistent with pancreatitis and an abnormally elevated serum amylase concentration. Common causes of biliary and pancreatic pain such as stones, stricture, or alcohol, can not be implicated, and previously the label of either an idiopathic or functional disorder was given to these patients.

In recent years it has been recognized that the symptoms produced in these patients may be due to a dysfunctioning sphincter of Oddi (Toouli 1984). A number of non-invasive investigations may help to support this diagnosis. Such tests include the morphine–neostigmine test, fatty meal sonography of the bile duct, secretin-stimulated estimation of pancreatic duct diameter, and radionuclide estimation of bile flow. However, the most objective investigation that is available for the diagnosis of this disorder is that of endoscopic sphincter of Oddi manometry.

The morphine–neostigmine test is a useful screening test for selecting patients who may be considered to have sphincter of Oddi dysfunction (Roberts-Thomson and Toouli 1985). The investigation has limited value as it is not specific enough to identify patients who will respond to therapy. Nevertheless, there is undoubtedly a group of patients with sphincter of Oddi dysfunction who are exquisitely sensitive to the administration of morphine and this test may select this subgroup of patients with dysfunction of the sphincter of Oddi. Morphine and neostigmine are administered intramuscularly and serum is withdrawn at hourly intervals for estimation of liver enzymes and amylase. In addition, the patient is asked to score the degree of pain experienced. A positive test is characterized by a reproduction of the pain plus elevation of liver enzyme or amylase in excess of double the upper limit of normal. The pain and enzyme elevation usually occur approximately 3–4 hours after the administration of morphine and neostigmine.

Fatty meal sonography of the bile duct is carried out by real-time ultrasonography (Darweesh, *et al.* 1988). The maximal diameter of the bile duct is measured at a fixed point adjacent to the site where the right hepatic artery crosses the common hepatic duct. Following the ingestion of a fatty meal, it is expected that normal changes in sphincter of Oddi motility will enhance bile flow into the duodenum and, hence, the diameter of the common hepatic duct should decrease. An increase in ductal diameter reflects a resistance to outflow which may characterize dysfunction of the sphincter of Oddi.

A similar investigation is undertaken for the pancreatic duct (Bolondi, Gaiani, Gullo, and Labo 1984). The diameter of the pancreatic duct is determined and should normally measure less than 1 mm. Following infusion of secretin at 1 unit/kg, there is an increase in ductal diameter followed by a rapid return to normal size within 30 minutes. If the ductal diameter remains dilated in excess of 1.5 mm in 30 minutes this suggests an increase in resistance to the outflow of pancreatic juice, consistent with dysfunction of the sphincter of Oddi.

The radionuclide technetium-99m DIDA can also be used to evaluate flow through the bile duct in post-cholecystectomy patients (Roberts-Thomson, Toouli, Blanchett, Lichtenstein, and Andrews 1986). Following its injection intravenously, the subject is positioned under a gamma-camera and continual recordings are made from the biliary tract and duodenum. In order to analyse flow, areas of interest are outlined and the counts per second within these areas are determined. The shape and slope of the curve of counts from the bile duct reflect flow through the biliary tree. Delay in outflow may represent a resistance across the sphincter of Oddi, due to sphincter of Oddi dysfunction.

Sphincter of Oddi manometry is, however, the most objective method for evaluating motility changes across the sphincter of Oddi. Accurate direct pressure measurements from the sphincter of Oddi became possible by miniaturization of manometry catheters and the development of fluid perfusion systems of low compliance (Arndorfer, Steff, Dodds, Linelan, and Hogan 1977). Polyethylene catheters with three lumens of 0.5 mm internal diameter, making up a catheter of 1.7 mm outer diameter, are used. Three side-holes are fashioned at 2 mm intervals starting at 10 mm from the distal tip. The three lumens record across a length of 5 mm from within the sphincter of Oddi. The catheter is 200 cm long and is perfused with deionized bubble-free water via a pneumo-hydraulic capillary system at a pressure of 750 mmHg. The volume of water perfused through the catheter is 0.125 ml/min and the whole system is capable of accurately recording pressure changes up to 300 mmHg/second (Toouli, Geenan, Hogan, Dodds and Arndorfer 1982). Recording from three lumens allows an evaluation of the sequencing of sphincter of Oddi contractions as well as determination of basal pressure, amplitude, and frequency of contractions. Using the above system, sphincter of Oddi motility may be measured either via introduction of a catheter through an endoscope (Geenen, Hogan, Dodds, Steward, and Arndorfer 1980) or at operation via introduction of the catheter through the cystic duct (Toouli *et al.* 1986; Fig. 14.2) or post-operatively in patients with T-tubes in order to study sphincter of Oddi physiology (Worthley *et al.* 1989).

The most common method of recording manometry is via an endoscope and the catheter is introduced through the biopsy channel of a duodenoscope (Fig. 14.3). The catheter is introduced into either the bile duct or the pancreatic duct via the duodenal papilla. It is then withdrawn so that all three recording posts are situated within the sphincter of Oddi segment. In order to assist with the positioning of the catheter across the sphincter, circular markings are placed on the catheter at 2 mm intervals from the most proximal hole for a total length of 12 mm. Recordings are made for approximately 3–10 minutes. Following an initial baseline recording, cholecystokinin-octapeptide is administered at a dose of 20 mg/kg in order to evaluate the response of cholecystokinin. The normal pressure profile of the

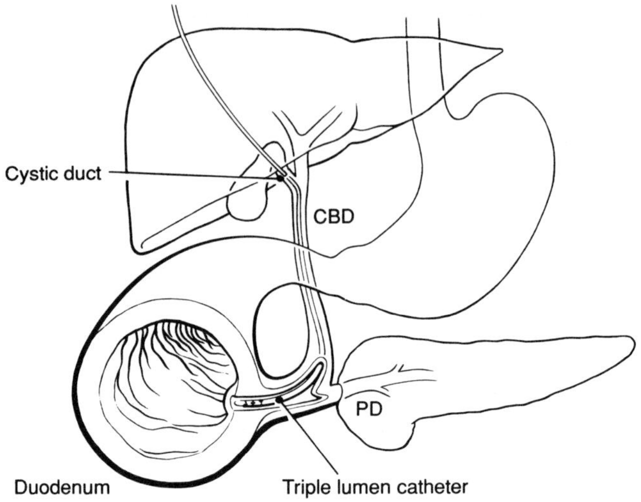

Fig. 14.2. Schematic diagram illustrating the method for measuring sphincter of Oddi pressures at operation. The triple lumen catheter is introduced via the cystic duct and positioned so that all three lumens record from the sphincter of Oddi. CBD, common bile duct; PD, pancreatic duct.

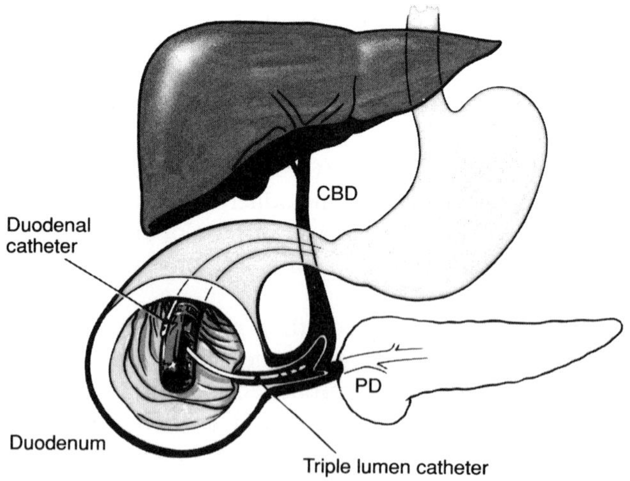

Fig. 14.3. Schematic diagram illustrating the endoscopic method for measuring sphincter of Oddi pressures. The triple lumen catheter is introduced into either the common bile duct (CBD) or pancreatic duct (PD) via the biopsy channel of the duodenoscope and positioned so that all three lumens record from the sphincter of Oddi. A separate catheter records duodenal pressures.

Table 14.1. Sphincter of Oddi manometry in 18 control patients.

	Median	Range	Abnormal
Basal Pressure (mmHg)	15	5–35	> 40
Amplitude (mmHg)	135	95–195	> 300
Frequency (*n*/min)	4	2–6	> 7
Sequences (%)			
Antegrade	80	12–100	
Simultaneous	13	0–50	
Retrograde	9	0–50	
Cholecystokinin-octapeptide (20 ng/kg)	Inhibition		Contraction

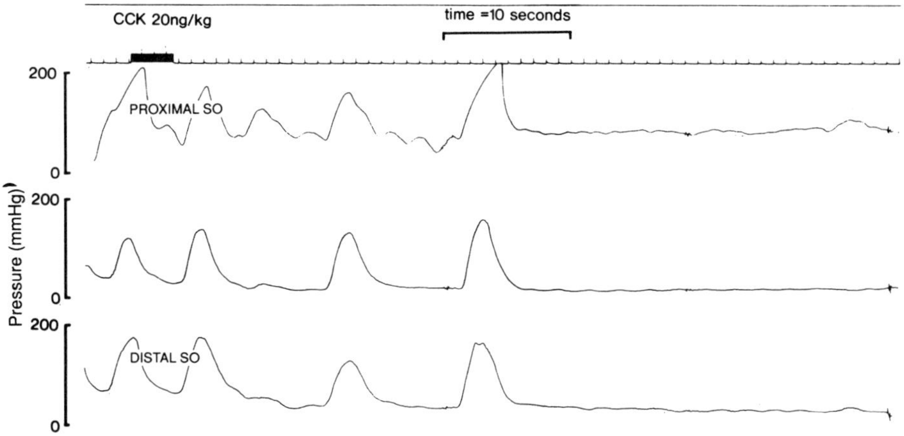

Fig. 14.4. Manometric recording from the sphincter of Oddi (SO) showing the normal phasic contractions superimposed on a modest basal pressure. Administration of cholecystokinin-octapeptide (CCK-OP, 20 ng/kg) produced inhibition of the phasic contractions.

sphincter of Oddi, as demonstrated by endoscopic manometry, is shown in Table 14.1. Cholecystokinin-octapeptide normally inhibits the sphincter of Oddi, phasic contractions, and decreases the basal pressure (Fig. 14.4).

Based on findings at endoscopic manometry, sphincter of Oddi dysfunction has been categorized into two major groups (Toouli, Roberts-Thomson, Dent, and Lee 1985).

Stenosis of the sphincter of Oddi

Manometrically this group of patients is characterized by an abnormally elevated sphincter of Oddi basal pressure (Fig. 14.5). The stenosis may be

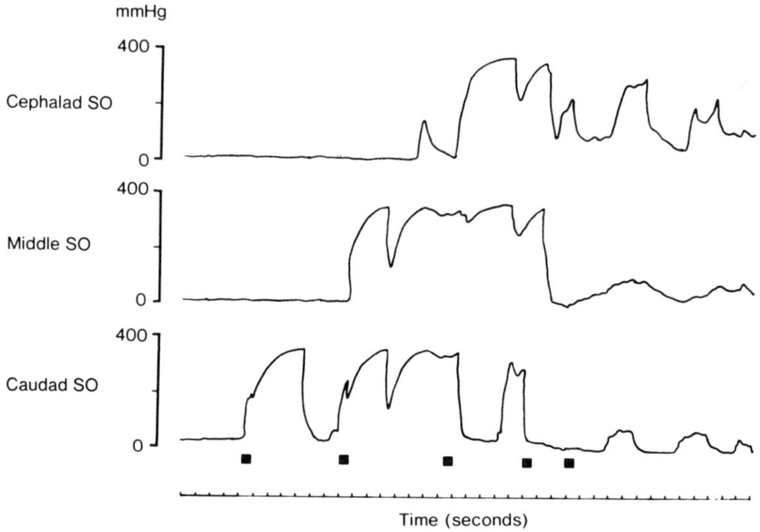

Fig. 14.5. Manometric recording from the sphincter of Oddi (SO) demonstrating a region of high basal pressure. The triple lumen catheter is withdrawn from the bile duct, across the sphincter, and into the duodenum in a stepwise fashion marked by the black squares. Hence the most caudal lumen records the high basal first, then the middle lumen, and subsequently the most cephalad lumen.

due to fibrotic changes in the sphincter or smooth muscle hyperplasia. To date, however, there has been no correlation of manometric with pathological findings.

Sphincter of Oddi dyskinesia

This group of patients exhibits a variety of manometric findings:

1. *Rapid phasic contraction frequency* Spontaneously occurring bursts of rapid contraction may be seen and are believed to reflect an irritable sphincter. The rapid contractions may produce transient obstruction to flow.

2. *Intermittent episodes of elevated pressure* This is similar to (1) and may be an associated finding. This may also reflect an irritable sphincter which develops spasm intermittently.

3. *Excessive retrograde contraction* In normal subjects the majority of sphincter of Oddi contractions are oriented in an antegrade direction. In some patients, however, the majority of contractions are retrograde. This observation is also evident in patients with gallbladder and common bile duct stones, and may result in a relative retardation of flow through the sphincter.

4. *Paradoxical response to cholecystokinin* Administration of a bolus dose of cholecystokinin-octapeptide normally produces inhibition of sphincter of Oddi phasic contractions. This action is thought to be mediated via non-adrenergic, non-cholinergic nerves to the sphincter of Oddi. A paradoxical response consists of sphincter contraction in place of inhibition and may be due to the direct effect of the hormone on the smooth muscle of the sphincter. This finding may be secondary to damage to the intrinsic neurons of the sphincter and may be a condition pathologically similar to achalasia of the oesophagus.

A recently completed prospective study has evaluated the effect of endoscopic sphincterotomy in the treatment of sphincter of Oddi dysfunction (Geenen, Hogan, Dodds, Toouli, and Venn 1989). This study has shown that in patients with manometrically diagnosed sphincter of Oddi stenosis, division of the sphincter of Oddi is associated with long-term cure. Similarly, in patients presenting with idiopathic recurrent pancreatitis and in whom a stenosis of the sphincter is demonstrable, surgical sphincteroplasty and pancreatic ductal septectomy is highly successful for the relief of symptoms (Moody, Becker, and Potts 1983). As a result of these studies, it is concluded that manometric evaluation of the sphincter provides objective assessment of sphincter motility and selects patients whose symptoms may resolve following division of the sphincter.

Conclusion

Results from motility studies of the biliary tract have demonstrated the presence of motility abnormalities in the gallbladder and sphincter of Oddi. These motility disorders account for the presence of acalculous biliary disease and produce significant symptomatology in a small percentage of people presenting with biliary-like pain. Recently reported prospective trials have shown that, following identification of these abnormalities, specific treatment is associated with significant long-term relief of symptoms.

References

Arndorfer, R.C., Steff, J.J., Dodds, W.J., Linelan, J.H., and Hogan, W.J. (1977). Improved infusion system for intraluminal esophageal manometry. *Gastroenterology* **73**, 23–7.

Bolondi, L., Gaiani, S., Gullo, L., and Labo, G. (1984). Secretin administration induces a dilatation of the main pancreatic duct. *Dig. Dis. Sci.* **29**, 802–8.

Darweesh, R.M.A., Dodds, W.J., Hogan, W.J., *et al.* (1988). Efficacy of quantitative hepatobiliary scintigraphy and fatty meal sonography for evaluating patients with suspected partial common bile duct obstruction. *Gastroenterology* **94**, 779–86.

Freeman, J.B., Cohen, W.N., and DenBesten, L. (1975). Cholecystokinin cholangiography and analysis of duodenal bile in the investigation of pain the right upper quadrant of the abdomen without gallstones. *Surg. Gynecol. Obstet.* **140**, 371–6.

Geenen, J.E., Hogan, W.J., Dodds, W.J., Steward, E.T., and Arndorfer, R.C. (1980). Intraluminal pressure recording from the human sphincter of Oddi. *Gastroenterology* **78**, 317–24.

Geenen, J.T., Hogan, W.J., Dodds, W.J., Toouli, J., and Venu, R.P. (1989). The efficacy of endoscopic sphincterotomy in post-cholecystectomy patients with sphincter of Oddi dysfunction. *N. Engl. J. Med.* **320**, 820–7.

Harvey, R.F. and Read, A.E. (1973). Effects of cholecystectomy on colonic motility and symptoms in patients with the irritable bowel syndrome. *Lancet* **i**, 1–3.

Hess, W. (1979). Physiology of the sphincter of Oddi. In *The papilla vateri and its diseases*. (ed. M. Classen, J. Geenen, and K. Kawai). *Proceedings of the International Workshop of the World Congress of Gastroenterology*, Madrid, 1978, pp. 14–21. Verlag Gerhard Witzhock, Kohn.

Moody, F.G., Becker, J.M., and Potts, J.R. (1983). Transduodenal sphincteroplasty and transampullary septectomy for post-cholecystectomy pain. *Ann. Surg.* **197**, 627–36.

Rhodes, M., Lennard, T.W.J., Farndon, J.R., and Taylor, R.M.R. (1988). Choleycstectomy (CCK) provocation test: long term follow-up after cholecystectomy. *Br. J. Surg.* **75**, 951–3.

Roberts-Thomson, I.C. and Toouli, J. (1985). Abnormal responses to morphine neostigmine in patients with undefined biliary type pain. *Gut* **26**, 1367–72.

Roberts-Thomson, I.C., Toouli, J., Blanchett, W., Lichtenstein, M., and Andrews, J.T. (1986). Assessment of bile flow by radioscintigraphy in patients with biliary type pain after cholecystectomy. *Aust. N. Z. J. Med.* **16**, 788–93.

Takahashi, I., Nakaya, M., Suzuki, T., and Itoh, Z. (1982). Postprandial changes in contractile activity and bile concentration in gallbladder of the dog. *Am. J. Physiol.* **6**, G365–G371.

Tondelli, P., Gyr, K., Stalder, G.A., and Allgower, M. (1979). The biliary tract. 1 Cholecystectomy. *Clin. Gastroenterol.* **8**, 487–505.

Toouli, J. (1984). Sphincter of Oddi motility. *Br. J. Surg.* **71**, 251–6.

Toouli, J., Roberts-Thomson, I.C., Dent, J., and Lee, J. (1985). Manometric disorders in patients with suspected sphincter of Oddi dysfunction. *Gastroenterology* **88**, 1243–50.

Toouli, J., Geenen, J.E., Hogan, W.J., Dodds, W.J., and Arndorder, R.C. (1982). Sphincter of Oddi motor activity: a comparison between patients with common bile duct stones and controls. *Gastroenterology* **82**, 111–7.

Toouli, J., Bushell, M., Stevenson, G., Dent, J., Wycherley, A., and Iannos, J. (1986). Gallbladder emptying in man related to fasting duodenal migrating motor contractions. *Aust. N. Z. J. Surg.* **56**, 147–51.

Wood, J.R. and Svanvik, J. (1983). Gallbladder water and electrolyte transport and its regulation. *Gut* **24**, 579–93.

Worthley, C.S., Baker, R.A., Iannos, J., Saccone, G.T.P., and Toouli, J. (1989). Human fasting and postprandial sphincter of Oddi motility. *Bri. J. Surg.* **76**, 709–14.

Yap, L., McGee, M.A., McKenzie, J., Wycherley, A., and Toouli, J. (1989). Acalculous biliary pain: diagnostic use of cholecystokinin cholescintography in the selection of patients for cholecystectomy. *Gastroenterology* **96**, A558.

15. Liver resection

Nagy A. Habib and Brian R. Davidson

Historical background

Elective resection of the liver for tumour was first reported in 1890 (Tiffany 1980) and by the end of the following decade more than 20 cases had been reported (Kenn 1899). Haemorrhage was the main cause of the high morbidity and mortality rates encountered by these early liver surgeons. In order to reduce this, techniques for atraumatic suturing and vascular inflow occlusion (Pringle's manoeuvre; Pringle 1908) were introduced at the beginning of this century. It was not, however, until there was a better understanding of the segmental anatomy of the liver in the 1950s that major resections could be seriously undertaken (Couinaud 1957). Lortat-Jacob and Robert (1952) were the first to describe a formal liver resection in which the right lobe bile duct and vessels were ligated along with the right hepatic vein before dividing the parenchyma. The technique of dividing the liver parenchyma by 'finger fracture' was first practised at the same time. This allowed the tissue to be divided whilst preserving the branches of the portal vein, hepatic artery, bile duct, and hepatic vein, which could be secured within the liver. Further refinements of this technique were subsequently described by Tung and Quang (1965). An alternative, and perhaps safer, approach has been practised which involves isolation of the vessels outside the liver substance, followed by temporary clamp occlusion until major structures are isolated within the liver substance (Bismuth 1982). It is the application of these techniques in recent years which has allowed extensive resections to be carried out with low morbidity and mortality rates.

Anatomy of the liver

Gross anatomy

Although the falciform ligament divides the liver morphologically into a right and left lobe, functionally the organ is divided into a right and a left liver by an imaginary line that stretches from the gallbladder fossa anteriorly and to the left side of the inferior vena cava posteriorly. Therefore, one can talk of 'two' livers, with excision of the right liver being called a right hepatectomy, and excision of the left liver as a left hepatectomy.

There is no communication between these livers, except outside the liver capsule. Each liver is divided into medial and lateral sectors. The right

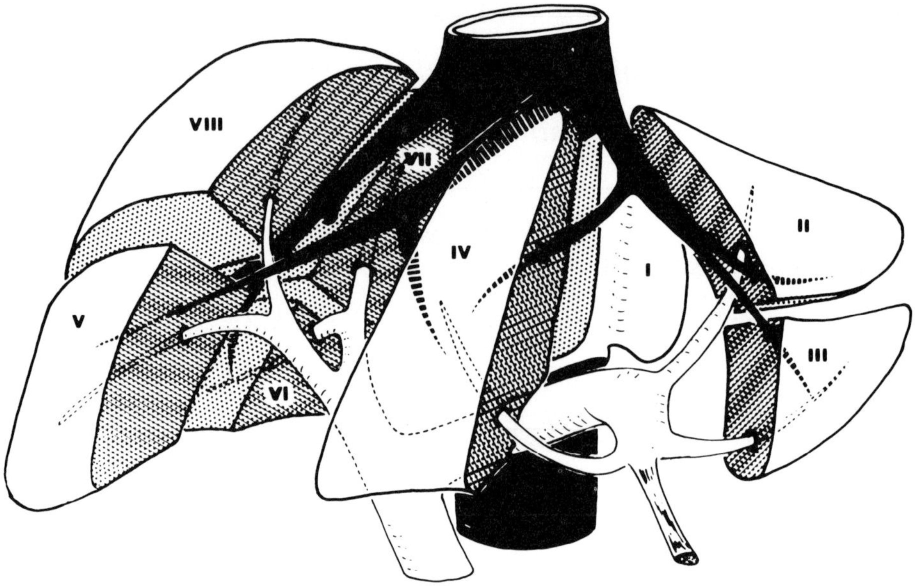

Fig. 15.1. Surgical anatomy of the liver.

medial and lateral sectors are divided by another imaginary line, between a point equidistant from the gallbladder fossa to the anterio-inferior angle of the liver anteriorly, to the inferior vena cava posteriorly. The left medial and lateral sectors of the liver are divided by the umbilical fissure. Each sector is divided into two segments. The entire liver, therefore, consists of four sectors and eight segments (Fig. 15.1). On the left side the medial sector is divided into a large anterior segment called the quadrate lobe (or segment four) and a smaller posterior segment called the caudate lobe (or segment one). The left lateral sector comprises a posterior segment two and an anterior segment three. The right medial sector is divided into an anterior-inferior segment five and a postero-superior segment eight, and the right lateral sector is divided into an antero-inferior segment six and a postero-superior segment seven.

Couinaud in his classification (Fig. 15.1) named the segments from one to eight in a clockwise direction starting from the caudate as one, swinging to the right to segments two and three, and coming to the quadrate lobe, which is segment four; on the left the segments are numbered five, six, and seven, and end at segment eight, which is just on the right aspect of the inferior vena cava.

Vascular supply

The blood supply of the right liver (i.e. segments five, six, seven, and eight) is from the right branch of the hepatic artery and the right branch of the portal vein. In some cases the arterial supply to the right liver may be from the superior mesenteric artery. The right branch of the hepatic artery and the portal vein divide into two sectorial branches. The branch to the anterio-medial sector divides to supply segments five and eight and the postero-lateral sector divides to supply segments six and seven.

On the left side, the left branch of the hepatic artery and the left branch of the portal vein run together along the posterior aspect of the quadrate lobe where they supply the quadrate lobe anteriorly and superiorly, and the caudate lobe inferiorly and posteriorly. On reaching the umbilical fissure they turn abruptly anteriorly. At the angle branches are given to segment two and, as they run anteriorly, branches are given to segments three and four.

Venous drainage of the liver is by three main hepatic veins. The right hepatic vein lies between the right medial and lateral sectors and drains the adjacent parts of segments five, six, seven, and eight. The medial hepatic vein runs along the imaginary line between the gallbladder and the inferior vena cava (the principal plane between the right and left liver) and drains the adjacent parts of segments four, five, and eight. The left hepatic vein runs between the left medial and lateral sectors, and drains segment two, three, and four. The medial and the left hepatic veins join together before entering the inferior vena cava. In about 30 per cent of patients, the right liver has two hepatic veins, the main vein and a right inferior hepatic vein which usually drains segments five and six. The caudate lobe drains directly into the inferior vena cava through three and five pairs of small veins.

Biliary drainage

Biliary drainage of the right and left livers is by the right and left main hepatic ducts which converge at the hilus to form the common hepatic duct. The caudate lobe is usually drained separately by one or more ducts which join the right or left main hepatic ducts. The main hepatic ducts form from the intrahepatic ducts whose branches correspond to those of the hepatic artery and portal vein. Within each segment of liver the branch of the bile duct tends to lie above that of the portal vein and hepatic artery.

Physiology of the liver

The normal liver has an enormous capacity to regenerate, making it possible successfully to resect up to 80 per cent of liver volume, leaving only two segments (for example, the left lateral sector comprising segments two and three). The right liver comprises 60 per cent of the liver parenchyma and the left liver comprises 40 per cent (segments two and three comprise 15 per cent and segment four 25 per cent). In patients with liver cirrhosis the liver has an impaired ability to regenerate. It is therefore very difficult in these patients to assess how much liver may be resected safely while avoiding post-operative liver failure. The severity of liver disease in patients with cirrhosis may be categorized using the Child's classification (Christensen, *et al.* 1984). The extent of liver resection which may safely be performed varies with this grading: the more severe the liver disease the smaller the resection which is feasible. As a general rule in patients with Child's grade A liver cirrhosis one can resect up to 50 per cent of liver parenchyma, Child's B up to 25 per cent, and Child's C up to 10 per cent. Recently other factors important to outcome have been suggested, such as the degree of inflammation in the non-tumoral liver parenchyma.

Pathology and the resection of liver lesions

Primary malignant liver tumours may be divided into those arising from the hepatocyte (hepatocellular carcinoma and fibrolamellar carcinoma), the bile duct epithelium (cholangiocarcinoma) and those from the endothelium (haemangiosarcoma). The most common malignant tumours found in the liver, however, are secondary cancers.

Hepatocellular carcinoma

This tumour shows a marked geographical variation in its incidence, being far more common in Africa and Far East Asia than in the West. It is strongly associated with liver cirrhosis and factors that may produce chronic liver disease such as hepatitis B virus (Sherman and Shafritz 1984), alcohol (Lee 1966), aflatoxin (Krishnamarchari, Nagarajan, Bhat, and Tilak 1975), anabolic steriods (Sweeney and Evans 1976), α_1-antitrypsin deficiency (Eriksson and Hagerstrand 1974), and the oral contraceptive pill (Davis, Portmann, Searle, Wright, and Williams 1975). It is associated with a very poor prognosis, with death in 3–4 months if untreated (Okuda, *et al.* 1984). Macroscopically, the tumour may form either discrete (massive/nodular) or diffuse (multifocal) lesions, usually within an obviously cirrhotic liver. Some lesions are well encapsulated. Microscopically, the diagnosis is usually based on the resemblance between the tumour cells and normal hepatocytes (abundant eosinophilic cytoplasm, polygonal cells, vesicular nucleus with a recognizable nucleolus). In general a poor correlation had been found between the cellular features and prognosis (Lai, Wu, Lam, and Todd 1979). This includes the presence or absence of bile pigment secretion, a feature pathognomonic of hepatocellular carcinoma. Hepatocellular carcinoma frequently metastasizes to other parts of the liver and to the lungs.

Bile duct cancer

Bile duct cancer (cholangiocarcinoma) is a rare form of tumour but its incidence may be on the increase (Broden, Ahliberg, Bengtsson, and Hellers 1978). These tumours mainly affect people aged 50–70 years and patients usually die within a year due to biliary obstruction, cholangitis, and liver failure. The aetiology is unknown. The lesions of a cholangiocarcinoma may be papillary, nodular, or diffuse, each type of lesion having different pathological features. Papillary tumours are mainly confined to the distal common bile duct. They grow into the lumen and are associated with sclerosis of the duct walls. Nodular cholangiocarcinomas form a small, well-circumscribed lesion projecting into the lumen in the upper half of the biliary tree. The diffuse lesion produces duct thickening over an extensive area with luminal narrowing and inflammation of the surrounding tissues.

Vascular tumours

Angiosarcoma is rare but is the main form of malignant liver tumour of endothelial origin. Exposure to chemical agents (arsenic, thorium dioxide, and vinyl chloride) has been implicated in its development. Multiple lesions are usually present, often associated with marked fibrosis.

Indications and contra-indications to liver resection for tumours

Surgery for liver tumours may be considered as either curative treatment, or for the palliation of symptoms. Both primary and secondary tumours may be considered for resection whether single or multiple if contained within a resectable area of the liver (see surgical anatomy).

Is the lesion technically resectable?

Liver tumours are generally considered to be resectable if there is no metastatic spread, either distant or to another area within the liver. Involvement of the inferior vena cava, the portal vein, or the main biliary tree are often considered to be contra-indications to surgery although some surgeons may consider resecting the diaphragm, synchronous metastases, and segments of the portal vein or inferior vena cava.

Will the patient survive the procedure?

An assessment of whether the patients will survive the procedure depends on an accurate history and examination of the patient before operation, with particular emphasis being placed on the patient's age, previous abdominal surgery, and a history of ischaemic heart or chronic respiratory disease. The extent of liver resection which can be carried out is very dependent on the function of the remaining segments or lobe of liver. This may be very difficult to assess before operation, but patients with hepatitis or cirrhosis are in great danger of post-operative liver failure. It is therefore advisable to biopsy the 'normal' liver, pre-operatively where an extensive resection is envisaged, to exclude the presence of liver cirrhosis.

Will the patient's quality or length of life be improved?

A judgement as to whether the patient's quality or length of life may be improved is perhaps the most difficult factor to assess. Surgery being undertaken to relieve symptoms, rather than for potential cure, can be justified only in centres where the morbidity and mortality rates of the procedure are minimal. The long-term results that have been reported for the treatment of different types of tumour should always be borne in mind before recommending resection (see long-term results).

Pre-operative investigations and preparation for liver surgery

The aim of the pre-operative investigations is to provide an accurate diagnosis, to stage the disease, to assess resectability, and to gauge the fitness of the patient for surgery. The standard pre-operative management of a patient should include the following investigations.

Ultrasonography

This non-invasive procedure allows the size and shape of a tumour to be measured and gives information on its consistency and its relationship to major vessels and bile ducts. The information is often complementary rather than an alternative to computer tomographic (CT) scanning.

CT scanning

This is the standard method of staging the tumour. It gives information on the site, size, and consistency of the tumour, allows other lesions in the liver to be detected, and provides information regarding the relationship of the tumour to major structures. Contrast enhancement of the scans provides additional information on the vascularity of the tumours and their relationship to blood vessels. Lipiodol, a contrast agent extracted from poppy seed oil, is retained by primary hepatocellular carcinomas and may be administered at hepatic angiography and subsequently used as a method of detecting occult tumour deposits in the liver by CT scanning. Figure 15.2 shows the typical appearance on CT scanning of a large hepatocellular carcinoma in the right lobe of the liver.

Hepatic angiography

This technique allows the vascularity of the tumours to be assessed. It also shows the vascular supply to the liver itself, as well as any congenital anomalies such as branches from the left gastric or the superior mesenteric arteries. The venous phase outlines the portal vein and may reveal occlusion, displacement, or encasement. The inferior vena cava is not well dem-

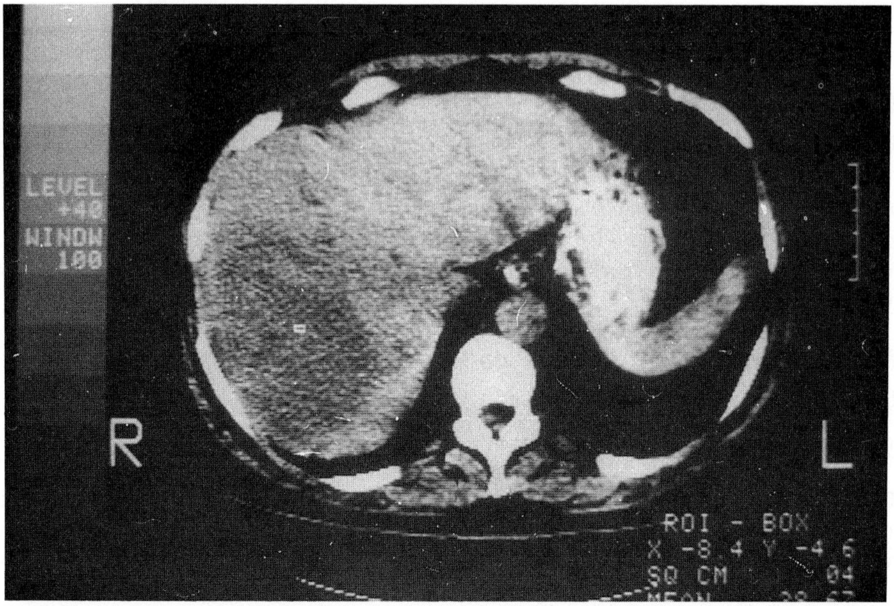

Fig. 15.2. Computed tomographic scan appearances of a primary liver cell cancer.

onstrated and inferior vena cavography or magnetic resonance imaging should be employed if invasion is considered to be a possibility.

Biopsy

Percutaneous biopsy of a lesion allows a definitive diagnosis to be obtained before operation. It may, however, rarely lead to tumour dissemination along the needle track and is, therefore, thought inadvisable by some (Thompson, Gibson, Czerniak, and Blumgart 1985). Biopsy guns which are presently under evaluation may avoid this complication. 'Normal liver' should be biopsied in patients the suspected of having liver cirrhosis since its presence will influence the extent of resection which may be carried out without producing post-operative liver insufficiency.

Investigations of liver function and underlying liver disease

Liver function tests give an indication of the depth of jaundice (bilirubin), hepatocellular dysfunction (transaminases), biliary obstruction (bilirubin and alkaline phosphatase), and synthetic function (albumin). Patients with poor liver function also fail adequately to synthesize clotting factors and should be commenced on vitamin K (10 mg intramuscularly twice daily) before operation with monitoring of their coagulation profiles. Serum should also be screened for the presence of hepatitis B or C virus antigens and, if present, whether there is replicating virus.

Tumour markers

The most useful markers are α-feto-protein which is insensitive but highly specific for the presence of primary liver cell tumour, and carcino-embryonic antigen which is often raised in the presence of hepatic metastases from gastrointestinal cancer. The carbohydrate antigens CA 19.9 and CA 50 may prove to be of value in differentiating benign from malignant biliary strictures (Itzkowitz 1986).

The search for extra-hepatic metastases

Tests should include a CT scan of the chest and a radio-isotope bone scan.

Endoscopic or percutaneous cholangiography

This is indicated in patients presenting with obstructive jaundice and enables any involvement of the biliary tree by tumour to be accurately assessed and pre-operative biliary drainage procedures to be performed. Pre-operative resolution of jaundice is likely to confer considerable benefit to the function of the residual liver following resection.

Routine investigations

A full blood count, urea and electrolytes, blood grouping, chest radiography, and electrocardiography (ECG) are mandatory. If there is a history of chronic respiratory problems then baseline respiratory function tests and arterial blood gas analysis should be performed.

Preparation for surgery

A fully informed consent is obtained for all procedures with adequate explanation of any possible complications. Eight units of blood is cross-matched for all patients undergoing liver surgery. If the patient is cirrhotic or has a coagulopathy, fresh frozen plasma is also required. All patients are given prophylactic antibiotics on induction (cefotaxime 2 g or cefuroxime 1.5 g with metronidazole 500 mg intravenously) along with two post-operative doses at 6 and 12 hours.

Operative techniques

Positioning the patient

The patient is positioned supine on the table but with rotation to the left by placing a wedge under the lower right chest. Elevation of the head of the table encourages the bowel to remain in the lower compartment of the abdomen.

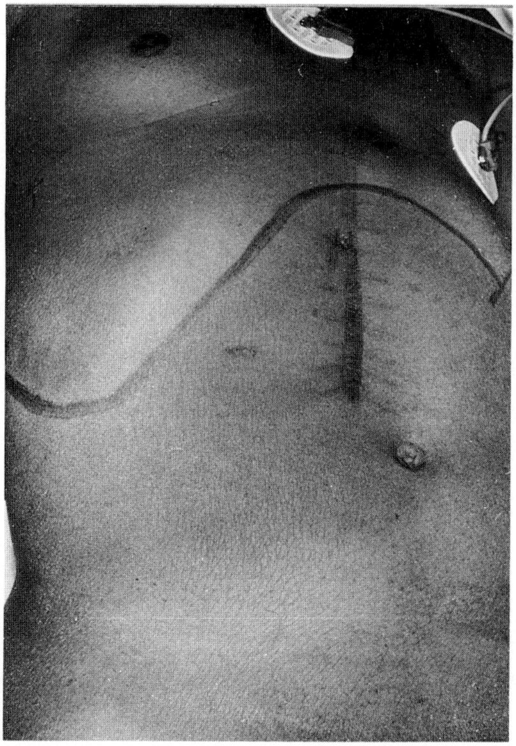

Fig. 15.3. The S incision.

Skin incision

Two incisions can be made.

S incision (Fig. 15.3)

This is suitable for patients with a wide sternal angle. It starts below the left costal margin by dividing the left rectus muscle and proceeds along the right costal margin through the right rectus, around the angle of the rib cage, and continuing upwards parallel to the ribs in the direction of the renal angle. The last part of the incision facilitates traction of the costal margin upwards with direct access to the vena cava and the hepatic veins.

Transverse incision with mid-line extension (Fig. 15.4)

This is preferred if the sternal angle is acute. A transverse incision is made at the level of the lower rib cage with extension towards the right renal angle and upwards in the mid-line to the xiphisternum. This incision is sometimes called the modified 'Mercedes Benz' incision and gives two flaps of anterior abdominal wall, which can be retracted by stitching to the skin over the

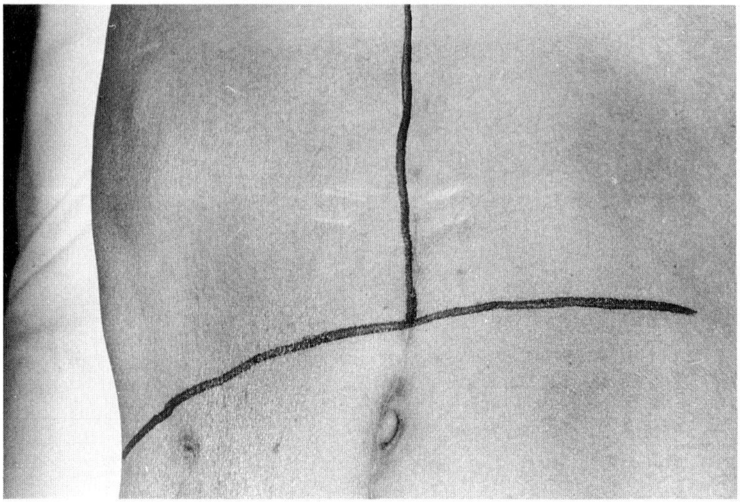

Fig. 15.4. Transverse incision with mid-line extension.

chest wall. Regardless of the choice of incision used, care is required at the right extremity of the incision not to open the right pleural space.

Rectraction

It is important to have good retraction of both right and left costal margins during the entire procedure. Fixed retractors are suitable for this purpose. Following retraction of the rib cage one can proceed to exploratory laparotomy and exclude the presence of findings that would contra-indicate liver resection.

Mobilisation of the liver

The falciform ligament, connecting the liver to the undersurface of the diaphragm, is divided in the antero-posterior direction using a cutting diathermy needle. Posteriorly the falciform ligament divides into two leaves, to the right and to the left. This point is at least 2 cm proximal to the hepatic veins or the supra-hepatic vena cava. At this stage one proceeds towards the left lobe of the liver by dividing the left triangular ligament, watching for a low insertion of a left subphrenic vein. To facilitate the incision of the left triangular ligament the stomach can be protected by positioning an abdominal pack between the left lobe of the liver and the stomach. Haemostasis is normally secured with diathermy.

After division of the left triangular ligament, mobilization of the left lobe is completed by incising the lesser omentum, being careful to avoid an aberrant left hepatic artery originating from the left gastric artery. Following mobilization of the left liver, the right leaf of the falciform ligament is divided along the right triangular ligament. This may be facilitated by the assistant's left hand rotating the liver towards the left and inferiorly. Mobilization of the inferior surface of the liver starts by dividing any adhesions between the liver or the gallbladder, large bowel, small bowel, or duodenum. The peritoneum between the inferior surface of the liver and the anterior surface of the right kidney is then divided and the incision proceeds towards the right to join the upper leaf of the right triangular ligament. At this stage of the dissection the assistant retracts with his or her right hand the inferior pole of the right liver upwards in the direction of the patient's left shoulder. It is this rotation of the liver that facilitates the posterior dissection, particularly in the bare area.

The peritoneum overlying the inferior vena cava is then divided and the right side of the liver is mobilized further. This is facilitated by the assistant retracting the right side of the liver upwards using the left hand. Any tissue remaining between the posterior surface of the liver and the posterior abdominal wall is divided, great care being taken not to damage the right adrenal vein as it enters the inferior vena cava. At this point attention is turned to the hilar dissection.

Hilar dissection

The foramen ovale is identified and a sling placed around the structures at the free edge of the lesser omentum in order to gain control of the hepatic pedicle in case of sudden bleeding (Pringle manoeuvre). Hilar dissection starts with mobilization of the gallbladder and cholecystectomy, leaving a long remnant of the cystic duct. The common bile duct is dissected free and retracted with a sling. Dissection of the left aspect of the hepatic pedicle exposes the common hepatic artery. The right and left dranches of the hepatic artery are dissected and retracted with slings. Retraction of the common bile duct to the right, and the hepatic artery to the left, allows the portal vein to be located in the space between these two structures. Dissection of the portal vein is undertaken cautiously with a blunt instrument, care being taken not to injure its small branches. Once the portal vein is dissected a sling is passed around so that good control of this structure can be achieved if necessary. Dissection of the portal vein towards the hilus exposes the right and left branches of the portal vein. The right branch of the portal vein may be more easily approached from the right aspect of the hepatic pedicle. To improve access the assistant rotates the hepatic pedicle so that its posterior aspect faces the right side of the patient. Great care is needed to avoid brances from the caudate lobe as they enter the right branch of the portal vein. The left branch of the portal vein may be more easily approached from the left of the hepatic pedicle.

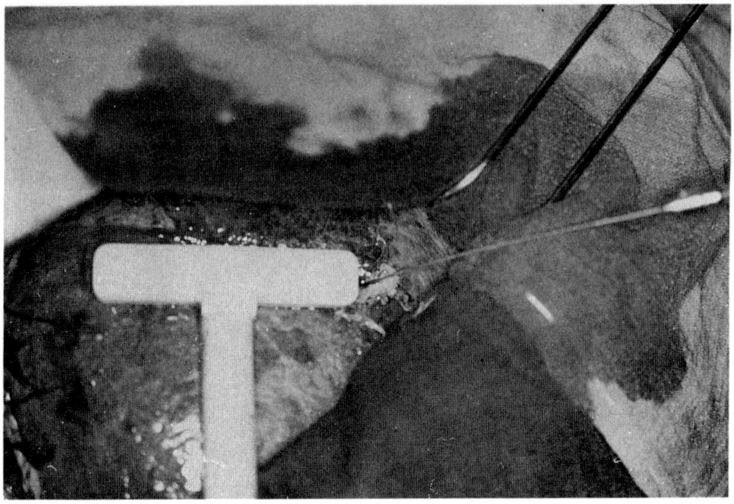

Fig. 15.5. Use of the intra-operative ultrasound probe.

Choice of hepatic resection

Following full mobilization of the liver an intra-operative ultrasound scan may be performed (Fig. 15.5). This helps to assess tumour spread and allows the main structures in the liver to be visualized, such as the course of the right, left, or middle hepatic veins. It is at this stage that the final decision is made as to whether it is justifiable to proceed with a liver resection and the type of resection to be performed.

Right hepatectomy

This procedure involves the removal of that portion of the liver to the right side of the imaginary line extending from the gallbladder fossa to the interior vena cava. Before performing the resection it is necessary to mobilize the liver fully and to gain control of the major vessels.

Inferior vena cava control

The infra-hepatic portion of the inferior vena cava is dissected by extending the incision of the posterior parietal peritoneum over the lateral aspect of the inferior vena cava, which may then be encircled by a sling. The supra-hepatic vena cava is also dissected by incising the overlying peritoneum. The tributaries of the right and left inferior phrenic veins into the inferior vena cava are avoided. Once the supra-hepatic vena cava has been isolated, caval control is achieved. If the cava has to be clamped during the operative procedure a significant drop in blood pressure will result. This may be minimized by the anaesthetist over-filling the vascular bed before clamping.

Dissection of the right hepatic vein

Before dissection of the right hepatic vein, the small veins to the caudate lobe are secured (see surgical anatomy). This is facilitated by the left hand of the assistant rotating the liver towards the patient's left side. The veins, of which there may be 2–6 pairs, are tied on the liver and transfixed on the side of the inferior vena cava. Bleeding from a missed caudate vein is a common cause of post-operative blood loss. After dissection and ligation of these small veins an accessory right inferior hepatic vein may be encountered (approximately 30 per cent of cases). It is important to recognize, dissect, and transfix this vein. Further cephalad dissection reveals the right hepatic vein which lies within a sheet of fibrous tissue. Division of this tissue enables dissection of the space between the right and left hepatic veins which is cautiously performed with a blunt instrument. If this plane cannot be readily dissected, no further mobilization of the right hepatic vein should be attempted, the vein being ligated following division of the liver parenchyma. If major haemorrhage occurs during dissection of the right hepatic vein a Pringle manoeuvre, along with clamping of the supra-hepatic and infra-hepatic vena cava, should be performed until the bleeding point can be arrested. The source of the haemorrhage may be isolated most readily by dividing and transfixing the right hepatic vein. Clamping of the vena cava is very important in this situation as the patient may die instantaneously from a massive air embolus rather than haemorrhage.

Vascular control before parenchymal resection

The right branch of the hepatic artery and the right branch of the portal vein are ligated with silk or linen. If division of these branches is postponed until a later stage then the decision to perform hepatectomy remains reversible. Having emptied the right liver of blood the right hepatic vein is tied in continuity with silk or linen, but is not divided outside the liver. Following ligation of the vessels to the right liver, division of the hepatic parenchyma is commenced.

Hepatic parenchymal resection

Following ligation of the right branches of the hepatic artery and the portal vein, a line of devascularization forms between the right and the left livers. The resection line is made 1 cm to the right of this demarcation line (right side of the patient). If possible the middle hepatic vein, which lies in this plane, should be preserved. It may be located using intra-operative ultra-sonography (Fig. 15.5). Resection commences by incising Glisson's capsule and proceeds by gently crushing the liver parenchyma with a haemostat. This technique allows separation of the parenchyma while the blood vessels

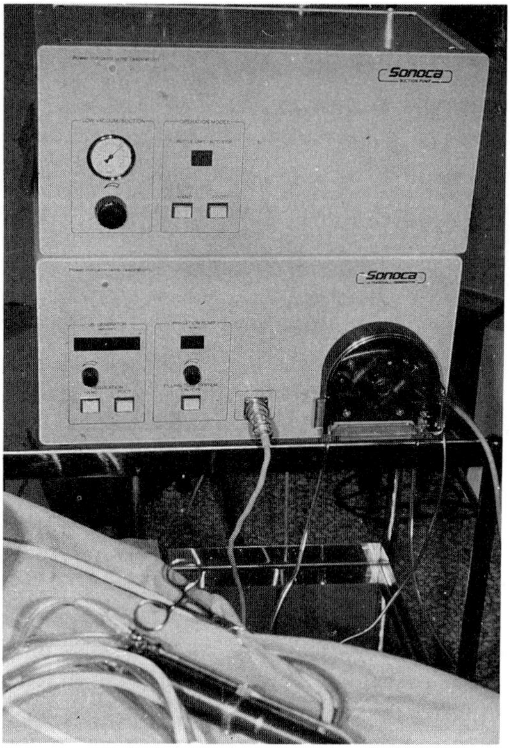

Fig. 15.6. The ultrasonic dissector.

and bile ducts remain intact. Alternatively the ultrasonic dissector may be used (Fig. 15.6). The remaining branches are either ligated or diathermied. If significant bleeding occurs from the liver parenchyma, the Pringle manoeuvre may be performed with release every 15 minutes for 2 minutes. The direction of liver division is important, being towards the right side of the inferior vena cava. The dissection is kept some distance from the hilus to prevent injury to the biliary confluence. The segmental blood supply to the right liver is secured within the liver parenchyma by transfixion. Once the level of the hilus is reached, the operator's left hand should be placed behind the right side of the liver at the site of insertion of the right caudate veins in the vena cava. By placing the fingers of the left hand in the groove formed by the inferior vena cava the operator will help the direction of the dissection and avoid damaging the middle or left hepatic veins. Branches from the middle hepatic vein are transfixed as bleeding at this stage may be difficult to control. When the posterior part of the liver is reached, the right hepatic vein is clamped and transfixed from within the liver parenchyma, and the right liver is removed.

Haemostasis

Time should be spent in securing all the bleeding points, usually by transfixion, following the hepatic resection. Sites which require special attention to haemostasis include the cut surface of the liver, the inferior phrenic veins as they enter the inferior vena cava, and the right triangular ligament. If difficulty is encountered in securing haemostasis from the cut surface of the liver this may be packed with gauze for 10 minutes, the upper and lower capsules of the liver may be approximated by suturing, the infra-red coagulator used or a haemostatic glue applied. Any biliary leak may be delineated by injecting methylene blue into the cystic duct following a Pringle manoeuvre, any area where the blue dye emerges being transfixed. If haemostasis is secured there is no need for drainage. Omentum and the hepatic flexure of the colon can be encouraged to occupy the place of the right liver. Rotation of the liver should be avoided by stitching back the falciform ligament.

Right hepatectomy extended to the quadrate lobe

This dissection was formerly called a right trisegmentectomy. It is mainly performed for tumour of the right side encroaching on the quadrate lobe (segment four) and involves resection of the right liver as described above along with the quadrate lobe. Dissection at the hilus in this situation must be carried out most carefully as the hilar structures are excised, except for the left branches of the hepatic artery and portal vein. The biliary convergence is excised and the left hepatic duct is anastomosed to a Roux-en-Y jejunal loop in order to establish biliary digestive continuity. Mobilization of the liver and ligation of the vascular structures is the same as that described for right hepatectomy. During parenchymal resection the dissection starts on the left side of the falciform ligament between segments three and four. This dissection must ensure that the vascular supply to segments two and three is preserved and proceeds towards the hilus and the right side of the inferior vena cava. It is essential to avoid ligation of the left hepatic vein posteriorly. The method of parenchymal resection is similar to that described for right hepatectomy. Every effort is made to leave the middle hepatic vein intact although this may not be possible.

Biliary digestive anastomosis

Biliary reconstruction following a right hepatectomy extended to the quadrate lobe may be performed by formation of a biliary enteric anastomosis between the left main hepatic duct and a Roux-en-Y jejunal loop. In the presence of a dilated left ductal system this anastomosis may be performed with a continuous 3/0 PDS® suture, but if the duct is not dilated then interrupted 5/0 PDS® sutures are more appropriate. If the caudate lobe is left *in situ*, its duct should be included in the biliary anastomosis.

Left lobectomy

This involves removal of segments two and three and constitutes one of the easier liver resections to perform. The initial steps of mobilizing the liver are as described for right hepatectomy. A sling is passed around the hepatic pedicle to enable a Pringle manoeuvre to be performed during the dissection but there is no need separately to identify the portal structures or to have slings around the vena cava. The hepatic resection is performed to the left of the falciform ligament. If the line of dissection moves to the right of this line the vascular supply to the quadrate lobe may be compromised. Following incision of the Glisson capsule, the liver parenchyma is crushed and ligated in an anterior–posterior direction. The main segmental supplies to segments two and three are tied successively (the arterial, portal, and biliary radicals). The left hepatic vein is ligated and divided within the substance of the liver and the middle hepatic vein is left intact.

Abdominal closure and drainage

If complete haemostasis is achieved the abdomen is closed without drainage and the cavity left after the liver resection is filled with greater omentum. Alternatively tube drains are placed in the residual cavity, and in the hepatorenal pouch, and these are removed on the fourth after day operation. Mass closure of the abdominal wall is carried out using 1 Nylon, followed by interrupted 2/0 Vicryl® sutures to the subcutaneous fat and subcuticular 2/0 Prolene® to skin.

Post-operative care

These procedures in experienced hands are possible with the minimum of trauma. Routine liver resections may be performed with blood loss of less than 1 litre and occasionally without intra-operative blood transfusion. In uncomplicated cases, anaesthesia can be reversed and the patient extubated on the operating table and transferred to the ward for post-operative care. If the procedure is prolonged or there are intra-operative difficulties then an initial period of intensive are monitoring is preferable.

Intravenous fluid

It is important to maintain the central venous pressure between 5 and 10 mmHg after operation and this is achieved by giving a combination of crystalloid and colloid solutions. Patients with liver cirrhosis should be treated initially with colloid, either in the form of plasma protein fraction of salt-poor albumin.

Ventilation

In most cases it is not necessary artificially to ventilate these patients post-operatively and it is sufficient to administer 40 per cent oxygen by mask. Physiotherapy in the immediate post-operative period is important to ensure lung expansion. Post-operative chest radiography should be carried out to exlude the occurrence of a right pneumothorax during mobilization of the right liver.

Renal function

It is important to maintain a urine output of approximately 40 ml per hour, and patients with obstructive jaundice or cirrhosis are routinely given a 'renal' dose of dopamine of 2–5 $\mu g\ kg^{-1}\ min^{-1}$. Oliguria in a post-operative patient who is normotensive, well hydrated, and with a normal central venous filling pressure should be treated with an initial fluid challenge and, if this is not successful, a bolus injection of 20 mg of frusemide.

Liver function

Patients in whom more than 50 per cent of the liver has been removed will develop a certain degree of liver failure. This is declared by an elevated prothrombin time, bilirubin, alkaline phosphatase, and aspartate transaminase. These parameters usually return to normal after 4–5 days. Patients with obstructive jaundice or liver cirrhosis are particularly susceptible to abnormalities of liver function. The patient should be actively supported with fluids, nutrition, and clotting factors until liver regeneration takes place (Bismuth, *et al.* 1983).

Complications

These can be divided into early (first 48 hours), intermediate (first week after operation), and late.

Early complications

The main early post-operative complications are haemorrhage and respiratory problems. Haemorrhage may declare itself post-operatively as a low blood pressure, central venous pressure, or urine output along with an increasing pulse rate and respiratory rate. The presence of a coagulopathy should always be suspected and any clotting abnormality corrected with fresh frozen plasma, before undergoing a further laparotomy. Bleeding is usually encountered from the transection line, the hepatic veins, or the caudate lobe veins. Respiratory problems usually arise from post-operative pulmonary atelectasis although a pneumothorax should always be excluded. Physiotherapy or bronchial aspiration may be necessary to treat collapse.

Intermediate complications

The commonest is post-operative liver failure. This may be due to the extent of resection of liver parenchyma, especially in a compromised liver (cirrhosis or obstruction). Active supportive therapy is given until liver regeneration occurs. Renal failure may arise as part of the hepato-renal syndrome associated with liver failure. This may be reversed with careful fluid replacement monitored by central venous pressure measurements and the administration of a renal dose of dopamine. If major problems are encountered with post-operative liver or kidney failure then the surgeon should seek help from a hepatologist or nephrologist.

Sepsis

Infective complications following a liver resection are similar to those following any major intra-abdominal surgery. In addition, a haematoma in the subphrenic cavity secondary to liver resection occasionally results in the development of a subphrenic abscess. Patients with ascites are in danger of developing infection within the ascitic fluid after operation.

Chyle leak

This occurs due to damage to the lymphatics at the liver hilus, and presents most frequently after the patient resumes dietary intake. The leak can reach enormous quantities and usually lasts for 3–4 days before resolution, fluid replacement being provided in the form of colloid.

Late complications

Liver resection is usually free from long-term complications due to the ability of the normal liver to regenerate. If these do occur they are usually attributable to tumour recurrence.

Survival following surgery for hepatocellular carcinoma

The two main complications of liver resection are haemorrhage and post-operative liver failure. Each is most commonly encountered in patients with hepatocellular carcinoma and liver cirrhosis. The reported operative mortality rate varies greatly from less than 5 per cent (Leese and Bismuth 1989) to almost 50 per cent (El-Domeiri, Huvos, Goldsmith, and Foote 1971). Many authors have highlighted the increased morbidity and mortality rates of surgery when liver cirrhosis is present (Sorenson, *et al.* 1979; Huguet and Mouiel 1983) and the risks may be stratified by the pre-operative liver function and the size of resection required. Long-term survival following successful resection is also variable. Smith reported a 28 per cent 2-year survival rate (Smith 1979) whereas Foster and Berman (1977) documented that 68 per cent of patients were alive after 2 years. More informative, perhaps, is the 5-year survival rate which may be as low as 4 per cent (Huguet and Mouiel 1983) or as high as 32 per cent (Iwatsuki and Starzl 1988).

Survival following surgery for liver metastases

Surgery is indicated in only a percentage of patients with liver metastases and, of these, patients with colorectal cancer appear most likely to benefit. The natural history of untreated colorectal cancer metastases has been investigated and 8–20 per cent of patients with untreated solitary metastases will be alive after 3 years (Wood, Gillis, and Blumgart 1976; Wagner, Adson, van Heerden, Adson, and Illstrup 1984). Surgery for solitary metastases, however, may be associated with a 30 per cent survival rate at 10 years (Adson and van Heerden 1980; Wilson and Adson 1976) and may be performed with a minimal morbidity and mortality (Iwatsuki, *et al.* 1988; Holm, Bradley, and Aldrete 1989). Unfortunately only about 5 per cent of patients with colorectal cancer develop a solitary metastasis, one in four of all patients presenting with liver metastases (Ridge and Daly 1985). Even when several metastases are present in one lobe of the liver, however, a 20–40 per cent 5-year survival rate may be obtained by surgical resection (Kortz, Meyers, Hanks, Schrimer, and Jones 1984; Butler, Attiyeh, and Daly 1986). These results would suggest that an active policy should be employed for the detection of surgical resection of liver metastases following surgery for colon cancer, but remains controversial.

Survival following surgery for cholangiocarcinoma

The survival rate of patients with cholangiocarcinoma is generally poor, independent of the form of treatment. A recent review of the results of surgical resection from a major centre showed an operative mortality rate in 22 patients of 23 per cent, but good palliation in survivors, with two patients surviving for more than 10 years (Bengmark, Ekberg, Evander, Klofer-Stahl, and Tranberg 1988). A more radical surgical approach to resection of these tumours has been employed and has shown encouraging early results with 10 of 13 patients resected surviving for between 13 and 35 months (Lygidakis, van der Heyde, van Dongen, Kromhout, Tytgat, and Huibregtse 1988). In patients who are not suitable for resection, palliative procedures may be considered with the possible options, including a segment-three biliary enteric anastomosis (Chio, Fan, Lai, and Wong 1988), endoscopic intubation (Deviere, Baize, de Toueuf, and Cremer 1988) and operative insertion of a U-tube (Terblanche, Kahn, Bornman, and Werner 1988). An alternative approach for tumours unsuitable for resection is liver transplantation. Ringe, Wittekind, Bechstein, Bunzendahl, and Pichlmayr (1989) reported a median survival of 7.5 months in transplanted patients with regional node involvement and 35 months if nodes were not involved. Starzl's results of transplantation for cholangiocarcinoma are similarly pessimistic with no patient surviving for more than 2 years (Iwatsaki *et al.* 1988).

Perspectives in liver surgery

Over the past decade liver resection has become established as the optimal method of management for primary liver cancers, bile duct cancers, and metastases in the liver. Although liver resection in the early days was considered a hazardous and heroic procedure, the currently reported morbidity and mortality rates are similar to those of other major abdominal operations. These results should encourage a more frequent performance of liver resections and the evaluation of adjuvant radiotherapy, chemotherapy, or immunotherapy.

References

Adson, M.A. and van Heerden, J.A. (1980). Major hepatic resections for metastatic colorectal cancer. *Ann. Surg.* **191**, 576–83.

Bengmark, S., Ekberg, H., Evander, A., Klofer-Stahl, B., and Tranberg, K.G. (1988). Major liver resection for hilar cholangiocarcinoma. *Ann. Surg.* **20**, 120–5.

Bismuth, H. (1982). Surgical anatomy and anatomical surgery of the liver. *World J. Surg.* **6**, 3–9.

Bismuth, H., Houssin, D., and Mazmanian, G. (1983). Postoperative liver insufficiency: prevention and management. *World J. Surg.* **7**, 505–50.

Broden, G., Ahliberg, J., Bengtsson, L., and Hellers, G. (1978). The incidence of carcinoma of the gallbladder and bile ducts in Sweden, 1958 to 1972. *Acta Chir. Scand. Suppl.* **482**, 24–5.

Butler, J., Attiyeh, F.F., and Daly, J.M. (1986). Hepatic resection for metastases of the colon and rectum. *Surg. Gyn. Obstet.* **162**, 109–13.

Choi, T.K., Fan, S.T., Lai, E.C. and Wong, J. (1988). Malignant hilar biliary obstruction treated by segmental bilioenteric anastomosis. *Surgery* **104**, 525–9.

Couinaud, C. (1957). *Etudes anatomiques et chirugicales*. Masson, Paris.

Christensen, E., Schlichting, P., Fauerholdt, L., *et al.* (1986). Prognostic value of Child Turcotte criteria in medically treated cirrhosis. *Hepatology* **4**, 430–5.

Davis, M., Portmann, B., Searle, M., Wright, R., and Williams, R. (1975). Histological evidence of a carcinoma in a hepatic tumour associated with oral contraceptives. *Br. Med. J.* **4**, 496–8.

Deviere, J., Baize, M., de Toueuf, J., and Cremer, M. (1988). Long term follow up of patients with hilar malignant stricture treated by endoscopic internal biliary drainage. *Gastrointest. Endosc.* **34**, 95–101.

El-Domeiri, A.A., Huvos, A.G., Goldsmith, H.S., and Foote, F.W. (1971). Primary malignant tumours of the liver. *Cancer* **27**, 7.

Eriksson, S. and Hagerstrand, I. (1974). Cirrhosis and malignant hepatoma in alpha$_1$ A T deficiency. *Acta Med. Scand.* **195**, 451–8.

Foster, J.H. and Berman, M.M. (1977). Solid liver tumours. In *Major problems in clinical surgery*, Vol. 22, W.B. Saunders, Philadelphia.

Holm, A., Bradley, E., and Aldrete, J.S. (1989). Hepatic resection of metastasis from colorectal cancer. Morbidity, mortality and pattern of recurrence. *Ann. Surg.* **209**, 428–34.

Huguet, C.I. and Mouiel, J. (1983). *Les tumeurs primitives du foie chez l'adulte.* Masson, Paris.

Itzkowitz, S. (1986). New carbohydrate tumour markers. *Gastroenterology* **90**, 491–4.

Iwatsuki, S. and Starzl, T.E. (1988). Personal experience with 411 hepatic resections. *Ann. Surg.* **208**, 421–34.

Iwatsuki, S., Starzl, T.E., Todd, D., *et al.* (1988). Experience in 1,000 liver transplants under cyclosporin-steroid therapy. *Transplant Proc.* **20** (Supplement 1), 489–504.

Keen, W.W. (1899). Report of a case of resection of the liver for the removal of a neoplasm with a table of twenty-six cases of resection of the liver for hepatic tumor. *Ann. Surg.* **30**, 267–83.

Kortz, W.J., Meyers, W.C., Hanks, J.B., Schrimer, B.D., and Jones, R.S. (1984). Hepatic resection for metastatic cancer. *Ann. Surg.* **199**, 182–6.

Krishnamarchari, K.A., Nagarajan, B., Bhat, R.U., and Tilak, T.B. (1975). Hepatitis due to aflatoxicosis. *Lancet* **ii**, 1061–3.

Lai, C.L., Wu, P.C., Lam, K.C., and Tood, D. (1979). Histologic prognostic indicators in hepatocellular carcinoma. *Cancer* **44**, 1677–83.

Lee, F.I. (1966). Cirrhosis and hepatoma in alcoholics. *Gut* **7**, 77–85.

Leese, T., Bismuth, H. (1989). Surgical management of space occupying lesions in the liver. *Baillière's Clin. Gastroenterol.* **3**, 253–77.

Lortat-Jacob, J.L. and Robert, H.G. (1952). Hepatectomie droite regle. *Presse Med.* **60**, 549–50.

Lygidakis, N.J., van der Heyde, M.N. van Dongen, R.J., Kromhout, J.G., Tytgat, G.N., and Huibregtse, K. (1988). Surgical approaches for unresectable primary carcinoma of the hepatic hilus. *Surg. Gynecol. Obstet.* **166**, 107–14.

Okuda, K., Obata, H., Nakajima, Y., *et al.* (1984). Prognosis of primary hepatocellular carcinoma. *Hepatology* **4**, 55–65.

Pringle, J.G. (1908). Notes on the arrest of hepatic hemorrhage due to trauma. *Ann. Surg.* **48**, 541–9.

Ridge, J.A. and Daly, J.M. (1985). Treatment of colorectal hepatic metastases. *Surg. Gynecol. Obstet.* **161**, 597–607.

Ringe, B., Wittekind, C., Bechstein, W.O., Bunzendahl, H., and Pichlmayr, R. (1989). The role of liver transplantation in hepatobiliary malignancy: a retrospective analysis of 95 patients with particular regard to tumor stage and recurrence. *Ann. Surg.* **1**, 88–98.

Sherman, M. and Shafritz, D.A. (1984). Hepatitis B virus and hepatocellular carcinoma: molecular biology and mechanistic considerations. *Semin. Liver Dis.* **4**, 98–109.

Smith, R. (1979). Tumours of the liver. *Ann. R. Coll. Surg. Engl.* **61**, 87–99.

Sorenson, T.I., Aronsen, K.F., Aune, S., *et al.* (1979). Results of hepatic resection for primary epithelial cancer in 31 adults. *Am. J. Surg.* **138**, 407.

Sweeney, E.C. and Evans, D.J. (1976). Hepatic lesions in patients treated with synthetic anabolic steroids. *J. Clin. Pathol.* **29**, 626–33.

Thompson, J.N., Gibson, R., Czerniak, A., and Blumgart, L.H. (1985). Focal liver lesions: a plan for management. *Br. Med. J.* **290**, 1643–5.

Terblanche, J., Kahn, D., Bornman, P.C., and Werner, D. (1988). The role of U tube palliative treatment in high bile duct carcinoma. *Surgery* **103**, 624–32.

Tiffany, L. (1890). The removal of a solid tumour from the liver by laparotomy. *M. Med. J.* **23**, 531.

Tung, T.T. and Quang, N.D. (1965). L'hepatectomie reglée par ligature vasculaire transparenchymateuse. *Presse Med.* **73**, 3015–17.

Wagner, J.S., Adson, M.A., van Heerden, J.A., Adson, M.H., and Illstrup, D.M. (1984). The natural history of hepatic metastases from colorectal cancer. *Ann. Surg.* **199**, 502–8.

Wilson, S.M. and Adson, M.A. (1976). Surgical treatment of hepatic metastases from colorectal cancers. *Arch. Surg.* **111**, 330–3.

Wood, C.B., Gillis, R., and Blumgart, L.H. (1976). A retrospective study of the natural history of patients with liver metastases from colorectal cancer. *Clin. Oncol.* **2**, 285–8.

16. Treatment of metastatic liver disease

Irving Taylor

The majority of patients with metastatic liver disease are unsuitable for any specific form of therapy. The presence of liver metastasis is a manifestation of widespread malignancy, and usually symptomatic treatment is all that is either required or possible. Nevertheless, there are some tumours which develop as occult liver metastases in the absence of malignancy elsewhere. This appears to be particularly the case with colorectal liver metastases and hence specific treatments have been advocated with possible survival benefit. This situation does not pertain either to other gastrointestinal malignancies which spread to the liver via the portal vein, or to tumours that disseminate via the systemic circulation, for example breast cancer, where extra-hepatic metastases are usually evident.

In this review emphasis is placed predominantly on the indications and treatment options available for colorectal liver metastases, although mention is made of specific treatments available for other primary sites.

Prognosis of liver metastases

In the case of some tumours (for example, pancreatic and gastric liver metastases), prognosis can be measured in terms of a few weeks and no specific treatment has been convincingly shown to prolong survival. For colorectal liver metastases the situation is clearer and more information is available, albeit from retrospective studies. Examples of published survival times for untreated colorectal liver metastases are provided in *Table 16.1*. However, more recent studies have indicated the importance of careful staging of the disease.

The extent of liver involvement is clearly a most important prognostic factor. Wagner, *et al.* (1984) in a careful retrospective study of 252 patients showed a variation in median survival of 10 months for extensive bilateral disease, compared with 15 months when confined to 1 lobe and 21 months for patients with solitary metastases. In addition, 21 per cent of 39 patients with solitary lesions survived for more than 3 years, whereas all patients with multiple disease were dead by 3 years.

Other authors have provided similar data. Neilson, Balslov, and Jensen (1971) found that patients with 'few' metastases had a median survival of 18

Table 16.1. Natural history of patients with colorectal liver metastases.

Reference	No. of patients	Survival (months)	
		Mean	Median
Pestana *et al.* (1964)	353	9	—
Swinton *et al.* (1967)	41	13	7
Jaffe *et al.* (1968)	177	—	5
Bengmark and Hafstrom (1969)	38	8	—
Cady *et al.* (1970)	269	13	—
Baden and Andersen (1975)	105	—	10
Fischerman *et al.* (1976)	49	7	6
Wood *et al.* (1976)	113	7	—
Dawson *et al.* (1986)	61	7	—

months compared with 5 months for those with multiple lesions. Wood (1984) in a prospective study of 101 patients found that 14 per cent of patients had a solitary lesion. In this group, two patients (16 per cent) survived at least 5 years. Goslin, *et al.* (1982) demonstrated that patients with three metastases or fewer had a median survival of 24 months compared with 10 months for patients with four or more lesions.

Other factors that influence survival in untreated patients include the histology of the primary tumour (well-differentiated liver secondaries are more favourable than poorly differentiated ones), extent of surgery to primary tumour (complete resection is superior to bypass), and obviously the presence of extra-hepatic involvement.

It is apparent that patients with a solitary metastasis, and no evidence of extra-hepatic disease, have a prolonged survival if left untreated. In the absence of clinical trials it is not possible to state unequivocally that resection of these lesions (particularly if asymptomatic) is necessarily beneficial to the patient in terms of prolongation of survival. Accordingly, strict criteria must be observed in determining whether a patient should be considered for major resection.

Symptomatic patients, abnormal liver chemistry, the percentage of hepatic replacement (PHR), and whether the disease is confined to the liver are the major prognostic factors, and these are important when evaluating treatment. Pettavel, Leyvraz, and Douglas (1984) have recommended a staging system which incorporates all these factors:

- Stage 1: PHR of less than 25 per cent
- Stage 2: PHR of 25–75 per cent
- Stage 3: PHR greater than 75 per cent.

This system, known as the Lausanne staging, also takes into account abnormal biochemistry and whether the patient is symptomatic.

Surgery

Improvements in surgical techniques, in anaesthesia, and in our understanding of surgical anatomy have resulted in more widespread acceptance and performance of resection for liver tumours. It should be remembered, however, that surgical feasibility alone does not necessarily justify its performance unless objective evidence exists to confirm efficacy.

Below are listed, in brief, some personal preferences with regard to resection of solitary (or localized) colorectal liver metastases:

1. A long subcostal (roof-top) incision usually provides adequate access.
2. A very careful laparotomy is required to exclude evidence of recurrent disease elsewhere.
3. Ligation of the appropriate hepatic veins from within the liver during the process of liver division is preferred.
4. The appropriate vascular and biliary structures are carefully dissected free and isolated at the porta hepatis. These are clamped but not ligated. Avascular demarcation is apparent and the liver substance is divided along the main scissural line.
5. Division of the liver is performed with a combination of incision, diathermy, suction, and finger fracture.
6. Adequate drainage is essential to avoid large haematoma formation.

Indications for surgery

In most series surgical resection has been confined mainly to colorectal liver metastases and occasional carcinoid tumours. This is certainly the experience of our unit in Southampton in recent years (Table 16.2). Occasionally gallbladder carcinoma requires a formal liver resection, but this is usually due to direct extension into the liver rather than to blood-borne metastases.

Ideally, the tumour should be solitary and confined to a single lobe. Attempts should be made to assess resectability before surgery. This involves ultrasonography and computed tomographic (CT) examination of the liver to exclude multiple metastases and evidence of extra-hepatic lymphadenopathy, particularly involving the porta hepatis. Hepatic artery angiography is a useful procedure for highlighting important anatomical variations, which may influence surgical resection. Evidence of portal vein involvement noted on the venous phase of the angiogram is most important in determining resectability. This does not, however, preclude resection

Table 16.2. Liver tumours seen in the university surgical unit, Southampton, 1982–8).

	No. of tumours	No. undergoing resection
Primary	14	4
Hepatoma	8	3
Cholangiocarcinoma	4	4
FNH	1	1
Benign adenoma	1	1
Cystadenocarcinoma		
Total	28	13
Secondary		
Colon	174	17
Breast	20	
Carcinoid	14	1
Unknown	13	
Stomach	10	
Pancreas	8	
Lung	4	
Ovary	3	
Oesophagus	2	
Prostate	2	
Gallbladder	2	1
Kidney	2	
Melanoma	1	
Appendix	1	
Meningioma	1	
Small bowel	1	
Total	258	19

FNH – Follicular Nodular Hyperplasia

since large tumours can push structures aside without necessarily invading them.

For patients with previous colorectal tumours, abdominal and pelvic CT scans are useful to ensure that local recurrence is not present. Similarly, chest radiography is obligatory.

At most, only about 10 per cent of patients will be considered suitable for resectional surgery. The majority of patients have extensive disease or evidence of metastases elsewhere, and so are not suitable for consideration. If a solitary small metastasis is noted on the free edge of the liver at the time of colorectal resection then it is reasonable to resect it synchronously, by means of a generous wedge excision. However, should a larger tumour be noted within the substance of the liver then resection should not be carried out at that time, although a biopsy, if possible, should be taken. Once the patient has recovered from colorectal surgery, further investigation of the liver is required to confirm the solitary nature of the lesion. Most surgeons would delay subsequent major resection of the liver for 2–3 months, during which time the patient should have recovered sufficiently to contemplate further surgery. In addition, if the metastases are particularly aggressive then further dissemination may be detectable which indicates that surgery is unnecessary.

Our own indications for major resection of colorectal liver metastases are as follows:

(1) patient generally fit, and normally under 70 years of age;

(2) either a solitary metastasis, or possibly two or three close together in one lobe with no evidence of disease in the remainder of liver, as shown by ultrasonographic scan and CT scan with contrast;

(3) no evidence of disease elsewhere in the peritoneal cavity evident at surgical resection of colorectal cancer or a CT scan of the pelvis;

(4) good liver function (biochemical and clinical) with no evidence of either jaundice or ascites;

(5) patient fully informed with an understanding of the implications of surgical resection.

Results of surgical resection

There are numerous reports in the literature of the results of surgical resection in selected patients with colorectal liver metastases. Interestingly, since Flanagan and Foster's important review in 1967 of 72 patients surviving hepatic resection, an increasing number of centres have reported small series. In the absence of controlled studies comparing resection with no treatment, we need to rely on such reports to determine the benefit of surgical resection. In Table 16.3 a selection of several studies is summarized. It is clear that the overall operative mortality rate for major resection should be about 5 per cent and that 3-year survival rates of approximately 40 per cent are achievable in selected patients.

Factors influencing outcome after resection

From a review of the available reports, several factors emerge as being important in influencing the results of overall survival following resection.

Extent of liver involvement

This is undoubtedly a major factor. Ekberg, *et al.* (1986) reported 72 patients; 35 had single metastases, 26 had widespread disease in one lobe, and 11 had

Table 16.3. Results of surgical resection for liver metastases.

Reference	No. of patients	No. of patients with metastases		Operative mortality rate (%)	Post-operative survival rate (%)		
		1–3	> 4		1 year	2–3 years	5 years
Attiyeh *et al.* (1978)	25	21	4	—	—	—	40
Wanebo *et al.* (1978)	25	25	—	10	92	—	28
Bengmark *et al.* (1982*b*)	39	—	—	5	—	23	—
Morrow and Grage (1982)	29	11	18	10	—	36	27
Logan *et al.* (1982)	19	12	—	5.3	—	63	—
Iwatsuki *et al.* (1983)	24	—	—	0	91	—	—
Fortner *et al.* (1984)	65	—	—	7	—	57	—
Cady and McDermott (1985)	23	18	5	11	—	—	40
Wagner *et al.* (1984)	67	—	—	4	—	—	25
Adson (1986)	39	—	—	5	—	40	24
Ekberg *et al.* (1986)	72	35	37	—	—	—	9

a large metastasis surrounded by small satellite lesions. The 5-year survival rate was 24 per cent for solitary lesions, 9 per cent for multiple, and 0 per cent for large metastases with satellite deposits. Other authors have experienced similar survival rates. There is little evidence to support the concept of resection of more than three metastases, to try to obtain survival benefit.

Dukes' classification of primary colorectal cancer

As might be expected, several studies have indicated that patients with initially Dukes' A or B colorectal cancer have a better survival rate following resection of liver metastases than patients with Dukes' C disease. Attiyeh, Wanebo, and Stearns (1978), for example, showed that in nine patients with an initially Dukes' A or B lesion there was a median survival time following hepatic resection of 108 months, compared with 24 months in 15 patients with Dukes' C disease.

Resection margin

This appears to be of great significance. Positive margins of resection and those with less than 1 cm between the cut edge and the carcinoma on the resected specimens have a markedly worse survival rate following resection.

This has been dramatically re-emphasized by Ekberg *et al.* (1986) who showed that resection margins were the only treatment variable that correlated with length of survival. In 27 patients with a margin greater than 1 cm, approximately 30 per cent survived for 5 years. However, all 12 patients with positive margins had died with recurrence by 31 months. Other authors have made similar observations (Cady and McDermott 1985; Rajpal, *et al.* 1982).

It is apparent that surgical resection, whether by the localized excision of a metastasis or major hepatectomy, should be accompanied by a generous margin of normal liver if the prognosis is to be improved.

Extra-hepatic metastases

The presence of extra-hepatic metastases, whether nodal or visceral, adversely influences prognosis to a marked degree. In Ekberg's series (1986) 12 patients were noted to have extra-hepatic disease and their survival rate was only 10 per cent at 3 years compared with 36 per cent in patients in whom no extra-hepatic spread was found.

Conclusion

In the presence of limited metastatic disease confined to one liver lobe (preferably solitary but no more than three), surgical resection is likely to be beneficial. This can not be stated categorically because there are no controlled studies to compare with untreated patients. Nevertheless, it would appear that 3-year survival rates of up to 40 per cent and 5-year survival rates approaching 25 per cent can be achieved with a low operative mortality rate. Selected patients with colorectal liver metastases fulfilling strict criteria should be offered this form of treatment.

Non-resectional treatment of liver tumours

The vast majority of patients with liver tumours (either primary or metastatic) are unsuitable for surgical resection. These patients are usually incurable but in an attempt to achieve worthwhile palliation and prolongation of survival several therapeutic modalities have been attempted: (1) systemic cytotoxic chemotherapy; (2) loco-regional approaches to the liver; and (3) miscellaneous other modalities.

Systemic cytotoxic chemotherapy

There is very little evidence to suggest that cytotoxic chemotherapy is of any benefit for patients with liver metastases. Most of the studies have concentrated on colorectal liver metastases, since none of the other gastrointestinal malignancies have documented objective remissions.

5-Fluorouracil (5-FU) has been the most widely investigated drug, and this has been used either alone or in combination with other agents. Examples of quoted response rates are shown in Table 16.4. In brief, response rates of approximately 20 per cent have been recorded with 5-FU alone and the combination regimens may improve this to 30 per cent, but there is a significant increase in toxicity. There have been no convincing reports of improvement in survival. In many of these studies it is not entirely clear how often the liver is the predominant area under study as opposed to other sites of metastases.

Ultimately, survival is the most objective criterion of efficacy. Rapaport and Bureleson (1970) reported a mean survival time from diagnosis of 11.6 months (median 8.5) in a series of 61 patients, which was stated to be better than a group of historical controls, although the tumour response rate was only 11 per cent.

The most impressive study of combination chemotherapy has been reported by Kemeny, *et al.* (1980). In a group of 77 patients treated with 5-FU, methyl CCNU®, vincristine, and streptozotocin a median survival time of 11 months was obtained. Many other studies have reported data from patients having various combinations of cytotoxic chemotherapy, but prospective randomized controlled trials are lacking, which makes interpretation of the data most difficult.

Loco-regional approaches for liver tumour

Both primary liver tumours and liver metastases obtain their blood supply from the hepatic artery. This has been demonstrated effectively both in animal models and in humans (Gelin, Lewis, and Nilsson 1968; Taylor, Bennet, and Sherriff 1979; Taylor 1981). Accordingly, attempts to deal with

Table 16.4. Response rates of systemic chemotherapy in colorectal metastases.

Reference	No. of patients	Drug(s)	Response rate(%)
Reitmeier *et al.* (1970)	20	5-FU	25
Moertel (1975)	69	Mitomycin C	12
	147	5 Fudr	22
	38	methyl CCNU	18
Frytak *et al.* (1975)	57	Doxorubicin	7
Baker *et al.* (1975)	128	5-FU + methyl CCNU	30
Kemeny *et al.* (1980)	74	5-FU + methyl CCNU + vincristine + streptozo-tocin	32
Shepard *et al.* (1985*a*)	20	5-FU + cisplatin	0

5-FU, 5-fluorouracil; 5-FUDR, 5-fluorodeoxyuridine.

tumours by loco-regional approaches have been attempted for more than 20 years, the largest experience being for colorectal liver metastases. Such approaches include: (1) hepatic artery ligation; (2) hepatic de-arterialization; (3) hepatic artery embolization; and (4) hepatic artery cytotoxic infusion.

Hepatic De-arterialization

Several approaches have been made to achieve satisfactory hepatic de-arterialization of liver tumours:

1. *Hepatic artery ligation* In this procedure the main hepatic artery is dissected free and ligated as close as possible to the liver.
2. *Hepatic de-arterialization* This is a more extensive undertaking whereby all connections to the liver except the common bile duct and portal vein in the hepatoduodenal ligament are ligated and divided.
3. *Hepatic artery embolization* This percutaneous procedure is achieved by injection of gelfoam, lamina dura, or spring coils into the main feeding arteries of the tumour.
4. *Transient hepatic de-arterialization* Hepatic de-arterialization is performed as in (2) but the hepatic artery is occluded intermittently to allow infusion chemotherapy.

Hepatic artery ligation/de-arterialization

Hepatic artery ligation has been advocated but the results are unsatisfactory. This is partly due to the fairly rapid development of a collateral circulation, soon after ligation, and also due to the development of portal perfusion into the tumours (Taylor *et al.* 1979).

Outcomes of de-arterialization have been similarly disappointing and, in addition, there is a significant mortality rate for this procedure. Almersjo, *et al.* (1972) carried out hepatic de-arterialization in a mixed group of patients with primary and secondary tumours. Their operative mortality rate was in excess of 20 per cent and mean survival was only 4–5 months. Although this was not a controlled study the conclusion was clearly that no survival benefit is likely to accrue from this extensive procedure. A summary of reports involving ligation and de-arterialization is given in Table 16.5.

An alternative proposition is repeated short-term arterial occlusion, advocated by Bengmark's group (Bengmark, *et al.* 1988). The rationale for this is not to cause tissue necrosis by ischaemia, which provides the stimulus for an alternative blood supply to develop, but to produce cytotoxic oxygen free radicals during short periods (about 60 minutes) of ischaemia. At laparotomy all arterial connections to the liver, except the hepatic artery are surgically divided. Strangulating strings of polyethylene are placed around the hepatic artery and exteriorized through a separate incision in the abdominal wall. By pulling the thin catheters an occlusion can be achieved at any time in the post-operative period. During the operation a catheter is also placed in the gastroduodenal artery for control of occlusion, and later infusion of cytotoxic drugs.

Twenty patients with liver tumours treated in this way have been reported (Dahl, *et al.* 1981). In patients with tumour localized to the liver, the median survival was 24 months and for patients with synchronous extra hepatic tumours it was 10 months. Some encouraging results have been obtained in patients with carcinoid tumour (Bengmark, *et al.* 1982*a*). Attempts are being made to improve the results of this technique with the use of an implantable device to produce transient occlusion (Persson, *et al.* 1989).

Hepatic artery ligation and distal arterial infusion

It is difficult to be clear about the benefit of this combination because of several factors. First, many reports are comprised of mixtures of primary and secondary hepatic tumours and there is, in addition, a lack of selection criteria or stratification for either the extent of liver involvement, or the use of prior or adjuvant systemic therapy. Second, it is unclear whether treatment is limited only to symptomatic patients, who may have more advanced disease.

A selection of publications is presented in Table 16.6. A randomized controlled trial has been reported in 24 patients with colorectal liver metastases (Taylor 1978). Patients were randomized to receive either: (1) no treatment; (2) hepatic artery ligation and distal perfusion and portal vein perfusion with 5-FU; or (3) hepatic artery ligation with distal perfusion and portal vein perfusion with 5-FU. Group 3 had a mean survival from treatment of 9.8 months which was longer than in the other two groups.

Table 16.5. Clinical studies on arterial ligation and de-arterialization.

Reference	Procedure	No. of patients		Operative mortality rate (%)	Survival (months)
		Primary	Secondary		
Almersjo *et al.* (1972)	De-arterialization	5	22	37	4.5
Fortner *et al.* (1973)	HAL + infusion	6	17	—	50% objective response
Mokka *et al.* (1975)	HAL + infusion	13	10	13%	8.9
Almersjo *et al.* (1976)	HAL (26) De-arterialization (14)	10	30	17.5	8
Dahl *et al.* (1981)	Transient de-arterialization + infusion	—	20	20	17
Petrelli *et al.* (1984)	HAL	—	97	2.0	9.5

HAL, hepatic artery ligation.

Table 16.6. Results of hepatic artery ligation/occlusion with distal hepatic arterial infusion.

Reference	No. of patients	Drug(s)	Response rate (%)	Median survival (months)
Fortner *et al.* (1973)	14	various 5-FU	50–78	—
Cuschieri *et al.* (1975)	12	5-FU	50	—
Patt *et al.* (1981)	55	FUDR + mitomycin C	43	11
Didolkar *et al.* (1985)	30	5-FU	97	17

5-FU, 5-fluorouracil; 5-FUDR, 5-fluorodeoxyuridine.

Hepatic artery ligation with portal vein infusion

In view of the compensatory haemodynamic changes which have been shown to occur following hepatic artery ligation, with an increase in portal vein perfusion, the combination of ligation/occlusion with portal vein cytotoxic perfusion has been performed.

Murray-Lyon, *et al.* (1970) described five patients in whom this procedure was carried out, all of whom derived symptomatic benefit and survived for between 10 and 20 months. Laufman, *et al.* (1984) described 19 patients with colorectal liver metastases treated with hepatic artery ligation and portal vein infusion of 5-FU and mitomycin C. A 63 per cent response rate was recorded with a median survival time from the start of treatment of 13 months. A larger series of 35 patients with synchronous multiple colorectal liver metastases has been reported with strict selection criteria (Taylor 1981). Patients with less than 20 per cent tumour involvement had a mean survival of 15 months with an overall median survival of 10 months.

Almersjo, *et al.* (1976) have reported some benefit in survival a series of 40 patients, with both primary and metastatic tumour, treated with ligation or de-arterialization, and 19 were also given intraportal 5-FU infusion.

Hepatic artery embolization

Hepatic artery embolization performed under radiological control is an alternative method of occluding hepatic arterial flow, without the necessity for laparotomy. The catheter is placed as close to the target area as possible. The most commonly used embolization materials have been Gelfoam, lamina dura, stainless steel coils, and Ivalon particles.

Chuang and Wallace (1981) described a mixed group of hepatic tumours in 47 patients who underwent embolization. A median survival time from treatment of 11.5 months was recorded and this was reported as an improvement over historical controls. Further encouraging early results have also been published (Chuang, *et al.* 1982). However, other studies have reported minimal, if any, survival benefit for non-endocrine tumours, such as colorectal metastases, and suggest that embolization be reserved for symptomatic relief only (Allison, Jordan, and Hennessy 1985; Campbell, *et al.* 1985). Indeed, a randomized trial has suggested that no survival benefit is obtained from embolization of colorectal liver metastases when compared with untreated controls (Hunt, Flowerdew, Birch, Mullee, and Taylor 1989). However, the technique is of proven benefit for the symptomatic treatment of carcinoid metastases.

Complications Most patients undergoing this procedure experience some pain in the right upper quadrant, fever, nausea, and vomiting for a few days — the post-embolization syndrome. Infection and liver abscess formation have been described but are rare. Nevertheless, it is probably wise to administer prophylactic antibiotics to cover the procedure.

Embolization with cytotoxic infusion

In a number of reported studies embolization has been combined with various drugs mixed with the material, a technique known as chemo-embolization.

The initial results of this approach have been particularly encouraging in patients with primary liver cancer. Yamada, *et al.* (1983) have described the results of 235 embolizations in 120 patients with unresectable hepatoma. Gelfoam embolus was mixed with mitomycin C or Adriamycin® with 75 per cent of the patients demonstrating an objective tumour reduction. The 1-year survival rate was 44 per cent, which compared well with that of hepatectomy (28 per cent) by the same group.

Other authors have combined embolization with intra-arterial infusion. Okamura, *et al.* (1982) infused Adriamycin into the hepatic artery, followed by Gelfoam embolization, in 62 patients with primary and six patients with metastatic liver lesions. The 1-year survival rate was 56 per cent.

Patt, *et al.* (1983) have reported Gelfoam embolization combined with intra-arterial 5-fluorodeoxyuridine or mitomycin C in 22 patients, but no apparent improvement in survival was achieved.

It should be noted that increasingly aggressive techniques of chemo-embolization are being described. In one recent series 89 patients with primary and secondary cancer have received lipiodol mixed with Adriamycin to occlude peripheral tumour vessels. Addition of central embolization was performed with gelatine sponge cubes (Shimamura, *et al.* 1988), and the authors documented extensive post-embolization necrosis in tumours of 5 cm or less in diameter. Unfortunately, the effect was temporary and no survival statistics were provided.

The use of this embolization technique for hepatic malignancies in children has also been described. Lipiodol together with Adriamycin, cisplatinum and 5-FU produced a marked decrease in tumour size and α-fetoprotein levels (Ogita, *et al.* 1987). Similar techniques have been described for the treatment of advanced carcinoid disease (Ahlman, *et al.* 1987) and islet cell tumours which have metastasized to the liver (Ajani, *et al.* 1988).

Infusion chemotherapy

Infusion chemotherapy into the hepatic artery has been used extensively for multiple liver metastases. With the development of implantable devices the emphasis has shifted to providing long-term infusion of suitable chemotherapeutic agents. For this form of therapy, suitable drugs should ideally

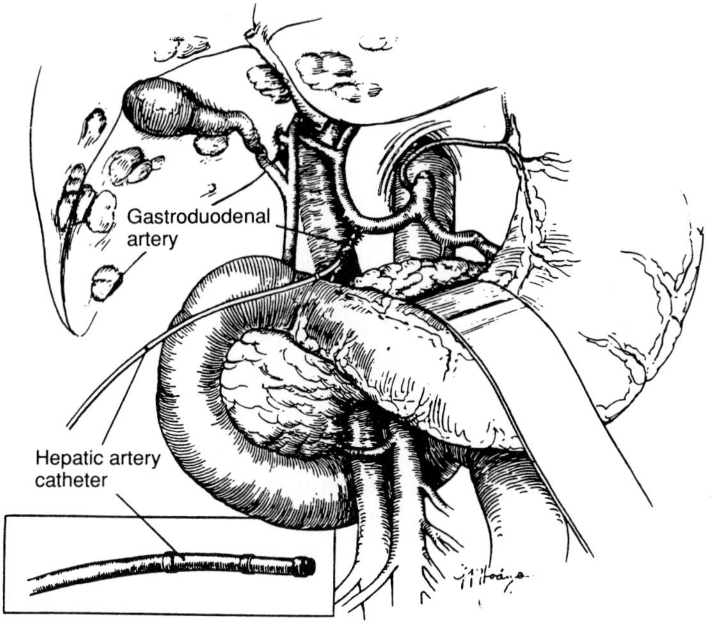

Fig. 16.1. Technique of hepatic artery cannulation.

have a short plasma half-life, high total body clearance, and efficient hepatic extraction (Elkman, Patlak, and Fenstermacher 1974; Ensminger and Gyves 1984).

The fluorinated pyrimidines have the greatest response rate when administered intravenously, and also the required theoretical pharmacokinetic properties for regional arterial infusion. They have accordingly been used either alone or in combination with other drugs in the vast majority of hepatic arterial infusion studies.

Techniques of infusion

The technique of hepatic arterial cannulation consists essentially of cannulating the gastroduodenal artery so that the tip of the catheter lies at its origin at the common hepatic artery. Following correct positioning the catheter is ligated in place so that it cannot become dislodged. Most of the available catheters have thickened rings around the end so that sutures can be snugly tied around them to prevent movement (Fig. 16.1).

The end of the catheter is then tunnelled through the abdominal wall until it is positioned in a subcutaneous pouch, for attachment either to a port with diaphragm, or an implantable continuous infusion device ('Infusaid' pump).

In the former case injections are administered percutaneously into the port through a diaphragm, with a special needle that allows penetration without subsequent leakage. Bolus injections are given at regular intervals or an external perfusion pump can be employed to deliver a fixed volume of the drug over a period of time.

Anatomical variations in hepatic arterial supply are frequent and can be troublesome. On occasions in which the right and left hepatic arteries originate too close to the gastroduodenal artery to permit mixing of drug and equal distribution to all areas of the liver, the gastroduodenal artery and right gastric artery are ligated. The splenic artery is also ligated and the catheter positioned at the junction of the splenic artery and coeliac axis. Occasionally, the right hepatic artery arises from the superior mesenteric artery, and in these circumstances two catheters may be required.

Results of infusional chemotherapy in liver metastases

Numerous studies have been reported on the use of both short-term and long-term arterial cytotoxic infusion in the treatment of colorectal liver metastases unsuitable for resection. In the review that follows the information is related totally to the results of treatment of liver metastases from primary colorectal cancer.

For short-term infusion, hepatic arterial catheters can be placed percutaneously, under radiological control, or at laparotomy via the gastroduodenal artery (Fig. 16.1). Chemotherapy had been given either as a bolus, or rapid infusion, or by continuous infusion using either external or implantable devices as described above.

In Table 16.7 a representative sample of the results of early studies of short-term infusion is given, and in Table 16.8 a number of studies utilizing long-term cytotoxic infusion is provided.

Despite the obvious problems in interpretation of such data from uncontrolled studies, the response rates following hepatic artery chemotherapy are consistently better than in previously reported studies of systemic chemotherapy. Nearly all studies of infusion therapy quote response rates in the region of 50–80 per cent. Sadly, randomized studies are few and far between. Grage, *et al.* (1979) randomized 74 patients with colorectal liver metastases to either hepatic arterial infusion or intravenous infusion of 5-FU. The arterial infusion group received only one 3-week course of arterial therapy, followed by the same subsequent intravenous therapy in both groups. In this study the response rate in the arterial therapy group (34 per cent) was not significantly higher than in the intravenous group (23 per cent), but in view of the short duration of hepatic arterial treatment this was not so unexpected.

Kemeny and Daly (1986) randomized 50 patients with colorectal liver metastases into either hepatic arterial or intravenous infusion of 5-FUDR. The response rate in the hepatic arterial group was 43 per cent compared

Table 16.7. Results of hepatic arterial infusion (short-term).

Reference	No. of patients	Drug(s)	Response rate (%)	Median survival (months)
Sullivan and Zurek (1965)	39	5-FU or methotrexate	62	—
Watkins *et al.* (1970)	82	FUDR	73	15
Ansfield *et al.* (1971)	53	5-FU	72	—
Cady and Oberfield (1974)	51	FUDR	50–70	11
Pettavel and Morgenthaler (1978)	52	5-FU/FUDR	81	—
Sundqvist *et al.* (1978)	15	5-FU	—	9
Oberfield *et al.* (1979)	48	5-FU/FUDR	54	—
Patt *et al.* (1981)	12	FUDR, mitomycin C	83	15

5-FU, 5-fluorouracil; 5-FUDR, 5-fluorodeoxyuridine.

Table 16.8. Results of hepatic arterial infusion (long-term).

				Median survival (months)	
Reference	No. of Patients	Drug(s)	Response rate (%)	From start of infusion	From diagnosis
Barone *et al.* (1982)	18	FUDR	56	12	—
Balch *et al.* (1983)	81	FUDR/mitomycin C	88	—	26
Weiss *et al.* (1983)	21	FUDR		13	17
Neiderhuber *et al.* (1984)	50	FUDR/mitomycin C	74–83	18	25
Schwartz *et al.* (1985)	18	FUDR	—	10	21
Shepard *et al.* (1985*b*)	62	FUDR/mitomycin, methotrexate	33	17	—
Trivisionno *et al.* (1986)	20	FUDR	50	11–29	—
Miller *et al.* (1988)	27	5-FU	28	9	—
Sterchi *et al.* (1989)	69	FUDR	48	18	—

5-FU, 5-fluorouracil; 5-FUDR, 5-fluorodeoxyuridine.

with 33 per cent, but survival figures cannot be interpreted because failure of systemic therapy led to cross-over to the arterial infusion group.

More recently, however, Chang, *et al.* (1987) reported a similar but non-cross-over, randomized study of hepatic arterial versus intravenous infusion of 5-FUDR in 64 patients with colorectal liver metastases. The response rate in the arterial therapy group was significantly higher (62 versus 17 per cent), but, most importantly, this was not translated into a significant overall survival benefit. However, patients treated with hepatic arterial infusion who had no known nodal involvement survived for longer than node-negative patients treated with systemic therapy. Daly, *et al.* (1987) have compared, in a randomized trial, hepatic arterial versus portal venous infusion of FUDR. A significant difference in response rates was observed even in this relatively small trial (50 versus 0 per cent). However, the cross-over trial design again prevents any comments on survival analysis.

Finally, the concept of isolated liver perfusion should be mentioned. Schwemmle, Link, and Rieck (1987) reported a median survival of 14 months for a group of 41 patients with a variety of liver metastases.

Analysis of survival data for long-term cytotoxic infusion is complicated by the variable presentation of survival times, either from the time of initial diagnosis of liver metastases or the commencement of infusion. Similarly, it is often not clear whether stratification of extent of liver involvement is included. For example, it is known that a major prognostic factor is the extent of liver involvement which should be taken into account in assessing survival. Accordingly, the comparison of results with either historical controls or computer models (Balch, *et al.* 1983; Weiss, *et al.* 1983) is probably not justified.

The majority of studies, however, seem to suggest that intra-hepatic chemotherapy is more effective than systemic chemotherapy. Certainly 'responders' have a better survival rate than 'non-responders' but this could be in spite of treatment rather than because of it.

Side-effects of arterial infusion

In most studies the systemic side-effects of arterial chemotherapy are reported to be reduced compared with intravenous administration. However, recent studies have emphasized the high incidence of 'local' toxic complications associated with long-term infusion regimens, particularly with FUDR. The most serious of these include chemical hepatitis, gastritis, peptic ulceration with haemorrhage, and sclerosing cholangitis. Various degrees of these complications have been reported in up to 50 per cent of patients undergoing long-term infusion with FUDR.

For successful intra-arterial chemotherapy, reliable devices are also important, and failure or complications arising from faulty technique should be considered. A comparison has been made between external catheters

(Hickman) and implantable catheters (ports). Although the complication rate was low for both, it was lower for the implantable device (Stanislav, *et al.* 1987). The complication rate was 1 per 507 patient days for Hickman catheters and 1 per 1450 patient days for the port. This, together with the longevity and diminished maintenance requirements, indicates that the implantable ports are superior.

Hepatic arterial infusion with microspheres

Attempts have been made to increase the concentration of drug with the liver and tumour by incorporating the drug with microspheres. There are of two types. In the first type, Adriamycin-loaded albumen microspheres are introduced selectively and are trapped in the first capillary bed encountered. Release of drug by diffusion and biodegradation of the albumen matrix should then occur, producing a high drug level in the target organ with minimal systemic exposure. Experimental studies have suggested that such an approach holds significant potential (McArdle, *et al.* 1988).

Another approach employs degradable starch microspheres (DSM). As mentioned above, the pharmacokinetics of arterial therapy is such that the concentration of drug achieved is dependent on hepatic arterial flow rate. Decreasing the hepatic arterial flow rate by 90 per cent should increase the arterial concentration of drug at a given dose by about 10-fold (Ensminger and Gyres 1984).

DSM are composed of polymers of hydrolysed potato starch bonded by epichlorohydrin, and are degraded by serum amylase, with a half-life of 20–30 minutes in humans. A transient flow reduction of up to 100 per cent following intra-arterial administration of DSM has been confirmed in humans (Dakhil, *et al.* 1982). Experimental studies in rats have demonstrated a 100 per cent increase in tumour uptake of 5-FU when given into the hepatic artery mixed with DSM (Flowerdew, *et al.* 1987*a*; Flowerdew, *et al.* 1987*b*).

Thus, there has been much interest in the use of DSM to enhance the benefits of regional chemotherapy of liver tumours. Aronsen, *et al.* (1979) reported on 12 patients with liver metastases treated with 5-FU and DSM, and documented a median survival time of 7 months. Pfeifle, Howell, and Bookstein (1985) undertook a pilot study of intra-arterial FUDR, doxorubicin, and mitomycin C with DSM. Seven patients with colorectal liver metastases had a median survival time of 10 months from diagnosis.

Hunt *et al.* (1989) have reported one of the very few randomized controlled trials in patients with multiple colorectal liver metastases which included a no-treatment control arm. Patients receiving intra-hepatic 5-FU and DSM appeared to have an improved overall survival rate compared no-treatment, but small numbers prevented statistical significance. However, the median survival time in patients with less than 50 per cent involvement was more than 21 months compared with 8 months in no-treatment controls. This form of therapy is interesting and deserves further assessment.

Miscellaneous other modalities

Several other specific forms of treatment have been utilized in patients with liver tumours, and require consideration.

Radiotherapy

External beam radiotherapy for both hepatoma and liver metastases is limited by the radiosensitivity of normal liver tissue. The maximum dose tolerated by the liver without inducing radiation hepatitis is in the range 30–35 Gy. This is unlikely to achieve any therapeutic benefit although valuable palliation may be attained (Borgeit, *et al.* 1981). It has been claimed, for example, to alleviate pain caused by significant liver metastases.

Radiotherapy combined with other therapeutic options may be more successful. Rotman, *et al.* (1986) combined external rediotherapy and concomitant intravenous 5-FU infusion in 27 patients with colorectal liver metastases. Median survival was 26 weeks.

An alternative approach is to use internal irradiation. This is provided by the administration of intra-arterial radioactive particles labelled to microspheres and has usually been in the form of ^{90}yttrium (^{90}Y) microspheres that emit pure β-particles. Experimental evidence in a rabbit model suggests that hepatic arterial ^{90}Y 17.5-μm microspheres are preferentially distributed to the tumour as opposed to the normal liver with high tumour/liver ratios (Chamberlain, *et al.* 1983).

Internal irradiation may also be combined with other therapies. Ariel and Padula (1978) used hepatic arterial 5-FU in addition to ^{90}Y microspheres, and reported mean survival times of 12–14 months in 65 symptomatic patients. Grady (1979) reported no appreciable improvement in survival with radioactive microspheres alone. It is unlikely that this form of therapy provides any worthwhile survival benefit in patients with liver tumours and there is evidence to suggest that radiation hepatitis is a common and serious complication.

Endocrine therapy

When liver metastases develop from primary tumours thought to be hormone dependent, appropriate endocrine therapy is indicated. Examples include tamoxifen in patients with breast malignancy, hydroxyprogesterone acetate in patients with kidney malignancy, and stilboestrol for prostatic malignancy.

Biological response modifiers

This approach is still relatively novel. However, a few partial responses in patients with liver tumours have been observed with interleukin 2/lymphokine activated killer cell (LAK) treatment and with interferon. However, such therapy is associated with significant side-effects and is not sufficiently evaluated to be considered for routine treatment.

Overall conclusions

Surgery offers the only hope of cure but this is possible in only a small proportion of patients. Loco-regional approaches remain the most likely treatments in those patients in whom the disease is confined to within the liver parenchyma. However, further studies and trials are necessary if these treatments are to demonstrate worthwhile benefit.

Newer therapies hold out some hope for improvement. Paramount amongst these are the biological response modifiers and effective cytotoxic chemotherapy.

Whilst awaiting newer and hopefully more effective treatment, it is important to assess and stage each patient accurately so that only those patients most likely to respond are treated. Wherever possible, treatments should be given in the context of clinical trials so that accurate information can be obtained. Finally, it should be remembered that, at best, most treatments are palliative and designed to prolong symptom-free survival.

References

Adson, M.A. (1986). Liver resection in primary and secondary liver cancer. In *Liver surgery* (ed. S. Bengmark and L.H. Blumgart) pp. 63–80. Churchill Livingstone, London.

Ahlman, H., Ahlund, L., Dahlstrom, A., *et al.* (1987). Use of a somatostatin analogue in association with surgery and hepatic arterial embolization in the treatment of the carcinoid syndrome. *Br. J. Cancer* **56**, 840–2.

Ajani, J.A., Carrasco, C.H., Charnsangave, J.C., *et al.* (1988). Islet cell tumours metastatic to the liver: effective palliation of sequential hepatic artery embolization. *Ann. Inter. Med.* **108**, 340–4.

Allison, D.J., Jordan, H., and Hennessy, O. (1985). Therapeutic embolization of the hepatic artery: a review of 75 procedures. *Lancet* **i**, 595–9.

Almersjo, O., Bengmark, S., Hafstrom, L., *et al.* (1976). Results of liver dearterialization combined with regional infusion of 5-fluorouracil for liver cancer. *Acta. Chir. Scand.* **142**, 131–8.

Almersjo, O., Bengmark, S., Rudenstam, C.J., *et al.* (1972). Evaluation of hepatic dearterialization in primary and secondary cancer of the liver. *Am. J. Surg.* **124**, 5–9.

Ansfield, F.J., Ramirez, G., Skibba, J.C., *et al.* (1971). Intrahepatic arterial infusion with 5-fluorouracil. *Cancer* **28**, 1147–51.

Ariel, I.M. and Padula, G. (1978). Treatment of symptomatic metastatic cancer to the liver from primary colon and rectal cancer by the intra-arterial administration of chemotherapy and radioactive isotopes. In *Progress in clinical cancer* (ed. A.M. Ariel) Vol. 7, pp. 247–54. Grune and Stratton, New York.

Aronsen, K.F., Hellekant, C., Holmberg, J., *et al.* (1979). Controlled blocking of hepatic artery flow with emzymatically degradable microspheres combined with oncolytic drugs. *Eur. Surg. Res.* **II**, 99–106.

Attiyeh, F.F., Wanebo, H.J., and Stearns, N.W. (1978). Hepatic resection for metastases from colorectal cancer. *Dis. Colon Rectum* **21**, 160–2.

Baden, H. and Andersen, B. (1975). Survival of patients with untreated liver metastases from cancer of the colon and rectum. *Scand. J. Gastroenterol.* **10**, 221–3.

Baker, L.H., Matter, R., Talley, R., *et al.* (1975). 5FU vs. 5FU and MeCCNU in gastrointestinal cancers. A phase III study of the Southwest Oncology Group. *Proc. Am. Soc. Clin. Oncol.* **16**, 229.

Balch, C.M., Urist, M.M., Soong, S., *et al.* (1983). A prospective phase II clinical trial of continuous RUDR regional chemotherapy for colorectal metastases to the liver using a totally implantable drug infusion pump. *Ann. Surg.* **198**, 567–73.

Barone, R.M., Byfield, J.E., Goldfarb, P.B., *et al.* (1982). Intra-arterial chemotherapy using an implantable infusion pump and liver irradiation for the treatment of liver metastases. *Cancer* **50**, 850–62.

Bengmark, S. and Hafstrom, L. (1969). The natural history of primary and secondary malignant tumours of the liver. I. The prognosis for patients with hepatic metastases from colonic and rectum carcinoma by laparotomy. *Cancer* **23**, 198–202.

Bengmark, S., Ericsson, M., Lunderqvist, A., *et al.* (1982*a*). Temporary liver dearterialization in patients with metastatic carcinoid disease. *World J. Surg.* **6**, 46–53.

Bengmark, S., Hafstrom, L., Jappsson, B., *et al.* (1982*b*). Metastatic disease in the liver from colorectal cancer: an appraisal of liver surgery. *World J. Surg.* **6**, 61–5.

Bengmark, S., Jeppsson, B., Lunderqvist, A., *et al.* (1988). Tumour calcification following repeated hepatic dearterialization in patients: a preliminary communication. *Br. J. Surg.* **75**, 525–6.

Borgeit, B.B., Gelber, R., Brady, L.W., *et al.* (1981). The palliation of hepatic metastases: results of the radiation therapy oncology group pilot study. *Int. J. Oncol. Biol. Phys.* **7**, 587–91.

Cady, B. and McDermott, W.V. (1985). Major hepatic resection for metachronous metastases from colon cancer. *Ann. Surg.* **201**, 204–9.

Cady, B. and Oberfield, R.A. (1974). Regional infusion chemotherapy of hepatic metastases from carcinoma of the colon. *Am. J. Surg.* **127**, 220–7.

Cady, B., Monson, D.O., and Swinton, N.W. (1970). Survival of patients after colonic resection for carcinoma with simultaneous liver metasteses. *Surg. Gynecol. Obstet.* **131**, 697–700.

Campbell, D.R., Mason, W.F., Flemming, B.K., *et al.* (1985). Therapeutic embolization of the hepatic artery. *J. Can. Assoc. Radiol.* **36**, 212–15.

Chamberlain, M.N., Gray, B.N., Heggie, J.C.P., *et al.* (1983). Hepatic metastases — a physiological approach to treatment. *Br. J. Surg.* **70**, 596–8.

Chang, A.E., Schneider, P.D., Sugarbaker, P.H., *et al.* (1987). A prospective randomized trial of regional versus systemic continuous 5-fluorodeoxyuridine chemotherapy in the treatment of colorectal liver metastases. *Ann. Surg.* **206**, 685–93.

Chuang, V.P. and Wallace, S. (1981). Hepatic artery embolization in the treatment of hepatic neoplasms. *Radiology* **104**, 51–8.

Chuang, V.P., Wallace, S., Soo, C.S., *et al.* (1982). Therapeutic ivalon embolization of hepatic tumours. *Am. J. Radiol.* **138**, 289–94.

Cuschieri, A., Swain, C., and Crosbie, R.B. (1975). Hepatic artery ligation and prolonged cytotoxic therapy in advanced primary and secondary liver tumours. *Proc. R. Soc. Med.* **68**, 678–80.

Dahl, E.P., Redlund, P.E., Tylen, U., *et al.* (1981). Transient hepatic dearterialization followed by regional intra-arterial 5-fluorouracil infusion as treatment for liver tumours. *Ann. Surg.* **193**, 82–8.

Dakhil, S., Ensminger, W., Cho, K., *et al.* (1982). Improved regional selectivity of hepatic arterial BCNU with degradable microspheres. *Cancer* **50**, 631–5.

Daly, J.M., Kemeny, N., Sigurdson, E., *et al.* (1987). Regional infusion for colorectal hepatic metastases. *Arch. Surg.* **122**, 1273–7.

Dawson, P.M., Habib, N.A., Peck, M., *et al.* (1986). Patient survival with liver metastases from colorectal cancer — a district hospital experience. *Eur. J. Surg. Oncol.* **12**, 131–3.

Didolkar, M.S., Elias, E.G., Whitley, N.O., *et al.* (1985). Unresectable hepatic metastases from carcinoma of the colon and rectum. *Surg. Gynecol. Obstet.* **160**, 429–36.

Ekberg, H., Tranberg, K.G., Andersson, R., *et al.* (1986). Determinants of survival in liver resection for colorectal secondaries. *Br. J. Surg.* **73**, 727–31.

Elkman, W.W., Patlak, C.S., and Fenstermacher, J.D. (1974). A critical evaluation of principles governing the advantages of intra-arterial infusions. *J. Pharmacol. Biopharmacol.* **2**, 257–85.

Ensminger, W.P. and Gyves, J.W. (1984). Regional cancer chemotherapy. *Cancer Treat. Rep.* **68**, 101–15.

Fischerman, K., Petersen, C.F., Lindkaer, J.S., *et al.* (1976). Survival among patients with liver metastases from cancer of the colon and rectum. *Scand. J. Gastroenterol.* **11**, 111–15.

Flanagan, L. and Foster, J.H. (1967). Hepatic resection for metastatic cancer. *Am. J. Surg.* **113**, 551–7.

Flowerdew, A.D.S., Richards, H.K., and Taylor, I. (1987*a*). Temporary blood flow stasis with degradable starch microspheres (DSM) for liver metastases in a rat model. *Gut* **28**, 1201–7.

Flowerdew, A.D.S., McLaran, M.I., Fleming, J.S., *et al.* (1987*b*). Liver tumour blood flow and responses to arterial embolization measured by dynamic hepatic scintigraphy. *Br. J. Cancer* **55**, 269–73.

Fortner, J.G., Mulcare, R.J., Solis, A., *et al.* (1973). Treatment of primary and secondary liver cancer by hepatic artery ligation and infusion chemotherapy. *Ann. Surg.* **178**, 162–72.

Fortner, J.G., Silva, J.S., Golbey, R.B., *et al.* (1984). Multivariate analysis of a personal series of 247 consecutive patients with liver metastases from colorectal cancer. *Ann. Surg.* **199**, 306–16.

Frytak, S., Moertel, C.G., Shutt, A.J., *et al.* (1975). Adriamycin therapy for advanced gastrointestinal cancer. *Cancer Chemother. Rep.* **59**, 405–9.

Gelin, L.E., Lewis, P.H., and Nilsson, L. (1968). Liver blood flow in man during abdominal surgery. II. The effect of hepatic artery occlusion on the blood flow through metastatic tumour nodules. *Acta Hepatol. Gastroenterol.* **15**, 21–4.

Goslin, R., Steele, G., Zamcheck, N., *et al.* (1982). Factors influencing survival in patients with hepatic metastases from adenocarcinoma of the colon and rectum. *Dis. Colon Rectum* **25**, 749–54.

Grady, E.D. (1979). Internal radiation therapy of hepatic cancer. *Dis. Colon Rectum* **22**, 371–5.

Grage, T.B., Vassilopoulos, P.P., Shingleton, W.W., *et al.* (1979). Results of a prospective randomized study of hepatic artery infusion with 5FU versus intravenous 5DU in patients with hepatic metastases from colorectal cancer. *Surgery* **86**, 550–5.

Hunt, T., Flowerdew, A., Birch, S., Mullee, M., and Taylor, I. (1989). Randomised controlled trial on the treatment of multiple colorectal liver metastases. *Gut* **30**, 1516 (Abstract).

Iwatsuki, S., Shaw, B.W., and Starzl, T.E. (1983). Experience with 150 liver resections. *Ann. Surg.* **197**, 247–9.

Jaffe, B.M., Donegan, W.L., Watson, F., *et al.* (1968). Factors influencing survival in patients with untreated hepatic metastases. *Surg. Gynecol. Obstet.* **127**, 1–11.

Kemeny, N. and Daly, J. (1986). Preliminary results of a randomized study of intrahepatic infusion versus systemic infusion of 5FUDR for metastatic colorectal carcinoma. *Recent Results Cancer Res.* **100**, 171–8.

Kemeny, N., Yagoda, A., Braun, D., *et al.* (1980). Therapy for metastatic colorectal carcinoma with a combination of methyl CCNU, 5-fluorouracil, vincristine, and streptozotocin (MOF-strep). *Cancer* **45**, 876–81.

Laufman, L.R., Nims, T.A., Guy, J.T., *et al.* (1984). Hepatic artery ligation and portal vein infusion for liver metastases from colon cancer. *J. Clin. Oncol.* **2**, 1382–9.

Logan, S.E., Meter, S.J., Kamming, K.P., *et al.* (1982). Hepatic resection of metastatic colorectal carcinoma. *Arch. Surg.* **117**, 25–8.

McArdle, C.S., Lewi, H., Hansell, D., *et al.* (1988). Cytotoxic-loaded albumen microspheres: a novel approach to regional chemotherapy. *Br. J. Surg.* **75**, 132–4.

Miller, R.C., Bukowski, R.M., Andersen, S., *et al.* (1988). Phase II evaluation of sequential hepatic artery infusion of 5-FU and hepatic irradiation in metastatic colorectal carcinoma. *J. Surg. Oncol.* **37**, 1–4.

Moertel, C.G. (1975). Clinical management of advanced gastrointestinal cancer. *Cancer* **36**, 675–82.

Mokka, R.E.M., Larmi, T.K., Huttunen, R., *et al.* (1975). Evaluation of the ligation of the hepatic artery and regional arterial chemotherapy in the treatment of primary and secondary cancer of the liver. *Ann. Chir. Gynecol. Fenn.* **64**, 347–52.

Morrow, C.E. and Grage, T.B. (1982). Hepatic resection for secondary neoplasms. *Surgery* **92**, 610–14.

Murray-Lyon, I.M., Parsons, V.A., Blendis, C.M., *et al.* (1970). Treatment of secondary hepatic tumours by ligation of hepatic artery and infusion of cytotoxic drugs. *Lancet* **ii**, 172–5.

Neiderhuber, E., Ensminger, W., Gyves, J., *et al.* (1984). Regional chemotherapy of colorectal cancer metastatic to the liver. *Cancer* **53**, 1336–43.

Neilson, J., Balslov, I., and Jensen, H.E. (1971). Carcinoma of the colon with liver metastases. Operative indications and prognosis. *Acta. Chir. Scand.* **137**, 463–5.

Oberfield, R.A., McCaffrey, J.A., Polio, J., *et al.* (1979). Prolonged and continuous percutaneous intra-arterial hepatic infusion chemotherapy in advanced metastatic liver adenocarcinoma from colorectal primary. *Cancer* **44**, 414–23.

Ogita, A., Tokiwa, K., Taniguchi, H., *et al.* (1987). Intra-arterial chemotherapy with lipid contract medium for hepatic malignancies in infants. *Cancer* **60**, 2886–90.

Okamura, J., Horikawa, S., Jujiyama, T., *et al.* (1982). An appraisal of transcatheter arterial embolization combined with transcatheter arterial infusion of chemotherapeutic agent for hepatic malignancies. *World J. Surg.* **6**, 352–7.

Patt, Y.Z., Chuang, V.P., Wallace, S., *et al.* (1981). The palliative role of hepatic arterial infusion and arterial occlusion in colorectal carcinoma metastatic to the liver. *Lancet* **i**, 349–50.

Patt, Y.Z., Peters, R.E., Chuang, U.B., *et al.* (1983). Effective re-treatment of patients with colorectal cancer and liver metastases. *Am. J. Med.* **75**, 237–40.

Persson, B.G., Nobin, A., Ahren, B., *et al.* (1989). Repeated hepatic ischaemia as a treatment for carcinoid liver metastases. *World J. Surg.* **13**, 307–12.

Pestana, C., Reitemeter, R.J., Moertel, C.G., *et al.* (1964). The natural history of carcinoma of the colon and rectum. *Am. J. Surg.* **108**, 826–9.

Petrelli, N.J., Barcewicz, P.A., Evans, J.T., *et al.* (1984). Hepatic artery ligation for liver metastases in colorectal carcinoma. *Cancer* **53**, 1347–53.

Pettavel, J. and Morgenthaler, F. (1978). Protracted arterial chemotherapy of liver tumours: an experience of 107 cases over a 12-year period. In *Progress in clinical cancer* (ed. I.M. Ariel) Vol. 17, pp. 217–33. Grune and Stratton, New York.

Pettavel, J., Leyvraz, S., and Douglas, P. (1984). The necessity for staging liver metastases and standardizing treatment response criteria. The case of secondaries of colorectal origin. In *Liver metastases* (ed. C.J.H. van de Welde and P.H. Sugarbaker) pp. 154–68. Martinus Nijhoff, Amsterdam.

Pfeifle, C.E., Howell, S.B., and Bookstein, J.J. (1985). Pilot study of intra-arterial floxuridine, mitomycin and doxorubicin in combination with degradable starch microspheres to treat primary and metastatic tumours of the liver. *Cancer Drug Deliv.* **2**, 305–11.

Rajpal, S., Desmahaptra, K.S., Ledesma, E.J., *et al.* (1982). Extensive resections of isolated metastasis from carcinoma of the colon and rectum. *Surg. Gynecol. Obstet.* **155**, 813–16.

Rapaport, A.H. and Bureleson, R.L. (1970). Survival of patients treated with systemic fluorouracil for hepatic metastases. *Surg. Gynecol. Obstet.* **130**, 773–7.

Reitmeier, R.S., Moertel, C.G., and Hahn, R.G. (1970). Combination chemotherapy in gastrointestinal cancer. *Cancer Res.* **30**, 1425–8.

Rotman, M., Kuruvilla, A.N., Choi, K., *et al.* (1986). Response of colorectal hepatic metastases to concomitant radiotherapy and intravenous infusion 5-fluorouracil. *Int. J. Radiat. Oncol. Biol. Phys.* **12**, 2179–87.

Schwartz, S.I., Jones, L.S., and McCune, L.S. (1985). Assessment of treatment of intrahepatic malignancies using chemotherapy via and implantable pump. *Ann. Surg.* **201**, 560–7.

Schwemmle, K., Link, K.H., and Rieck, B. (1987). Rationale and indications for perfusion in liver tumours: current data. *World J. Surg.* **II**, 534–40.

Shepard, K.V., Faintuch, J., Bitran, J.D., *et al.* (1985*a*). Treatment of metastatic colorectal carcinoma with cisplatinum and 5-FU. *Cancer Treat. Rep.* **69**, 123–4.

Shepard, K.V., Levin, B., Karl, R.C., *et al.* (1985*b*). Therapy for metastatic colorectal cancer with hepatic artery infusion chemotherapy using a subcutaneous implanted pump. *J. Clin. Oncol.* **3**, 161–9.

Shimamura, Y., Gunven, P., Takenaka, Y., *et al.* (1988). Combined peripheral and central chemoembolization of liver tumours: experience with lipiodol–doxorubicin and gelatin sponge. *Cancer* **61**, 238–42.

Stanislav, G.V., Fitzgibbons, R.J., Bailey, R.T., *et al.* (1987). Reliability of implantable central venous access devices in patients with cancer. *Arch. Surg.* **122**, 1280–3.

Sterchi, J.M., Richards, F., White, D.R., *et al.* (1989). Chemoinfusion of the hepatic artery for metastases to the liver. *Surg. Gynecol. Obstet.* **168**, 291–5.

Sullivan, R.D. and Zurek, W.Z. (1965). Chemotherapy for liver cancer by protracted ambulatory infusion. *J. Am. Med. Assoc.* **194**, 481–6.

Sundqvist, K., Hafstrom, L., Jonsson, R.E., *et al.* (1978). Treatment of liver cancer with regional intra-arterial 5-FU infusion. *Am. J. Surg.* **136**, 328–31.

Swinton, N.W., Samaan, S., and Rosenthal, D. (1967). Cancer of the rectum and sigmoid. *Surg. Clin. North Am.* **47**, 657–62.

Taylor, I. (1978). Cytotoxic perfusion for colorectal liver metastases. *Br. J. Surg.* **65**, 109–14.

Taylor, I. (1981). Studies on the treatment and prevention of colorectal liver metastases. *Ann. R. Coll. Surg.* **63**, 270–6.

Taylor, I., Bennet, R., and Sherriff, S. (1979). The blood supply of colorectal liver metastases. *Br. J. Cancer* **39**, 749–56.

Trivisionno, D.P., Riether, R.D., Sheets, J.A., *et al.* (1986). Follow-up on a prospective study of continuous hepatic perfusion with implantable pump. *Dis. Colon Rectum* **29**, 691–3.

Wagner, J.S., Adson, M.A., van Heerden, J.A., *et al.* (1984). The natural history of hepatic metastases from colorectal cancer. *Ann. Surg.* **199**, 502–8.

Wanebo, H.J.J., Semoglou, C., Attiyeh, F., *et al.* (1978). Surgical management of patients with primary operable colorectal cancer and synchronous liver metastases. *Am. J. Surg.* **135**, 81–5.

Watkins, E., Khazei, A.M., and Nahra, K.S. (1970). Surgical basis for arterial infusion chemotherapy of disseminated carcinoma of the liver. *Surg. Gynecol. Obstet.* **130**, 580–605.

Weiss, G.R., Garnick, M.B., Osteen, R.T., *et al.* (1983). Long-term hepatic arterial infusion of 5-FUDR for liver metastases using an implantable infusion pump. *J. Clin. Oncol.* **1**, 337–44.

Wood, C.B. (1984). Natural history of liver metastases. In *Liver metastases* (ed. C.J.H. van de Welde and P.H. Sugarbaker) pp. 47–54. Martinus Nijhoff, Amsterdam.

Wood, C.B., Gillis, C.R., and Blumgart, L.H. (1976). A retrospective study of the natural history of patients with liver metastases from colorectal cancer. *Clin. Oncol.* **2**, 285–8.

Yamada, R., Sato, M., Kawabata, M., *et al.* (1983). Hepatic artery embolization in 120 patients with unresectable hepatoma. *Radiology* **148**, 397–401.

17. Hepatocellular carcinoma

Chue-Shue Lee

Biological behaviour

From clinical observations of the outcome of surgically treated hepatocellular carcinoma (HCC) in patients with asymptomatic small tumours (Lee, Sung, Hwang, Sheu, Chen, Lin, and Beasley 1986; Lee, Hwang, Beasley, Hsu, Lee, and Lin 1988), HCC can be classified into two varieties. Type I, also known as slow-growing HCC, appears grossly as a round, encapsulated, and mostly solitary mass, having a homogeneous appearance on its cut surface. Histologically, the cancer cells are confined within the mass. This type represents approximately 20 per cent of surgically treated patients with asymptomatic, small HCC. Type II, also called rapid-growing HCC, can have grossly either a round or irregular outline, with or without a capsule. It appears frequently to be heterogeneous on the cut surface of the tumour. Evidence of tumour invasion can be observed in most cases, in satellite nodules surrounding the main tumour, in portal or hepatic veins, in bile ducts, in intrahepatic spread (where the tumour is manifested as multiple lesions), and even in distant metastases in lung, bone, and soft tissue.

Histologically, two outcomes are possible: either the cancer cells expand outside the capsule of the tumour, or the boundary between the cancer cells and the normal liver tissues is ill defined. This type constitutes about 80 per cent of surgically treated patients with small HCC. Whereas long-term survival can be achieved in most patients with type I disease, recurrence of tumour is the most likely outcome in those with type II.

Characteristics

The association of post-necrotic liver cirrhosis with HCC is frequent; at autopsy it has been estimated at 88 per cent (Lee *et al.* 1988). Post-necrotic liver cirrhosis is caused by either the hepatitis B virus, prevalent in areas such as Taiwan, Hong Kong, China, and South Africa, or the non-A, non-B hepatitis virus, prevalent in areas such as Japan. Clinical serological studies of hepatitis B virus surface antigen (HBsAg) using radio-immunoassay indicate that as many as 91 per cent of patients with HCC are HBsAg carriers (Chen and Sung 1977). Furthermore, the male:female ratio of HCC is approximately 6:1, despite the fact that the incidence of HBsAg carriers among the general population in Taiwan is about 17 per cent, affecting both sexes equally. Moreover, the average age of patients is about 48 years (Lee *et al.* 1986) and, finally, vulnerability to HCC is hereditary, as illustrated by the fact that at least 11 per cent of patients have family members also affected by HCC (Lee *et al.* 1986).

Therefore, post-necrotic liver cirrhosis, the presence of HBsAg, males over 40 years in age, and a family history of HCC are the factors conducive to the development of HCC. The secretion of embryogenic protein (α-fetoprotein, AFP) is an important characteristic in patients with HCC; about two-thirds of these patients can be observed to have an abnormally elevated serum AFP of greater than 20 ng/ml (Lee *et al.* 1986).

Incidence

HCC is second only to lung cancer as the chief cause of death from malignant disease among the male population of Taiwan. Beasley, Hwang, Lin, and Chien (1981) reported that the yearly incidence of HCC is about 0.5 per cent among the high-risk groups — HBsAg carriers and men over 40 years old.

Clinical manifestations

The clinical symptoms and signs of symptomatic HCC mainly depend upon the location, size, and invasiveness of the tumours, as well as the degree of portal hypertension and liver cirrhosis. The most frequent symptom is the dull pain which originates from stretching of Glisson's capsule adjacent to the lesion, and presents either in the epigastrium or the right hypochondrium. Another frequent sign of HCC, provided the tumour is located in the inferior surface of the liver, is a palpable mass moving with respiration, either in the epigastrium or the right hypochondrium.

Hepatomegaly is also an obvious sign of HCC when tumours are located deep inside the liver. The least frequent signs of HCC are low-grade fever, diarrhoea, anorexia, and the loss of body-weight. If the tumour were to extrude from the surface of the liver, either internal bleeding due to spontaneous rupture of the tumour into the peritoneal cavity, or persistent pain in the right flank or shoulder, due to the direct malignant invasion of the parietal peritoneum or the diaphragm, may occur. If the lesion invades the bile ducts, it may then give rise to obstructive jaundice, caused by haemobilia (icteric-type HCC). If the tumour invades the portal vein or the hepatic vein, or the hepatic arterial and venous systems, resulting in an arterio-venous fistula, signs of portal hypertension may appear or be aggravated.

Finally, other signs, which are common in patients with HCC, include palmar erythema, gynaecomastia, splenomegaly, and spider angiomata on the forechest, oesophageal varices, and ascites.

Subclinical detection

Through periodic examination of high-risk individuals (males over 40 years who have liver cirrhosis, who are HBsAg carriers, and have a family history of HCC) using serum AFP and/or hepatic sonographic examination, subclinical asymptomatic HCC can usually be detected by screening. However, screening by serum AFP examination alone usually misses about one-third of such cases. If the tumour size is less than 1.0 cm in diameter or the tumour is located on the subphrenic surface, or just beneath the rib, or on the edge of the liver, hepatic sonographic examination often overlooks the tumour.

Diagnosis

Using hepatic sonography, computed tomography (CT), and hepatic angiography, tumours can be identified and then localized. Subclinical HCC should be differentiated from benign hepatic lesions, such as regenerating nodules, cysts, and haemangioma; while symptomatic large HCC requires differentiation from benign entities such as polycystic liver, huge haemangiomata, and inflammatory masses (hepatic amoebiasis, hepatic tuberculoma, hepatic actinomycosis). Malignant hepatic tumours to be distinguished from HCC include cholangiocarcinoma, metastatic liver tumour, gallbladder cancer, and various kinds of sarcoma.

Hepatic sonography can differentiate a cyst from a solid tumour easily and can, for example, demonstrate features peculiar to amoebic disease such as 'mouse biting' around the edge of the tumour and an island in the centre of the lesion. Sonography cannot, however, differentiate between benign and malignant tumours. To ameliorate this deficiency a hepatic CT scan, with and without contrast, can be used to differentiate hepatic haemangioma from hepatic solid tumours (Fig. 17.1). The immediate but persistent appearance of high-density contrast media on a CT scan indicates the presence of haemangioma, while a relatively low density inside the hepatic tumour, in contrast to the surrounding normal liver tissue, indicates the presence of a solid hepatic tumour.

Hepatic angiography does what CT scan cannot; a hepatic regenerating nodule not associated with a tumour, which 'stains' on hepatic angiography, can be differentiated from a malignant hepatic tumour with staining. Huge haemangiomas of the liver are sometimes difficult to diagnose but the characteristic appearance of a 'cotton ball' on the hepatic angiogram may serve as a guide. A chronic inflammatory mass of the liver is the most difficult to diagnose and usually requires an exploratory laparotomy for a histological diagnosis.

Clinically, it is difficult to distinguish HCC from cholangiocarcinoma,

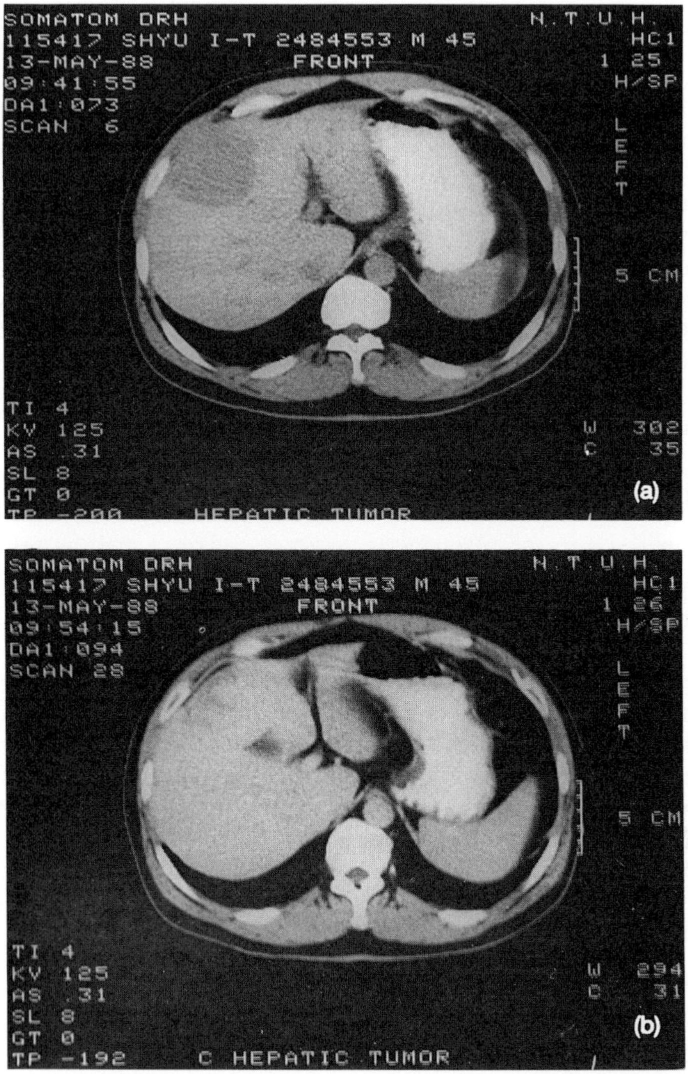

Fig. 17.1. (a) Computed tomographic scan showing hypodense lesion of the liver. (b) The above hypodense lesion is filled with contrast medium, indicating a haemangioma.

metastatic liver tumour, gallbladder cancer, and sarcoma, because all four malignant tumours show tumour staining at hepatic angiography. Needle biopsy of the lesion without exploratory laparotomy is contra-indicated. Tumour implantation may occur around the needle tract and even spread to the peritoneal cavity. An association with liver cirrhosis, HBsAg, a family history of HCC, abnormal elevation of serum AFP, occasional elevation of serum carcinoembrygenic antigen (CEA) of more than 10 ng/ml, and the lack of regional lymph node metastasis support the diagnosis of HCC.

In comparison, normal serum AFP, elevated serum CEA, and regional lymph node metastasis in association with a diagnosis of tumour within the liver are characteristic features of chloangiocarcinoma and gallbladder cancer. Elevated serum AFP can also be observed in metastatic liver cancer, provided the diagnosis of the primary lesion has been substantiated. Sarcomas of the liver require exploratory laparotomy for diagnosis.

Surgical treatment

Indication

Infiltrating tumours, multiple tumours, distant metastases, or decompensated liver reserve are contra-indications to surgical treatment. Palliative resection is considered in the treatment of patients with HCC with tumours that adhere to the parietal peritoneum or diaphragm, tumours that have satellite nodules, tumours that have invaded portal or hepatic veins, and tumours that have invaded the bile ducts, because early tumour recurrence is the usual outcome. However, long-term survival can occur in patients undergoing resection for spontaneously ruptured HCC, indicating that shed malignant cells of such lesions do not always survive in the peritoneal cavity. An unequal size of two HCC lesions usually indicates multiple HCC, whereas two equally sized HCC tumours indicate a synchronous origin. Long-term survival can be achieved after resection in the latter cases.

Anatomy

The liver is composed of two lobes; the right consists of half of the anterior segment and half of the posterior segment, which is further divided into the superior segments and the inferior segments, respectively (segments five, six, seven, and eight). The triangular-shaped left lobe is composed of the caudate segment (segment one), the superior segment (segment two), the inferior segment (segment three), and the median segment (segment four).

Each segment is nourished by the hepatic artery and the portal vein, bile being secreted into the bile ducts. The two vessels and the duct closely parallel each other. Knowledge of the direction of one gives information regarding the site of other structures. The portal vein branches at the extra-hepatic hilar area; the left portal vein then divides into two branches which enter the caudate and the median segments, respectively. Each branch further divides into inferior branches. The right portal vein divides immediately into anterior and posterior branches after entering the liver, with further divisions into superior and inferior branches, respectively.

The outflow of the liver comprises the left hepatic vein which collects blood from segments two, three, four, and the right hepatic vein, which collects blood from the anterior and posterior hepatic veins. The outflow of segment one usually drains directly into the vena cava.

Incision

The inverted T-shaped incision over the epigastrium, i.e. a vertical incision which starts from the xiphoid process down to the mid-point between the xyphoid process and the umbilicus, and a horizontal incision superior to the first incision [Fig. 17.2(a)] are adequate for resection of a tumour located anywhere in the left lobe. A long subcostal incision, beginning from the xiphoid process and extending the right flank area or to a left subcostal incision, is adequate for standard right hepatectomy and for resection of tumour located in the anterior, lateral, or inferior surface or the right lobe of the liver [Fig. 17.2(b)].

The right thoraco-abdominal incision is needed for partial hepatectomy for tumours located at the posterior segment and beneath the dome of the diaphragm [Fig. 17.2(c)]. Incision of the falciform ligament and the triangular ligament of either the right or the left lobe is needed to mobilize the liver for wider exposure, and easier resection is facilitated by adequate retraction.

Surgical technique

Controlled resection in the non-cirrhotic liver by extra-hepatic approach

A pre-operative hepatic angiogram to ensure that the right hepatic artery originates from either the common hapatic artery or the superior mesenteric artery should be available.

Standard right hepatectomy can be achieved, at the extra-hepatic hilar area, by division of the right hepatic artery, the right portal vein, and the right bile ducts. The first step, total occlusion of the inflow of the right lobe, while drastically minimizing blood loss during hepatic resection, demonstrates the appropriate resection line following discoloration of the liver surface.

The second step is finger dissection, or a fracture technique, for liver resection. The dissection begins with the intrahepatic identification and ligation of the anterior and posterior hepatic veins, followed by the intrahepatic control of tributaries which drain into the vena cava. The cut surface of the liver, after meticulous haemostasis by suture ligation, is managed by mattress sutures with the anterior surface approximated as far as possible to the posterior surface.

The third step requires that two large silicone drain tubes, one placed in the subphrenic space and the other placed in the subhepatic space, be used

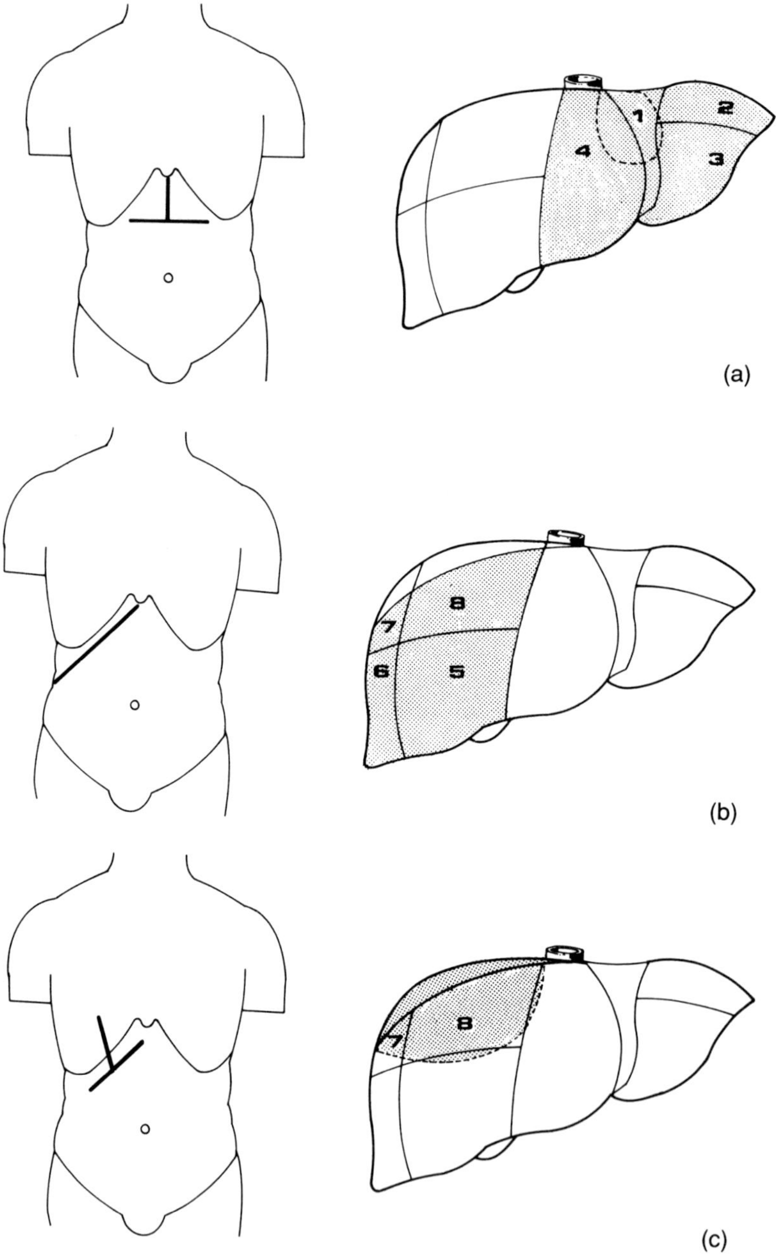

Fig. 17.2. (a) An inverted T-shape incision wound is applied for small hepatocellular carcinoma (HCC) located at either segment one, segment two, segment three, or segment four. (b) A subcostal incision is applied for small HCC located at either segment five, segment six, part of segment seven, or part of segment eight. (c) A thoraco-abdominal incision is applied for small HCC located at either part of segment seven or part of segment eight.

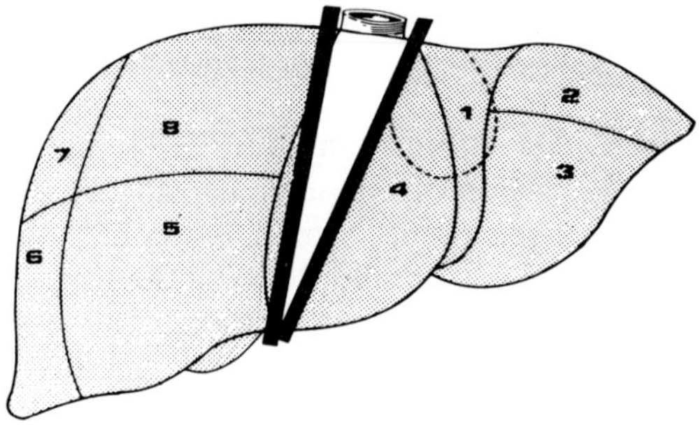

FIg. 17.3. Lin's hepatic clamp is applied to the left side of the liver for small hepatocellular carcinomas (HCC) located at either segment two, segment three, or segment four. The clamp is applied to the right side of the liver for small HCC located at either segment five or segment six, seven, or eight.

for drainage. Standard left hepatectomy is undertaken in a similar fashion. The last step is wound closure in layers.

Intrahepatic approach

Following mobilization of the right lobe of the liver, the hilar area is directly visualized. The entry of the right bile duct to the liver can be seen. A 1-cm incision is made 2 cm away from the hilum, applied perpendicular to the direction of the right hepatic duct over the inferior surface of the right lobe of the liver. Finger fracture dissection is undertaken for resection. The triads of the right portal vein, the right hepatic artery, and the right bile ducts can be identified easily by palpation, usually 2 cm beneath the liver surface. After total occlusion of the inflow of the triads, the resection is continued as for an extra-hepatic approach.

Inflow block by Lin's hepatic clamp

If the tumour is located on either side, Lin's hepatic clamp can be applied during right or left atypical hepatectomy (Fig. 17.3). Inflow and outflow of the right or the left liver should be blocked simultaneously so that the finger dissection technique can be applied during hepatic resection.

Resection in the cirrhotic liver

To preserve liver reserve as much as possible and to prevent possible hepatic failure, only limited hepatic resection may be applicable in the cirrhotic liver. The inflow of the right or the left liver can be blocked by Lin's hepatic clamp, temporary clamping of the common hepatic artery, or the Pringle manoeuvre, after which the resection line can be drawn with the tumour located at the centre of the resected specimen.

Consideration should be given to anatomical structures of the inflow and the outflow tracts which are close to the tumour. Interference with the inflow and outflow of the remnant of liver should be avoided as much as possible.

The finger fracture dissection technique is actually a three-layered method. We begin with division of Glisson's capsule by cautery, after which the second layer of the liver tissue, which is about 2 cm in thickness, is crushed either vertically or horizontally, leaving the tiny vessels and the bile ducts for further ligation or electrocoagulation. The entire resection line which surrounds the tumour should be completed before proceeding to the third layer resection. The third layer of the liver tissue is composed of larger vessels, bile ducts, and fragile liver tissue, which can be easily removed by using the index finger as a knife for repeated dissection. Usually the vessels and the bile ducts can be preserved by palpation. All the vessels and bile ducts can be easily identified and doubly ligated. This dissection technique usually takes about 20–40 minutes to complete.

Extent of hepatic resection

Extended standard right hepatectomy with resection of about 80 per cent of the liver, and preservation of the lateral segment of the left lobe of the liver, will not usually lead to hepatic failure, if applied only in the non-cirrhotic liver. The non-cirrhotic liver has the ability rapidly to regenerate to almost original liver size. There is, however, no regenerational capacity present in the cirrhotic liver, and in order to prevent the likelihood of hepatic failure only a limited hepatic resection is feasible (Lin and Chen 1965; Lin, Lee, Chen, Liau, and Lin 1979). In general, the weight of the resected specimen should not exceed 350 g (about a quarter of the entire cirrhotic organ), and liver reserve assessment by the 45-minute bromsulphthalein retention rate should be less than 34 per cent.

Complications

In my experience, operative mortality and hospital mortality rates are 3 per cent (Lee *et al.* 1986). Massive intra-operative blood loss is the main cause of death at operation, while ruptured oesophageal varices, sepsis, and myocardial infarction are the most common causes of hospital mortality. The worst complications of hepatic failure can be avoided if one strictly observes the rules regarding the extent of hepatic resection and patient selection. Post-operative complications include pleural effusion in the right chest cavity (10 per cent), bile leakage (4 per cent), subphrenic abscess (4 per cent), and upper gastrointestinal bleeding due to gastritis.

Prognosis and outcome

The 5-year survival rate for symptomatic HCC after surgical treatment is, depending on the biological behaviour of HCC, between 3 and 20 per cent (Lin 1970; Fortner, Kim, Maclean, Barrett, Iwatsukis, Turn Ball, Howland,

and Beattie 1978; Lee, Wong, and Ong 1982; Okuda 1980), while that of asymptomatic small HCC is about 50 per cent (Lee *et al.* 1988).

Other treatment modalities

Trans-arterial embolization, systemic or regional chemotherapy, and even radiotherapy have been proven to be limited therapeutic options. The clinical difficulties encountered in performing prospective randomized controlled studies, and the variable natural course of HCC, compound problems when drawing definite conclusions regarding other treatment modalities.

Prevention

In connection with hepatitis B virus infection, there must exist some unknown aetiological factors for the formation of HCC, since not all HBsAg carriers develop malignancy. Widespread immunization with anti-hepatitis B vaccine in the next generation holds the most promise for the elimination of HCC.

References

Beasley, R.P., Hwang, L.Y., Lin, C.C., and Chien, C.S. (1981). Hepatocellular carcinoma and hepatitis B virus — A prospective study 22 707 men in Taiwan. *Lancet* **ii**, 1129–32.

Chen, D.S. and Sung, J.L. (1977). Serum alphafetoprotein on hepatocellular carcinoma. *Cancer*, **40**, 779–83.

Fortner, J.G., Kim, D.K., Maclean, B.J., Barrett, M.K., Iwatsuki, F., Turnbull, A.D., Howland, W.S., and Beattie, E.J. Jr. (1978). Major hepatic resection for neoplasia — personal experience in 108 patients. *Annals of Surgery*, **188**, 363–71.

Lee, N.W., Wong, J., and Ong, G.B. (1982). The surgical management of primary carcinoma of the liver. *World J. Surg.* **6**, 66–75.

Lee, C.S., Hwang, L.Y., Beasley, R.P., Hsu, H.C., Lee, H.S., and Lin, T.Y. (1988). Prognostic significance of histologic findings in resected small hepatocellular carcinoma. *Acta Chir. Scand*, **154**, 199–203.

Lee, C.S., Sung, J.L., Hwang, L.Y., Sheu, J.C., Chen, D.S., Lin T.Y., and Beasley, R.P. (1986). Surgical treatment of 109 patients with symptomatic and asymptomatic hepatocellular carcinoma. *Surgery*. **99**, 481–490.

Lin, T.Y. (1970). Primary cancer of the liver — Quadrennial Review. *Scand. J. Gastroenterol* (*suppl.*), **6**, 223–4.

Lin, T.Y. and Chen, C.C. (1965). Metabolic function and regeneration of cirrhotic and noncirrhotic livers after hepatic lobectomy in man. *Annals of Surgery*, **162**, 959–72.

Lin, T.Y., Lee, C.S., Chen, C.C., Liau, K.Y., and Lin, W.S.J. (1979). Regeneration of human liver after hepatic lobectomy studied by repeated liver scanning and repeated needle biopsy. *Annals of Surgery*, **190**, 48–53.

Okuda, K. (1980). Liver cancer study group of Japan: primary liver cancer in Japan. *Cancer*. **45**, 2663–9.

18. Screening for gastrointestinal malignancy

W.M. Thomas and Jack D. Hardcastle

Principles of screening

The rationale of screening for malignant disease is the premise that the development of a malignant focus is followed by a well-defined progression of the disease, each step reducing the prospect of long-term survival. A screening programme is therefore likely to be most successful in a disease which typically presents at an advanced clinicopathological stage, and where there is evidence that treatment instigated when the disease is localized results in an improved prognosis. Moreover, where identification and removal of a pre-malignant entity is possible, the prospect of reducing the incidence of a malignant condition is introduced.

Clearly there are benefits and disadvantages of any screening programme. Potential benefits include an improved prognosis, less radical treatment, and a possible treatment-cost benefit.

Disadvantages include the possibility of a longer period of psychological morbidity for those with disease not influenced by treatment, hazards introduced by the screening test, over-treatment and, unless the screening test is highly specific and sensitive, the danger of investigating many healthy individuals and of reassuring some individuals who are harbouring asymptomatic disease.

Before mass population screening programmes are introduced it is essential that the frequency and mortality rates of the disease, in that society, justify the considerable financial commitment involved.

There are important practical differences in the approach to the surveillance of individuals at particular risk of developing malignancy. Well-defined high-risk groups for the development of malignancy, at each site within the gastrointestinal tract, are known and will be dealt with in the appropriate sections. Mass population screening refers to screening where the only identifiable risk factors are age or sex; it is this form of screening that is most likely to influence overall mortality rates of the common gastrointestinal malignancies.

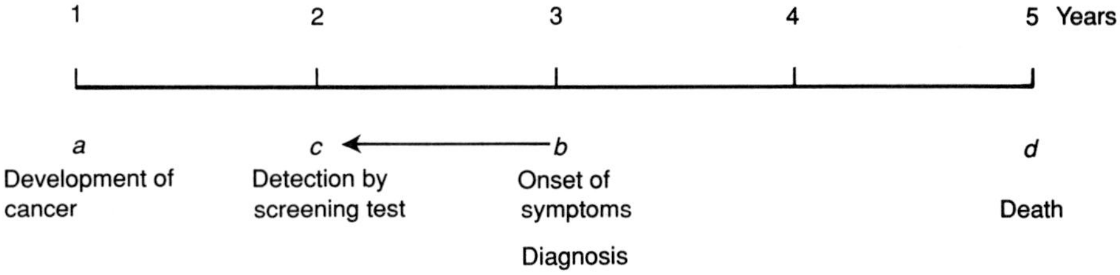

Fig. 18.1. Lead time bias.

Screening biases

The assessment of mass population screening without a controlled trial is difficult, principally because of a range of biases introduced whenever a screening test is made generally available.

Lead time bias

This term refers to the phenomenon whereby the pre-symptomatic diagnosis of a disease confers an apparent improvement in long-term survival.

In the example given (Fig. 18.1) the development of a carcinoma, at point *a* in time, is followed by an asymptomatic phase (the sojourn time) before the onset of symptoms and diagnosis at point *b*. Death at point *d* results in a survival time from diagnosis of 2 years — by moving the diagnosis back to point *c* (i.e. reducing the sojourn time) there is an *apparent* improvement of 1 year in survival, even if the time from development of cancer to death is the same.

Length bias

Slow-growing, less aggressive cancers are likely to have a longer pre-symptomatic phase than more aggressive anaplastic tumours; thus screening at any one point in time will detect a disproportionately greater number of these less aggressive cancers. An improved prognosis for tumours detected by screening may reflect their more favourable biological behaviour and be quite independent of pre-symptomatic detection.

Volunteer bias

The recruitment of volunteers into a screening programme may affect the interpretation of the programme in two ways, either enhancing or reducing its true efficacy.

In the first instance, comparison of mortality rates in a health-conscious group of volunteers offered screening, with those of the average population, introduces a bias in favour of the screened group who may have an inherently better prognosis from the disease. On the other hand, if a volunteer cohort is randomized into groups, which are screened or not screened, the difference in mortality between the groups would be expected to be less than the difference observed had a more typical, non-selected population been recruited.

Undoubtedly, the best way to allow for these biases is by means of a randomized controlled trial in which the test group (comprising individuals who accepted the screening test, those who refused the test, and those in whom malignant disease was missed by the test) are compared with an age- and sex-matched control group, which has not been screened and is not aware of the potential advantages of screening.

Purists will argue that all screening strategies should be subject to this rigorous analysis. However, many of the screening programmes which have already been instigated world-wide (for example, the gastric screening programme in Japan) are considered to have had such a profound effect on the course of the disease, and to have educated the public to such an extent, that future randomized controlled trials are both unethical and impractical. Nevertheless, in conditions where there is no proven mortality advantage for screening (for example, colorectal cancer screening), it is essential that the requisite studies be completed before mass population screening is introduced.

Three main sites of gastrointestinal malignancy have been subject to mass population screening programmes or controlled trials. They are the oesophagus, the stomach, and the colorectum.

Carcinoma of the oesophagus

Background

Oesophageal carcinoma is subject to marked regional variation in incidence. Whilst endemic in certain well-demarcated areas throughout the world, it is a relatively uncommon cause of cancer morbidity and mortality in most of western Europe and North America. In England and Wales there are 2800 new cases diagnosed every year in male patients, accounting for 2 per cent of all cancer registrations (Office of Population Censuses and Surveys 1988). The disease is less common in the female population. However, its aggressive nature is reflected in the fact that it is responsible for 4 per cent of cancer deaths in males and 3 per cent of cancer deaths in females.

The USA is recognized as a low-risk area with an incidence of about 9000 new cases diagnosed every year. High-risk areas include parts of Iran, China, and Africa, where incidence rates are as much as 20 times greater than those reported in western Europe. Carcinoma of the oesophagus is the commonest cancer in South Africa (McGlashan 1988). It is not surprising, therefore, that most reports of mass population screening have emanated from Asia, the Far East, and South Africa; often screening has targeted those at particular risk.

High-risk groups

Barrett's oesophagus

Although initially thought to be a tubular intrathoracic stomach, it is now accepted that the condition described by Barrett in 1950 refers to a columnar lined oesophagus. It is acknowledged that the condition predisposes to the development of lower oesophageal adenocarcinoma. However, the precise risk is difficult to quantify, largely because of inconsistencies in the definition of Barrett's oesophagus, and the uncertainty that lower oesophageal adenocarcinomas are not in fact carcinomas of the stomach which have extended into the oesophagus. Robertson, Mayberry, Nicholson, James, and Atkinson (1988) described four carcinomas arising in 56 patients with Barrett's oesophagus at a rate of 1 for every 56 patient years of follow-up, whilst Spreckler, *et al.* (1984) described an incidence of 1 per 175 patient years of follow-up.

The necessity for long-term follow-up of patients with Barrett's oesophagus remains contentious. Gillen and Hennessy (1989) have suggested that there is little benefit in providing surveillance for elderly patients with short segments of columnar lined oesophagus, although regular endoscopic screening should be offered to younger patients, those with extensive metaplastic epithelium, and, in particular, those with dysphasia.

Tylosis

This rare syndrome, inherited in an autosomal dominant fashion, comprises pathological thickening of the skin on the palms and soles and an associated high susceptibility to oesophageal cancer. It has been calculated that the risk of oesophageal cancer exceeds 90 per cent by the age of 65 years. Harper, Harper and Havel-Evans 1970; Munoz and Crespi 1983).

Achalasia

It has been proposed that malignancy, in association with this motor oesophageal disorder, is secondary to stasis of oesophageal contents. The risk of malignant change increases with time, patients typically presenting with carcinoma at least 20 years after the onset of symptoms of achalasia.

Caustic strictures

Again, long-standing stasis and inflammation is regarded as the basis for the malignant potential of this condition. The overall life-time risk is reported to be of the order of 3.5 per cent (Hopkins and Postlewait 1981).

In general, the risk of malignancy in individuals belonging to one of the high-risk groups justifies long-term endoscopic follow-up, a strategy that includes routine biopsy and cytology for the assessment of dysplastic changes.

Mass population screening

Endoscopic screening, as described for the high-risk groups, offers a very accurate assessment of the oesophageal mucosa. However, in those countries with a high incidence of oesophageal malignancy amongst the general population the mainstay of screening has been the cytological examination of oesophageal smears. The method of sample collection varies from using a swallowed inflatable balloon to scrape the oesophageal lining (Shu 1983), to an expandable brush pulled up the oesophagus by a string (Nabeya 1983). Shu reviewed the extensive experience of the Chinese who introduced the balloon sampling technique in the early 1960s, and before 1979 more than half a million people had been screened. It is claimed that the technique has an accuracy of approximately 90 per cent for the diagnosis of carcinoma of the oesophagus, reliably distinguishing malignant change from benign conditions.

Throughout geographical areas of China the cancer detection rate has varied from zero to 1.9 per cent amongst those who underwent cytological examination. Of the cancers detected, more than 70 per cent were described as being minimally invasive. The study has enabled the progression of dysplastic changes to be monitored. It is of interest that the incidence of severe dysplasia in the Chinese provinces reflects the incidence of carcinoma, with the average age of patients with severe dysplasia being approximately 8 years less than that of patients with carcinoma.

Nevertheless, a screening study of high-risk subjects with oesophagitis in Iran (Crespi, *et al.* 1979) has failed to demonstrate the slow progression of dysplasia to malignancy suggested by the Chinese study. In the Iranian study the average age of patients with dysplasia was very similar to the average age of patients with carcinoma. This suggests that there are regional differences in the nature of oesophageal malignancy. The slow-growing tumours, predominant in the Chinese population, would be expected to have a better prognosis.

Unfortunately, it is not possible objectively to measure the effect of mass population screening independently of the screening biases described above, as the necessary studies have not been completed. Experience from the regions with a high prevalence of the disease, in particular the reports of the massive screening programmes in China, suggest that cytological methods of screening for oesophageal cancer are practical and probably provide the only means of improving the prognosis from this disease in the short term.

Carcinoma of the stomach

Background

During the twentieth century there has been a modest decline in the incidence of gastric cancer throughout most of the developed world. Despite this, more than 12 500 new cases of gastric carcinoma are recorded in the UK every year, the disease accounting for approximately 10 per cent of all cancer registrations (Office of Population Censuses and Surveys 1988; Registrar General 1987). As in the case of oesophageal carcinoma a marked international variation is evident. The disease is particularly common in Japan where the incidence rates are four times higher than those of the UK (Hirayama 1971). Finland, Iceland, and Chile also have high incidence rates whilst there appears to be a relative sparing of Australians, New Zealanders, and US caucasians (Wynder, Konet, Dungal, and Segi 1963). Migrant studies have suggested that environmental factors are responsible for the variations described.

The disease is uncommon before the age of 40 years and increases steadily in incidence into the seventh decade. Males are affected twice as commonly as females overall. The prognosis from the disease is depressingly poor. The overall 5-year survival rate in England and Wales is approximately 10 per cent (Office of Population Censuses and Surveys 1983).

High-risk groups

Pernicious anaemia

Stockbrugger, *et al.* (1983) screened 80 patients with pernicious anaemia; 33 were found to have mucosal dysplasia and one patient was found to have a carcinoma. Despite its long-established association with gastric cancer, the precise risk remains unknown and no firm recommendations regarding surveillance can be made.

Familial adenomatous polyposis

This autosomal dominant condition is associated with a neoplastic risk in the upper as well as the lower gastrointestinal tract, those affected with upper gastrointestinal disease typically having duodenal adenomas. It appears that there is an associated risk of malignancy and that upper gastrointestinal endoscopy may have a role in long-term surveillance.

Previous gastric surgery

The excess risk of developing gastric cancer in patients who have undergone previous gastric surgery for benign disease remains debatable, Caygill, Hill, Kirkham, and Northfield (1986) studied almost 4500 patients undergoing such surgery and described a three-fold increased risk of gastric cancer at 20 years of follow-up. Clark, Ward, McDonald, and Tovey (1983), Farrands, Blake, Anseel, Cotton, and Hardcastle (1983*b*), and Perez, Narayanan, Russell, and Becker (1984) all reported an excess gastric cancer rate in patients having previous gastric surgery. However, Fischer, Graem, and Jenson (1983) failed to demonstrate this phenomenon in a follow-up study of 1000 patients. Logan and Langman (1983) have examined the prospect of screening patients post-operatively, concluding that long-term surveillance is not warranted.

Mass population screening

Early gastric cancer

In 1962, the Japanese Society for Gastrointestinal Endoscopy (Murakami 1971) defined early gastric cancer (EGC) as an invasive carcinoma limited to the submucosa or mucosa with or without lymph node metastases. The pre-eminence of the Japanese as the world leaders in gastric cancer screening has ensured the acceptance of this term. The experience in Japan is that a screening programme can successfully identify gastric malignancy at this stage. Only 5–10 per cent of symptomatic cases of gastric carcinoma in Europe and the US satisfy the definition of EGC (Adashek, Sanger, and Longmire 1979; du Pont, Lee, Burton, and Cohn 1978).

The Japanese screening programme

A national gastric cancer screening programme was instituted in Japan in 1960. The method of screening has been double contrast radiology, most of the screening being performed in mobile fluoroscopy units. There is evidence that the test is highly sensitive if 10 films are taken of each subject (Ichikawa 1971), but in most screening programmes six-film examinations are performed. This is estimated to have a sensitivity of 90 per cent for gastric cancer and maintains cost-effectiveness together with reducing radiation hazards (Hirayama 1978). The yield of neoplastic disease has been between one and two carcinomas for every 1000 examinations (Kaneko, *et al.* 1977), with 40–50 per cent being EGCs. This compares with a rate for EGC of 25 per cent in a group of patients presenting to a Japanese surgical clinic (Okui and Tejima 1980; Kaibara, *et al.* 1981). It is estimated that the optimal rescreen period is 3 years (Kohrogi 1987).

In the absence of a randomized controlled trial, the precise impact of the screening study on mortality rates from gastric cancer in Japan is unknown. However, a case-control study performed in Nose Town, Osaka (Oshima, *et al.* 1986) has suggested that screening reduces the likelihood of dying from gastric cancer by 40 per cent in males and by 60 per cent in females.

In a follow-up study of 18 000 screened people, Muir, Choi, and Schiftlers (1981) reported a decrease of approximately 25 per cent in gastric cancer deaths when compared with the expected deaths calculated from the sex- and age-specific rates amongst the general population.

There can be little doubt that the diagnosis of EGC offers one of the most favourable prognostic indicators to an individual, with evidence from the

Japanese studies of 5-year survival rates in excess of 90 per cent. Data from the Osaka Cancer Registry demonstrated an improvement in the overall 5-year survival rate from 17.3 per cent between 1965 and 1969 to 23.7 per cent between 1975 and 1979. It is now gradually being accepted, however, that much of this improvement is secondary to lifestyle changes, particularly the alteration in dietary habits away from the traditional Japanese fare of highly preserved foods.

Symptom screening

Oleagoitea, *et al.* (1986) and de Dombal, *et al.* (1988) have demonstrated that between 70 and 90 per cent of patients presenting with EGC have dyspeptic symptoms. This raises the possibility of screening for EGC by one of the simplest and cheapest means available, that is by a symptom questionnaire.

The yield of investigation of dyspepsia has been reported by Allum, Hallissey, Dorrell, Low, and Fielding (1986); in a group of 683 patients over the age of 40 years who presented to their general practitioners (family doctors) with dyspepsia (thus not strictly a screening programme) 93 per cent of the patients proceeded to further investigation which included endoscopy. Fifteen patients (2 per cent) had gastric cancer, 10 of whom were suitable for radical resection. Seven oesophageal cancers were also detected.

Harrison and Morris (1988, 1990) have further evaluated the prospects of this type of screening. They sent symptom questionnaires to 4279 patients aged 50–75 years. More than 88 per cent of those contacted returned completed questionnaires, demonstrating that this form of screening is most acceptable to the general population. However, dyspeptic symptoms were identified in a high proportion (33 per cent) of the screenees, and a drop in compliance was noted at each subsequent part of evaluation (72 per cent attended the dyspepsia clinic, and 84 per cent of those invited for gastroscopy attended).

At the time of analysis 599 gastroscopies had been performed; three carcinomas were diagnosed (two of which were EGCs). A surprisingly large proportion of individuals had 'pre-malignant' conditions: 5 per cent had a Barrett's oesophagus and 13.5 per cent had intestinal metaplasia.

In conclusion, gastric carcinoma screening has probably had a favourable effect on the long-term survival rate of patients screened in the Japanese programme, although the precise contribution of screening to the evident mortality reduction is unknown. There is no justification for similar mass population screening in low-risk western societies but simpler methods, such as symptomatic screening, require further evaluation. The case for endoscopic screening of high-risk subjects remains contentious with no clear advantage for aggressive follow-up regimens.

Colorectal carcinoma

Background

Colorectal carcinoma is essentially a disease of the western developed nations, having its highest incidence in north-west Europe, the US, Canada, and New Zealand. Amongst the economically developed nations, only Japan escapes with a low incidence, a regional variation that may reflect dietary factors.

In England and Wales the disease is responsible for 17 300 deaths per annum (Office of Population Censuses and Surveys 1988) and is second only to carcinoma of the lung and breast in women as a cause of death from malignant disease. In the US, there are approximately 155 000 new cases of, and more than 60 000 deaths from, the disease every year (Silverberg, Boring, and Squires 1990). In Australia, the absolute number of colorectal cancer deaths is rising rapidly, with little improvement in mortality rates (Dent, MacDonald, Chapius, and Goulston 1981; Rohan and McMichael 1981).

High-risk groups

Ulcerative colitis

Crohn and Rosenberg (1925) and Bargan (1928) recognized the malignant potential of ulcerative colitis. It is now acknowledged that the malignant risk is related both to the extent of the disease and to its duration. Overall, patients with extensive colitis run a 1 in 200 risk of developing carcinoma for each year of follow-up between 10 and 20 years. Thereafter, the risk increases to 1 in 60 per year (Lennard-Jones, Morson, Ritchie, Shove, and Williams 1977).

The polyposis syndromes

The polyposis syndromes, such as familial adenomatous polyposis and Gardner's syndrome, generally have an autosomal dominant mode of expression, thus affecting 50 per cent of offspring with a condition which confers a 100 per cent risk of developing colorectal cancer.

The cancer family syndrome

In this syndrome individuals are affected at a younger age and there is a high proportion of right-sided colonic cancers. There is an associated risk of other malignancies, in particular carcinoma of the breast, ovary, and endometrium.

Family history

It appears that the first-degree relatives of average-risk patients with colorectal cancer are at an increased risk of developing the disease, the risk being between three and eight times that of the general population (Lovett 1976; Duncan and Kyle 1982).

Clearly the relative risk varies in each of the known high-risk groups and this affects the frequency of surveillance. There is no doubt that those at risk of having familial adenomatous polyposis should undergo large bowel endoscopy from their early teens. There are also grounds for regular colonoscopic surveillance of patients with long-standing ulcerative colitis, at which time multiple biopsies are useful in assessing the degree of mucosal dysplasia. The frequency of colonoscopic examinations remains undecided, a situation similar to that for family history surveillance.

Mass population screening

The great majority of colorectal cancer cases occur sporadically in patients not belonging to one of the known high-risk groups. Amongst this population, the only identifiable risk factor is age; approximately two new cases of colorectal cancer are diagnosed annually per 100 000 population under the age of 40 years, but above this age the incidence rises rapidly. In the age range of 65–74 years the rate is approximately 250 per 100 000 per year (Office of Population Censuses and Surveys 1988). Most colorectal cancer screening has, therefore, targeted the population over the age of 45 years.

Symptom questionnaire

The results of questionnaire screening for colorectal carcinoma have been disappointing. Farrands and Hardcastle (1984) invited 1533 subjects between the ages of 45 and 74 years to complete a postal questionnaire. Only 34 per cent complied with the request, and of these a quarter reported at least one symptom of lower gastrointestinal disease and underwent a barium enema examination. The only neoplastic condition identified was one patient with an adenoma. Silman, *et al.* (1983) demonstrated that specificity could be increased by more precise wording. They emphasized the importance of the symptom of dark red rectal bleeding. Nevertheless, it appears that this form of screening lacks both sensitivity and specificity for malignant disease and that, unlike gastric cancer, colorectàl malignancy is essentially asymptomatic in its early stages.

Rigid sigmoidoscopy

Screening for recto-sigmoid cancers by rigid sigmoidoscopy has been widespread practice in the US where such examinations have been offered as part of health insurance plans. The data from these studies are open to marked volunteer bias and must be interpreted with some caution. Gilbertson and Nelms (1978) detected 25 recto-sigmoid cancers at rigid sigmoidoscopy in 21 158 asymptomatic subjects. Follow-up examinations in this cohort revealed a further 13 cancers, all at Dukes' stage A. The main claim of this study is an estimated 60 per cent reduction in the incidence of rectal cancers achieved by the removal of rectal adenomas, although subsequent reanalysis has indicated that the true reduction in incidence is considerably lower.

As a means of screening, rigid sigmoidoscopy has been largely superseded by the use of flexible large bowel endoscopy.

Flexible sigmoidoscopy

It would appear that of the endoscopic techniques available, fibre-optic flexible sigmoidoscopy offers the most promising means of large bowel cancer screening. Post-mortem studies have demonstrated that 70 per cent of all colonic tumours occur within the distal 60 cm of the colorectum, and of those polyps demonstrating a malignant focus, more than 90 per cent would theoretically be detectable by flexible sigmoidoscopy (Gillespie, *et al.* 1979). No randomized data are available to evaluate the potential mortality advantage, but in a screening study of 900 subjects aged over 44 years using left-sided colonoscopy after a phosphate enema, Foley, *et al.* (1988) detected six carcinomas and 163 adenomatous polyps. Only three of the patients with carcinoma had positive faecal occult blood tests. Wherry in 1981 described a series of 417 asymptomatic subjects over the age of 50 years who underwent standard flexible sigmoidoscopy. A total of 73 polyps (some metaplastic) were identified in 52 patients. However, in only 5.5 per cent of cases were the polyps adenomatous and greater than 1 cm in diameter.

These studies highlight one of the potential problems of endoscopic screening. When a large number of small adenomatous polyps is detected, only a very small proportion of may be expected to undergo malignant transformation, but, having been detected, subject the individual to life-long endoscopic surveillance.

Moreover, there is no evidence to suggest that this method of screening would be acceptable to the population as a whole — reported studies have relied on volunteers.

Colonoscopy

This procedure, generally accepted as offering the most accurate assessment of the large bowel mucosa, has no role in mass population screening, but may be indicated in the surveillance of those at particularly high risk of colorectal malignancy.

Faecal occult blood tests

Faecal occult blood tests offer a simple, cheap method of screening which can be easily distributed to the population at large and which requires no specialist skills for interpretation. Unlike other forms of gastrointestinal cancer screening, faecal occult blood testing is the subject of rigorous clinical evaluation in the form of randomized controlled trials.

The prospect of mass population screening by faecal occult blood testing was raised by Greegor in 1967. He documented seven cases of asymptomatic colonic cancer detected using a simple chemical stool test for occult blood.

The rationale for faecal blood testing is that subclinical blood loss is greater in patients with colorectal cancer than in healthy individuals. Quantitative estimates of faecal haemoglobin concentration either using a chromium-50 labelled red cell technique or by estimation of faecal porphyrins (Ebaugh, Clemens, Rodnan, and Peterson 1958; Schwartz, Dahl, Ellefson, and Ahlquist 1983) have demonstrated that healthy blood loss varies from about 0.5 to 1.2 ml per day. In terms of faecal haemoglobin concentrations these values suggest an upper limit of normal of 2.0 mg of haemoglobin per g stool. Ahlquist, McGill, Schwartz, Taylor, and Owen (1985) demonstrated significantly higher faecal haemoglobin levels in patients with gastrointestinal cancer. In 30 patients with colonic cancer the median faecal haemoglobin level was approximately 6 mg/g stool, but with a wide range. It was evident from the study that bleeding also occurs from a range of benign gastrointestinal diseases, such as diverticular disease, and that no clear separation of those with gastrointestinal malignancy was possible on the basis of faecal haemoglobin concentrations. Thus, one of the potential limitations of faecal occult blood screening is already evident: tests of high sensitivity for carcinoma have a correspondingly low specificity.

Simple, qualitative estimation of faecal occult blood is available by means of tests that depend on the chemical or immunological characteristics of haemoglobin. The chemical tests generally involve a phenolic oxidation of the substrate (in most cases guaiac gum). These tests are liable to interference from ingested animal haemoglobin and also from vegetables high in peroxidase activity. The immunological tests are more expensive and complex, but specifically detect human haemoglobin.

Trials of faecal occult blood screening

Haemoccult, a guaiac based test which has been the subject of most evaluation in the randomized trials world-wide, is known to have a relatively high threshold for faecal blood, making it a highly specific but rather insensitive test for colorectal malignancy (St. John, McHutchinson, Deacon, Alexeyeff, and Young 1988).

A series of randomized controlled studies is in progress world-wide. There are differences in the methods of recruitment, test interpretation, and follow-up but, nevertheless, the basic factors relating to the efficacy of faecal occult blood screening have been addressed. These are compliance, positivity rate, sensitivity and specificity of the test, and the ability to detect pre-symptomatic disease at an early clinicopathological stage.

Compliance

Perhaps the major determinant of the success of a screening programme is its acceptance by the target population. This is of particular relevance to faecal occult blood screening where the very nature of the test may deter many individuals.

In practice it appears that acceptable screening uptake may be achieved, but there are wide variations between populations. Moreover, the method of recruitment may have a major influence on compliance.

In the New York screening study (Winawer, *et al.* 1980; Flehinger, Herbert, Winawer, and Miller 1988), many subjects were enrolled from health-conscious volunteers attending their physicians for a regular health check. Amongst these, 70 per cent completed faecal occult blood testing, and amongst a second group attending for a particular health problem, compliance was even better at 80 per cent. It is noticeable, however, that there has been a dramatic decline in compliance for rescreening, only 35 per cent of those attending for health checks completing tests at 4 years, and fewer than 20 per cent of those with a particular health problem completing the tests at 1 year.

In terms of true mass population screening, the compliance from European studies is more relevant. Kewenter, Haglind, and Svanrik (1987) and Kewenter, Bjork, Haglind, Smith, Svanvik, and Ahren (1988) have studied 27 700 subjects between 60 and 64 years of age in Gotenborg, Sweden. Invitation was postal and applied to a randomly selected population, there being no volunteer bias. At the initial round of screening 66 per cent of subjects returned completed tests.

In Funen, Denmark, Kronberg, Fenger, Sondergaard, Pederson, and Olsen (1987) and Krouberg, Fenger, Olsen, Beck, and Sondergaard (1989) have reported a compliance rate of 67 per cent, achieved with the use of a reminder letter and personal telephone calls to the non-responders.

Compliance in the Nottingham, UK, screening study (Farrands, Chamberlain and Hardcastle 1983*a*; Hardcastle, Armitage, Chamberlain, Amar, James, and Balfour 1986; Hardcastle, *et al.* 1989) was particularly poor in the early years when only 35 per cent of the randomly selected population completed the tests. However, with a relatively simple modification of the method of recruitment, compliance has improved and currently uptake levels of 62 per cent are being achieved; overall compliance in this study stands at 53 per cent. Moderate variations according to age and sex have been described, compliance being greatest in men aged 55–69 years and in women aged 50–69 years. Farrands and Hardcastle (1984) found that acceptors of screening in the Nottingham study had more positive attitudes towards preventive medicine than refusals. Interestingly, inclusion of an educational leaflet made no difference (Pye *et al.* 1988) but the wording of the letter of invitation was important; in particular, a personal letter of invitation from the subject's own general practitioner substantially increased compliance.

In the Burgundy region of France different methods of recruitment have been examined. Overall, a compliance rate of 52.2 per cent has been achieved (J. Fairne, personal communication). This contrasts with compliance rates of about 20 per cent in smaller studies from other French districts. The compliance was particularly poor (36 per cent) amongst those asked to buy the tests from local pharmacies, even though participants were reimbursed.

Positivity rate, secondary investigation

In any screening study it is essential to minimize the false-positive rate whilst maintaining an acceptable sensitivity for the disease. Secondary investigations are expensive, induce anxiety, and are potentially hazardous.

Two factors have important practical implications in the rate of positive faecal occult blood tests when Haemoccult is used. As described previously, the test may be affected by the ingestion of red meat and vegetables with high peroxidase levels. Second, rehydration of the test card before interpretation (in an effort to improve sensitivity) increases the rate of positive reactions.

The influence of dietary factors has been examined in the Nottingham study (Thomas, Pye, Hardcastle, Chamberlain, and Charnley 1989), where subjects with positive tests on an unrestricted diet have been retested following a diet free of red meat and low in vegetable peroxidase. The rate of positive reactions has been reduced from 3.4 to 1.5 per cent using this regimen. There remains, however, some concern that some asymptomatic cancers may be missed at the second screen.

In the Danish study (Kronberg *et al.* 1989), where dietary restriction is enforced at the initial invitation to screen, 1.04 per cent have exhibited positive tests.

The effect of rehydration has been examined in the Swedish trial (Kewenter *et al.* 1988) and in a study from Minnesota (Mandel, *et al.* 1989). In Minnesota the sensitivity of Haemoccult for cancer is estimated to have risen from 80.8 per cent without rehydration to 92.2 per cent following rehydration, but this has corresponded with a marked increase in the rate of positive reactions from 2.4 to 9.8 per cent; colonoscopic examination of almost a tenth of the population aged between 50 and 74 years is clearly not a feasible option for most institutions. In the Swedish trial rehydration increased the rate of positive reaction from 1.9 to 5.8 per cent.

Sensitivity and specificity

There are methodological problems in assessing the sensitivity of any mass population screening procedure. Ideally the screening test should be compared with a 'gold standard' accepted as being the most sensitive means of detecting the condition in question. In the case of Haemoccult screening this would involve a comparison of the faecal occult blood test with colonoscopy; however, the vast numbers of people requiring investigation in such a study makes this approach logistically impossible. Moreover, there are ethical considerations; given the low expected detection rate (2.0–3.0 per 1000 persons screened), can we justify the inconvenience, discomfort, and potential hazards of mass population colonoscopy?

The calculation of sensitivity has therefore been based on the diagnosis of carcinomas in those people who have had a negative test in the interval before a retest (usually at 2 years). Such 'interval' cancers are assumed to have been missed at the initial screen.

In the Funen trial (Kronberg *et al.* 1989), a total of 90 cancers has been diagnosed in the group who completed the Haemoccult tests. Of these, 50 had positive test reactions and 40 had negative tests, presenting later with colorectal symptoms. Thus in this study the sensitivity of Haemoccult for asymptomatic cancers is 50/90 (55.6 per cent).

Using a similar method of analysis as that employed in Denmark, Kewenter *et al.* (1988) reported an overall interval cancer rate of 31.4 per cent from Gothenberg (sensitivity for carcinoma, 68.6 per cent), although this involved a variable period for rescreening of between 12 and 24 months. The striking feature of this study is the particularly low sensitivity of Haemoccult for cancer when test card rehydration was not used; of 18 cancers diagnosed in this group, 14 were interval cancers and assumed to have been missed by Haemoccult. It must be emphasized that this low sensitivity of 22.2 per cent is at odds with other screening trials.

In the report by Hardcastle *et al.* (1989) the sensitivity of faecal occult blood testing for carcinoma has been estimated as 65 per cent. A different method of calculation of sensitivity was also examined based on incidence rates of colorectal cancer. The reported incidence of interval cancers is 0.25 per 1000 person-years which can be compared with a control group incidence of 0.72 per 1000 person-years. If the underlying incidence in those screened is the same as that in the control group, this would suggest that with an interval of 2 years screening will detect 65 per cent of those cancers expected to present during that time period (i.e. a sensitivity for carcinoma of 65 per cent). However, in this study the observed incidence in those who declined the test invitation was higher (0.92/1000 person-years) and this might mean that the screened group has a lower incidence than the controls, in which case the sensitivity of 2-year screening would be 55 per cent.

There is evidence, particularly from the Funen and Nottingham trials, that the site of the tumour has an important bearing on test sensitivity, with high sensitivity for sigmoid cancers and a poor sensitivity for rectal and caecal tumours.

The specificity of a test is calculated from the number of people with a

Table 18.1. Stage distribution of cancers detected in the Nottingham trial of faecal occult blood screening.

Stage	Test Group (offered Haemoccult)				Control (not approached)
	Screen-detected	Interval	Non-responder	Total	
A	40 (53)	6 (27)	10 (12)	56 (31)	13 (11)
B	20 (26)	4 (18)	30 (36)	54 (30)	40 (32)
C	13 (17)	6 (27)	16 (19)	35 (19)	40 (32)
D	3 (4)	6 (27)	25 (30)	34 (19)	26 (21)
Not staged	—	—	2	2	4
Total	76	22	83	181	123

Values in parenthesis are percentages.

negative test who do not have the disease. The specificity of Haemoccult for colorectal neoplasia (carcinoma or adenoma) is excellent: more than 99.0 per cent in the European series.

Pre-symptomatic colorectal neoplasia

Ultimately, the success or otherwise of faecal occult blood screening will be judged by the effect of screening on colorectal cancer mortality rates. However, follow-up information regarding mortality from the randomized trials is not yet available. In the meantime we can look to the yield of pre-symptomatic disease, and in particular to the pathological stage distribution of the screen-detected cancers, for an interim assessment.

Evidence from the ongoing trials leaves no doubt that asymptomatic cancers can be diagnosed following the detection of faecal occult blood and that such cancers tend to be at a less advanced clinicopathological stage than those diagnosed in the corresponding control groups. In Nottingham, where 76 asymptomatic cancers have been diagnosed in the group completing screening, 40 (52.6 per cent) were at Dukes' stage A and only three (3.9 per cent) had liver metastases at the time of surgery. By comparison, 13 (10.6 per cent) of the 123 cancers in the control group were at stage A and 26 (21.1 per cent) had distant metastases. In the evaluation of the screening programme, however, it is essential to consider not only the screen-detected cancers but also those missed by the test (intervals), and those diagnosed in the subjects who refused screening (the non-responders). When this is done (Table 18.1) it is evident that, although the proportion of stage A cancers remains favourable in the test group, the number of stage D cancers is similar in the test and control groups, suggesting that an improvement in mortality rates cannot be expected in the near future and emphasizing the requirement for long-term follow-up.

It is becoming increasingly apparent that the interim results from all the major trials are remarkably similar, especially from the European series. Kronberg *et al.* (1989) have detected 50 cancers on screening; 26 (52.0 per cent) were at stage A compared with nine (7.8 per cent) of 115 control group cancers. The favourable stage distribution of screen-detected cancers is also seen in the reports from Minnesota and New York.

An important further consideration is the detection of a large number of potentially malignant colorectal adenomas. Hardcastle *et al.* (1989) have identified a total of 432 such polyps, 79 (18.3 per cent) of which were 2 cm or larger in diameter, and consequently at particular risk of malignant transformation. The long-term sequelae of the endoscopic removal of these malignant precursors have yet to be evaluated but it is possible that their removal, particularly if large dysplastic adenomas, will be reflected in a decline in colorectal cancer incidence rates in the screened group over the forthcoming years.

Clearly these results are encouraging, but a note of caution is necessary. Already in the Nottingham trial there is evidence of a length bias, with fewer screen-detected tumours being poorly differentiated in comparison with those in the control group. Moreover, it is too early to determine the effect that screening may have had on colorectal cancer survival rates. This will only be possible following an adequate period of follow up.

Prospects for screening at other sites

Screening strategies for malignancy at other sites are less well defined than for the common sites of gastrointestinal cancers as discussed above. The reasons are two-fold; first, the lower frequency of these malignancies makes justification of screening more contentious, and, second, attempts at screening have been frustrated by lack of suitable tests.

The particularly dismal prognosis of pancreatic cancer has motivated some groups to look to pre-symptomatic diagnosis and treatment of the disease. Pagnuzzi, *et al.* (1988) evaluated the role of the tumour-associated antigens CA 19–9 and CA 50 in the diagnosis of pancreatic–biliary cancers; in patients with pancreatic cancers they demonstrated a sensitivity of 84.6 and 80.7 per cent for CA 19–9 and CA 50, respectively, with corresponding specificity values of 92.4 and 88.5 per cent.

Similarly encouraging results have been reported by others (Ritts, del Villano, Go, Herberman, Klug, and Zurawski 1984; del Favero, *et al.* 1986; Haglund *et al.* 1986; Steinberg, *et al.* 1986). However, in a study of 866 subjects with no clinical evidence of malignancy and admitted to an internal medicine unit for benign disease, prospective evaluation of antigen determinations revealed that elevated CA 19–9 levels were present in 117 (13.5 per cent) and that 115 had false-positive elevations, usually in association with benign hepato-biliary disease, but also commonly with a wide range of conditions such as cardiovascular disease and neurological disorders.

In the case of primary hepatocellular carcinoma, which in some African and Eastern countries represents one of the commonest causes of cancer fatality, it is likely that primary preventive measures — in particular hepatitis immunization — provide the best prospect of reducing mortality rates in the long term. Nevertheless, screening programmes for resectable hepatocellular cancers based on AFP estimations are being evaluated (Sun, *et al.* 1987); if successful, these may provide a means of improving survival rates, particularly in the short term, bearing in mind that any beneficial effects of infant hepatitis vaccination will take decades to become apparent.

References

Adashek, K., Sanger, J., and Longmire, W.P. (1979). Cancer of the stomach. Review of consecutive ten year intervals. *Ann. Surg.* **00**, 6–10.

Ahlquist, D.A., McGill, D.B., Schwartz, S., Taylor, W.F., and Owen, R.A. (1985). Fecal blood levels in health and disease. *N. Engl. J. Med.* **312**, 1422–8.

Allum, W.H., Hallissey, M.T., Dorrell, A., Low, J., and Fielding, J.W.L. (1986). Programme for early detection of gastric cancer. *Br. Med. J.* **293**, 541.

Bargan, J.A. (1928). Chronic ulcerative colitis associated with malignant disease. *Arch. Surg.* **17**, 561.

Barrett, R. (1950). Chronic peptic ulcer of the oesophagus and oesophagitis. *Br. J. Surg.* **38**, 175–82.

Caygill, C.P.J., Hill, M.J., Kirkham, J.S., and Northfield, T.C. (1986). Mortality from gastric cancer following gastric surgery for peptic ulcer. *Lancet* **i**, 929–32.

Clark, C.G., Ward, M.W.N., McDonald, A.M., and Tovey, F.I. (1983). The incidence of gastric stump cancer. *World J. Surg.* **7**, 236–40.

Crespi, M., Grassi, A., Armin, G., *et al.* (1979). Oesophageal lesions in northern Iran: a premalignant condition. *Lancet* **ii**, 217–21.

Crohn, B.B. and Rosenberg, H. (1925). Sigmoidoscopic picture of chronic ulcerative colitis. *Am. J. Med. Sci.* **170**, 220.

De Dombal, F.T., Thompson, H., Williams, G.T., *et al.* (1988). The BSG early gastric cancer survey. A further report, *Gut* **29**, A724.

Del Favero, G., Fabris, C., Plebani, M., *et al.* (1986). CA 19–9 and carcinoembryonic antigen in pancreatic cancer diagnosis. *Cancer* **57**, 1576–9.

Dent, O.F., MacDonald, L., Chapius, P.H., and Goulston, K. (1981). Colorectal cancer in Australia; 1908–1978. *Med. J. Aust.* **2**, 415–16.

Duncan, J.L. and Kyle, J. (1982). Family incidence of carcinoma of the colon and rectum in north-east Scotland. *Gut* **23**, 169–71.

du Pont, J.B., Lee, J.R., Burton, G.R., and Cohn, I. (1978). Adenocarcinoma of the stomach: review of 1497 cases. *Cancer* **41**, 941–7.

Ebaugh, F.G., Clemens, T., Rodnan, G., and Peterson, R.E. (1958). Quantitative measurement of gastrointestinal blood loss. *Am. J. Med.* **25**, 169–81.

Farrands, P.A., and Hardcastle, J.D. (1984). Colorectal screening by a self-completion questionnaire. *Gut* **25**, 445–7.

Farrands, P.A., Chamberlain, J., and Hardcastle, J.D. (1983*a*). Factors affecting compliance of screening for colorectal cancer. *J. Exp. Clin. Cancer Res. a* **2**, 45.

Farrands, P.A., Blake, J.R.S., Anseel, J.D., Cotton, R.E., and Hardcastle, J.D. (1983*b*). Endocsopic review of patients who have had gastric surgery. *Br. Med. J. b* **286**, 755–8.

Fischer, A.M., Graem, N., and Jenson, O.M. (1983). Risk of gastric cancer after Billroth II resections for duodenal ulcer. *Br. J. Surg.* **70**, 552–4.

Flehinger, B.J., Herbert, E., Winawer, S.J., and Miller, D.G. (1988). Screening for colorectal cancer with faecal occult blood test and sigmoidoscopy: preliminary report of the colon project of Memorial Sloan-Kettering Cancer Center and PMI-Strang Clinic. In *Screening for gastrointestinal cancer* (ed. J. Chamberlain and A.B. Miller) pp. 9–16. Hans Huber, Stuttgart.

Foley, D.P., Dunne, P., Ryan, T.D., *et al.* (1988). Left-colonoscopy highlights the failure of Haemoccult to detect colorectal neoplasia. *Gut* **29**, A1483.

Gilbertson, V.A. and Nelms, J.M. (1978). The prevention of invasive cancer of the rectum. *Cancer* **41**, 1137–9.

Gillen, P. and Hennessy, T.P.J. (1989). Barrett's oesophagus. In *Reflex oesophagitis* (ed. T.P.J. Hennessy, A. Cuschieri, and J.R. Bennett). Butterworth, London.

Gillespie, P.E., Chambers, T.J., Chan, K., *et al.* (1979). Colonic adenomas colonoscopic survey. *Gut* **20**, 240–5.

Greegor, D.H. (1967). Diagnosis of large bowel cancer in the asymptomatic patient. *J.A.M.A.* **12**, 123–5.

Haglund, C., Roberts, P.J., Kuusela, P., Scheimin, R.M., Makela, O., and Jalanko, H. (1986). Evaluation of CA 19–9 as a serum tumour market in pancreatic cancer. *Br. J. Cancer* **53**, 197–203.

Hardcastle, J.D., Armitage, N.C., Chamberlain, J., Amar, S.S., James, P.D., and Balfour, T.W. (1986). Fecal occult blood screening for colorectal cancer in the general population. *Cancer* **58**, 183–9.

Hardcastle, J.D., Thomas, W.M., Chamberlain, J., *et al.* (1989). Randomised, controlled trial of faecal occult blood screening for colorectal cancer: results for the first 107 349 subjects. *Lancet* **i**, 1160–4.

Harper, P.S., Harper, R.M.J., and Havel-Evans, A.W. (1970). Carcinoma of the oesophagus with tylosis. *Q. J. Med.* **39**, 317.

Harrison, J.D. and Morris, D.L. (1988). Early results of a population based screening programme for gastric cancer. *Gut* **29**, A702.

Harrison, J.D. and Morris, D.L. (1990). Screening for gastric cancer by gastroscopy of dyspeptic subjects identified by a dyspepsia questionnaire. *Br. J. Surg.* **77**, A698.

Hirayama, T. (1971). Epidemiology of stomach cancer. *GANN Monograph on Cancer Research* **11**, 3–19.

Hirayama, T. (1978). Outline of stomach cancer screening in Japan. *UICC Technical Reports* **40**, 264–78.

Hopkins, R.A. and Postlewait, R.W. (1981). Caustic burns and carcinoma of the oesophagus. *Ann. Surg.* **194**, 146–8.

Ichikawa, H. (1971). Detectability of early gastric cancer with indirect fluorodiography. *GANN Monograph on Cancer Research* **11**, 27–43.

Kaibara, N., Kawagudi, H., Nishidoi, N., *et al.* (1981). Significance of mass survey for gastric cancer from the standpoint of surgery. *Am. J. Surg.* **140**, 543–5.

Kaneko, E., Nakamura, T., Umeda, N., *et al.* (1977). Outcome of gastric carcinoma detected by gastric mass survey in Japan. *Gut* **18**, 626–30.

Kewenter, J. Haglind, E., and Svanvik, J. (1987). Fecal occult blood screening for colorectal cancer: the Swedish experience. In *Causation and prevention of colorectal cancer. Proceedings of the workshop of the European Organisation for Cooperation in Cancer Prevention Studies (ECP)* (ed. J. Faivre and M.J. Hill) Excerpta Medica, Amsterdam.

Kewenter, J., Bjork, S., Haglind, E., Smith, L., Svanvik, J., and Ahren, C. (1988). Screening and rescreening for colorectal cancer: a controlled trial of faecal occult blood testing in 27 700 subjects. *Cancer* **63**, 645–51.

Kohrogi, N. (1987). A study on the efficiency of gastric cancer screening with special reference to the appropriate frequency of screening. *Fukuoka Igaku Zasshi* **78**, 67–81.

Kronberg, O., Fenger, C., Olsen, J., Bech, K., and Sondergaard, O. (1989). Repeated screening for colorectal cancer with fecal occult blood tests. A prospective randomised study at Funen, Denmark. *Scand. J. Gastroenterol.* **24**, 599–606.

Kronberg, O., Fenger, C., Sondergaard, O., Pederson, K.M., and Olsen, J. (1987). Initial mass screening for colorectal cancer with fecal occult blood test. *Scand. J. Gastroenterol.* **22**, 677–86.

Lennard-Jones, J.E., Morson, B.C., Ritchie, J.K., Shove, D.C., and Williams, C.B. (1977). Cancer in colitis: assessment of the individual risk by clinical and histological criteria. *Gastroenterology* **73**, 1280–9.

Logan, R.F. and Langman, M.J.S. (1983). Screening for gastric cancer after surgery. *Lancet* **ii**, 667–70.

Lovett, E. (1976). Family studies in cancer of the colon and rectum. *Br. J. Surg.* **63**, 13–18.

Mandel, J.S., Bond, J.H., Bradley, M., *et al.* (1989). Sensitivity, specificity and positive predictivity of the Hemoccult test in screening for colorectal cancers. *Gastroenterology* **97**, 597–600.

McGlashan, N.D. (1988). Oesophageal cancer in the black peoples of South Africa 1980–1982. *S. Afr. J. Sci.* **84**, 92.

Muir C.S., Choi, N.W., and Schiftlers, E. (1981). Time trends in cancer mortality in some countries: their possible causes and significance. *Skandia International Symposia* Almquist and Wiskell International, Stockholm.

Munoz, N. and Crespi, M. (1983). High risk conditions and precancerous conditions of the oesophagus. In *Precancerous lesions of the gastrointestinal tract* (ed. P. Sherlock, B.C. Morson, L. Barbara, *et al.*) Raven Press, New York.

Murakami, T. (1971). Pathomorphological diagnosis: definition and gross classification of early gastric cancer. *GANN Monograph on Cancer Research* **11**, 53–5.

Nabeya, K. (1983). Markers of cancer risk in the esophagus and surveillance of high risk groups. In *Precancerous lesions of the gastrointestinal tract* (ed. P. Sherlock, B.C. Morson, L. Barbara *et al.*) Raven Press, New York.

Office of Population Censuses and Surveys (1983). *Monitor* HMSO, London.

Office of Population Censuses and Surveys (1988). Cancer statistics: registrations in England and Wales 1984. HMSO, London.

Okui, K. and Tejima, H. (1980). Evaluation of gastric mass survey. *Acta Chir. Scand.* **146**, 185–7.

Oleagoitea, J.M., Echevarria, A., Santidrian, J.I., *et al.* (1986). Early gastric cancer. *Br. J. Surg.* **73**, 884–6.

Oshima, A., Hirata, N., Ubukata, T., *et al.* (1986). Evaluation of a mass screening program for stomach cancer with a case — control study design. *Int. J. Cancer* **38**, 829–33.

Paganuzzi, M., Onetto, M., Marroni, P., *et al.* (1988). CA 19–9 and CA 50 in benign and malignant pancreatic and biliary disease. *Cancer* **61**, 2100–8.
Perez, D., Narayanan, N.C., Russell, J.C., and Becker, D.R. (1984). Gastric carcinoma after peptic ulcer surgery. *Am. Surg.* **50**, 538–40.
Pye, G., *et al.* (1988). A comparison of methods for increasing compliance within a general practitioner workload. *J. Epidemiol. Community Health* **42**, 66–71.
Registrar General (1987). *Annual Report for Scotland 1987* HMSO, London.
Ritts, R.E., del Villano, B.C., Go, V.L.W., Herberman, R.B., Klug, T.L., and Zurawski, V.R. (1984). Initial clinical evaluation of an imunoradiometric assay for CA 19-19 using the NCI serum bank. *Int. J. Cancer* **33**, 339–45.
Robertson, C.S., Mayberry, J.F., Nicholson, D.A., James, P.D., and Atkinson, M. (1988). Value of endoscopic survillance in the detection of neoplastic changes in Barrett's oesophagus. *Br. J. Surg.* **75**, 760–3.
Rohan, R. and McMichael, A.J. (1981). Alimentary tract cancer mortality in Australia 1908–1978. *Med. J. Aust.* **1**, 232.
Schwartz, S., Dahl, J., Ellefson, M., and Ahlquist, D. (1983). The HemoQuant test: a specific and quantitative determination of heme (hemoglobin) in feces and other materials. *Clin. Chem.* **29**, 6061–7.
Shu, Y.J. (1983). Cytopathology of the esophagus. An over-view of esophageal cytopathology in China. *Acta Cytol.* **27**, 7–16.
Silman, A.J., Mitchel, P., Nicholls, R.J., *et al.* (1983). Self reported dark red bleeding as a marker comparable with occult blood testing in screening for large bowel neoplasms. *Br. J. Surg.* **70**, 721–4.
Silverberg, E., Boring, C.C., and Squires, T.S. (1990). Cancer statistics 1990. *CA* **40**, 9–26.
Spreckler, S.J., Robbins, A.H., Rubins, H.B., *et al.* (1984). Adenocarcinoma and Barrett's oesophagus. An over-rated risk? *Gastroenterology* **87**, 927–33.
Steinberg, W.M., Gelfand, R., Anderson, K.K., *et al.* (1986). Comparison of the sensitivity and specificity of the CA 19–9 and carcinoembryonic antigen assays in detecting cancer of the pancreas. *Gastroenterology* **90**, 343–9.
St. John, D.J.B., McHutchinson, J.G., Deacon, M., Alexeyeff, M., and Young, G.P. (1988). Detection of colorectal pathology: comparison of Haemoccult and HemoQuant tests for occult blood. *Gastroenterology* **94**, 445 (Abstract).
Stockbrugger, R.W., Merion, G.G., Beilby, J.O.W., *et al.* (1983). Gastroscopic screening in 80 patients with pernicious anaemia. *Gut* **24**, 1141–7.
Sun, T., Yu, H., Hsia, C., *et al.* (1987). Evaluation of sero-survey trials for the early detection of hepato-cellular carcinoma in areas of high prevalence. In *Screening for gastrointestinal cancer* (ed. Chamberlain and Miller) Hans Huber, Stuttgart.
Thomas, W.M., Pye, G., Hardcastle, J.D., Chamberlain, J., and Charnley, R.M. (1989). Haemoccult screening for colorectal cancer: the role of dietary restriction and selective three month rescreening. *Br. J. Surg.* **76**, 976–8.
Winawer, S.J., Andrews, M., Flehinger, B. *et al.* (1980). Progress report on controlled trial of faecal occult blood testing for the detection of colorectal neoplasia. *Cancer* **45**, 2959–64.
Wherry, D.C. (1981). Screening for colorectal neoplasia in asymptomatic patients using flexible fibreoptic sigmoidoscopy. *Dis. Colon Rectum* **24**, 521–5.
Wynder, E.L., Konet, J., Dungal, N., and Segi, M. (1963). An epidemiological investigation of gastric cancer. *Cancer* **16**, 1461–96.

19. Surgery for inflammatory bowel disease

John H. Pemberton

Inflammatory bowel disease is a medical problem until it becomes resistant to conservative management; surgery is then required. Experience with surgery for inflammatory bowel disease has broadened as prognosis has improved; the better the results, the earlier patients tend to be referred which, in turn, facilitates the improved results. The rationale and aims of surgery for chronic ulcerative colitis and for Crohn's disease differ; surgery is curative for ulcerative colitis while for Crohn's disease surgery is only a management option. The key words in surgery for Crohn's are 'conserve bowel'. Indeed, the latest advance in surgery for Crohn's disease does not even resect the disease.

The aims of this chapter are to describe the classic and new operative approaches for patients with Chron's disease and chronic ulcerative colitis, detail their rationale, describe results, and assess the impact of operations on quality of life.

Surgery for Crohn's disease

The proper perspective for any discussion of surgery for Crohn's disease is maintained by remembering that the disease cannot be cured by surgery. When to be aggressive (by removing disease, the surgeon restores health and decreases doses of medication) and when to be conservative (the surgeon removes bowel, causes nutritional debility as well as sometimes creating the need for a stoma) are central issues. The aim of the surgeon should probably be to deal with the patient's presenting problem as simply as possible by conserving bowel, while striving to improve the quality of life.

Indications

Importantly, indications for operation in patients with Crohn's disease are rarely absolute except when free gas, an abscess, or uncontrolled bleeding is present. Obstruction and fistulae (entero-entero, entero-colic, entero-vesicle, entero-cutaneous) are the most common indications for surgery. In addition, severe peri-anal disease often prompts proctectomy.

Surgery for gastroduodenal Crohn's disease

Gastro-enterostomy and truncal vagotomy is the treatment of choice for patients with intractable gastroduodenal Crohn's disease. Gastro-enterostomy alone results in ulcerations at the anastomosis; or is it perhaps recurrent Crohn's disease? (Nugent, Richmond, and Park 1977; Ross, Fazio, and Farmer 1983). Alternatively, a short but severe stricture in 'burned out' Crohn's disease of the duodenum could be treated by strictureplasty (Alexander-Williams 1983).

Small bowel Crohn's disease

There are two interesting debates in surgery for small bowel Crohn's disease: the importance of microscopically free margins, and resection versus strictureplasty. Pennington, Hamilton, Bayless, and Cameron (1980) examined the margins of resection in patients with small bowel Crohn's disease; they found no correlation between the presence of inflammation and recurrence of disease. Wolff, Blatt, Frydenberg, Weiland, and Ilstrup (1983), however, found a significantly higher rate of recurrence of Crohn's disease if the margins of resections were involved by inflammation, compared with historical controls (control 45 per cent versus involved margin 90 per cent). As is usual in controversies where results of studies are completely opposite, the studies are nearly always retrospective and, as such, suffer the complexities of inexact and incomplete definitions of terms and of patients. Likely, the truth lies between the radical resectors, such as Bergman and Krause (1977), proponents of the moderately radical resection, Wolff and colleagues (1983), the moderately conservative resectors such as Pennington and others (1980), and those who advocate radically conservative resection, such as Alexander-Williams (1983).

A good rule to follow might be this: in a previously unoperated patient with active small bowel Crohn's disease, a margin of 3–5 cm should be sought proximally and distally. If the margins are involved by Crohn's-specific inflammation (mucosal infiltration by inflammatory cells or ulceration) then an additional 3–5 cm of margin should be sought. If the margin is still positive then the anastomosis should be performed without further resection. In a patient previously operated on, a margin of 2 cm should be sought. If positive, a further 2 cm should be resected and no more.

Strictureplasty

Introduced by Lee and Papaionnou (1982), and popularized by Alexander-Williams (1983) and others (Fazio and Galandiuk 1985; Sayfan, Wilson, Allan, Andrews, and Alexander-Williams 1989), strictureplasty, in selected patients with multiple areas of involvement by Crohn's disease throughout the small bowel (skip lesions), is a valuable addition to the Crohn's surgeon's armamentarium. The secret of this procedure, one that flies in the

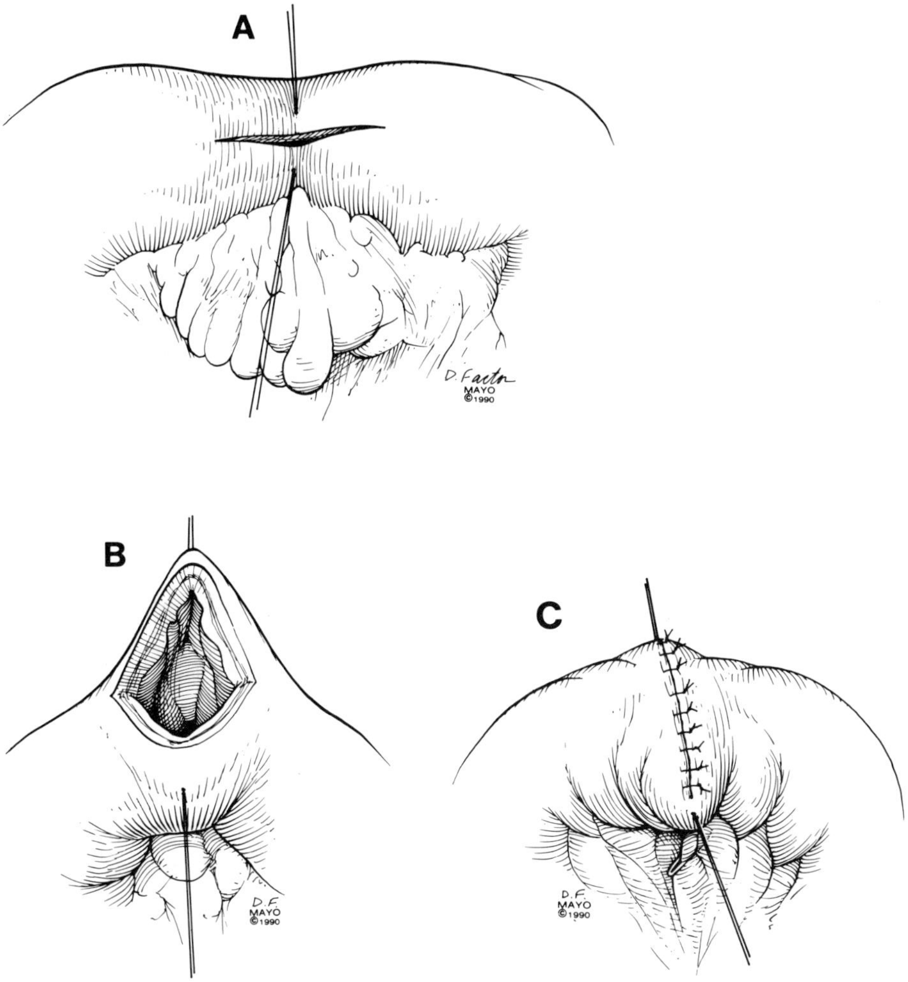

FIg. 19.1. Diagram of the strictureplasty operation. (A) A longitudinal incision is made throughout the length of the strictured segment. (B) The incision is opened transversely. (C) The incision is closed transversely using a single layer of interrupted sutures in a manner similar to the Weinberg modification of the Heineke–Mikulicz pyloroplasty.

face of conventional surgical wisdom, is that it is performed in segments of bowel involved by *burned out* disease. It is an elegantly simple but bold solution to the problem of conserving bowel; a simple longitudinal incision through the stricture with transverse, single-layer closure (similar to the Heineke-Mikulicz pyloroplasty) is all that is done (Fig. 19.1). Alexander-Williams (1983), Sayfan and colleagues (1989), Fazio (1990*a*), and Pritchard, *et al.* (1990) have reported good to excellent results; there is surprisingly little morbidity from the procedure. In the series from the Lahey Clinic (Pritchard *et al.* 1990), 1 of 13 patients had a pelvic abscess post-operatively during 2 years of follow-up. Four patients required reoperation for reobstruction, three of whom needed new strictureplasties and one required resection of an old strictureplasty site. The Cleveland experience was similar, but the morbidity rate was higher (16 per cent), including three entero-cutaneous fistulae and two intra-abdominal abscesses among 30 patients (Fazio 1990*a*). In our experience, strictureplasty was preferred 35 times in 14 patients without mortality. There was one small bowel obstruction, no fistulae or abscesses, and one patient required reoperation for a new stricture at a site remote from the previous strictureplasties (Wolff, *et al.* 1987).

It seems, then, that strictureplasty, in Fazio's words, is the 'emerging conservative operation for high risk Crohn's patients with chronic bowel obstruction' (Fazio 1990*a*). The perfect patient for this approach is one who has symptoms of chronic obstruction and who has multiple skip areas of fibrotic disease.

Whether to bypass diseased segments of small bowel is an argument that is passé. This operation is reserved for especially difficult situations, such as ileo-caecal disease with a densely adherent retroperitoneal abscess. Otherwise, bypass is not useful in the management of Crohn's disease.

Colonic Crohn's disease

Segmental resection of the colon

Segmental resection is performed in patients with ileo-caecal Crohn's (ileo-ascending or transverse colostomy) and is the treatment of choice. In general, however, segmental resection of colonic Crohn's disease is associated with high rates of recurrence. The best rule to follow is to resect all colon proximal to the site of disease. The scenario most appropriate for segmental resection, however, is the one where there is ileo-colonic disease *and* isolated sigmoid involvement; in this situation, ileo-colostomy and segmental resection of the sigmoid colon should be performed.

Abdominal colectomy and ileo-rectostomy

There is no question that for patients with colonic Crohn's disease *and* rectal sparing, colectomy and ileo-rectostomy is the procedure of choice (Farnell, van Heerden, Beart, and Weiland 1980; Farnell and Adson 1985) (Fig. 19.2). This statement is made with full knowledge that Goligher (1985) has observed that up to 70 per cent of such patients will require proctectomy at some point for recurrent disease. Moreover, Lefton, Farmer, and Fazio (1975) from Cleveland reported that only 50 per cent of patients have satisfactory long-term results.

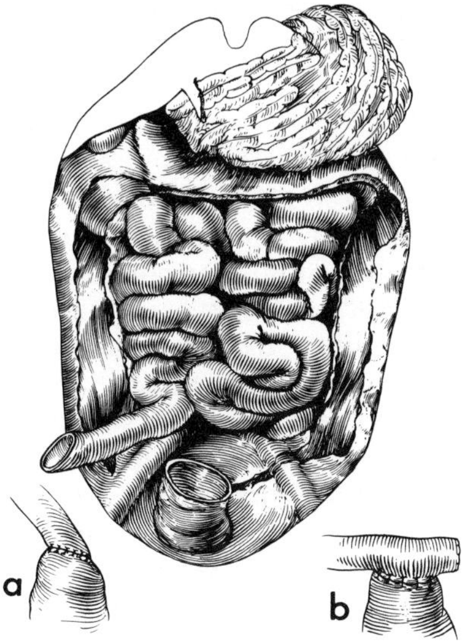

Fig. 19.2. Ileo-rectostomy. An abdominal colectomy has been completed, the specimen removed, and the bowel is ready for the anastomosis. The anastomosis is performed either end to end (a) or side to end (b). [Reproduced from Farnell and Adson (1985) by kind permission of Year Book Medical Publishers, Chicago.]

The usefulness of a diverting ileostomy after ileo-rectostomy is debatable but in general, in the USA, a protecting stoma is not used; if the surgeon decides one is indicated because the anastomosis was performed to a diseased rectum, then the ileo-rectostomy should not have been performed in the first place.

Proctectomy and ileostomy

If the rectum is not spared and/or if the patient has severe anal involvement by Crohn's disease, then proctectomy and ileostomy is the procedure of choice. The mortality rate is less than 2 per cent (Lock, Fazio, Farmer, Jagelman, Lavery, and Weakley 1981*b*). This operation has a major impact, of course, on lifestyle; the patients are incontinent and must wear a stomal appliance at all times. However, patients are relieved of symptoms and of having to take heavy doses of steroids; in general, they recover quickly and do very well. The biggest problem after proctectomy for Crohn's disease is a non-healing perineal wound which occurs in up to one-third of the patients (Wolff 1990). To some extent, the incidence of this time-consuming and bothersome complication may perhaps be lowered by judicious proctectomy (sparing as much of the levator ani muscles as possible), closure of the levators and subcutaneous tissues, and drainage by catheters placed on either side of the perineal incision.

Anorectal Crohn's disease

Involvement of the anorectum by Crohn's disease will be the *initial* manifestation of disease in about 7 per cent of patients (Fazio 1990*b*). The spectrum of involvement is vast, from a single healed secondary site to a destroyed anal canal. Fistulae (simple or complex) and fissures (which are often painless but are characteristically huge and have over-hanging skin edges) often smolder, controlled by metronidazole and sometimes other anti-inflammatory medications. It is important, of course, to determine the status of the proximal bowel in patients presenting with anal Crohn's disease. If active disease is present proximally there may be some benefit to the *anal* disease if the proximal diesease is resected (Fazio 1990*b*; Wolff 1990). Although proximal diversion by a sigmoid colostomy will mitigate anal disease, as soon as bowel continuity is restored the disease recurs (McIlrath 1971). Occasionally, a simple recto-vaginal fistula may be repaired successfully provided the rectum and anal canal are free from granularity, oedema, and ulceration. Patients undergoing this procedure should be diverted.

Recurrence

Recurrence rates in patients with Crohn's disease are extraordinarily high — so high, in fact, that recurrence may not be the right word: recrudescence of disease may be a better term. Major factors which influence recurrence rates include: (i) age; (ii) site of initial disease; (iii) previous disease; and (iv) positive margins.

Stahlgren and Ferguson (1961) and deDombal, Burton, and Goligher (1971) found that the younger the patient the sooner the disease recurred. Moreover, a shorter symptom course before operation favoured recurrence (Goligher 1980). Patients with pure ileal or pure colonic Crohn's disease have a lower rate of recurrence than patients with ileo-colonic disease; the rates of recurrence are 32 per cent for colonic Crohn's, 38 per cent for ileal Crohn's, and 50 per cent for ileo-colonic disease (Lock, Farmer, Fazio, Jagelman, Lavery, and Weakley 1981*a*). Moveover, patients with Crohn's disease of the anus are at high risk of recurrence (Gump, Sakellariadis, Wolff, and Broell 1972). Hellers (1979) has found that the rate of recurrence after one operation was 30 per cent at 5 years and 50 per cent at 10 years. After two operations, the rate of recurrence rose to 50 per cent at 5 years and 65 per cent at 10 years. The controversies of positive margins were considered earlier.

Comment

The whole gastrointestinal tract from mouth to anus is at risk for developing the sequelae of Crohn's disease. Moreover, because the disease is infrequently cured by surgery, recurs predictably, and operations sometimes result in an ileostomy and loss of the anus, surgery should be conservative. On the other hand, symptoms are relieved and patients return to active lives. Importantly, patients with Crohn's disease do not relate their quality of life to whether or not an operation was required in the past, but rather to the *activity of the disease* (Farmer and Michener 1979); if the disease is palliated by operation, the quality of life improves. In addition, we found that patients with Crohn's disease and a Brooke ileostomy were satisfied with their life style (93 per cent) and took part actively in the activities of daily life (Pemberton, Phillips, Dozois, and Wendorf 1985). The proper attitude for the surgeon to assume in dealing with Crohn's disease is, therefore, to be conservative but not retiring when advising operations for the disease. The goal is to improve the quality of life, and this is eminently achievable.

Surgery for chronic ulcerative colitis

Chronic ulcerative colitis is a non-specific, inflammatory disease of the colon and is, by definition, curable if the colon is removed. The standard approach in this country has been proctocolectomy with an abdominal ileostomy; the operation eliminates the colonic disease effectively but results in an incontinent stoma. Because the disease does not recur in the small bowel, alternatives to standard abdominal ileostomy have been introduced, the general goal of such alternative surgery being to control enteric content. Our hypothesis is that if control of enteric output is achieved, quality of life improves. The ideal surgical approach that provides control should be based on two criteria: all disease must be removed, yet the pathway for defaecation must be retained.

In this section, the alternative operations for patients with chronic ulcerative colitis are described, advantages and problems detailed, and future applications discussed.

Indications for operation

Certainly the most common indication for operation in patients with ulcerative colitis remains intractability. One rule to follow is that the *patient* determines when symptoms are sufficiently bothersome to prompt an operation. In contrast, if dysplasia or radiographic and colonoscopic evidence of malignancy is found, surgery must be recommended strongly. The other common indications are actually complications of the disease including toxicity, haemorrhage, perforation, and unremitting extra-intestinal manifestations.

Proctocolectomy with Brooke ileostomy

The *aim* of the operation is to remove all diseased bowel and to establish a well-functioning stoma, the output of which is managed by an appliance.

The *rationale* for the operation is that proctocolectomy 'cures' the disease, the stoma is easy to manage, the rate of complication is low, and the long-term functional results are good.

Patient selection

Importantly, unlike other alternative operations, patients of any body habitus and any age are candidates for this operation. Of course, a large paniculus makes construction of the stoma hazardous, and obese patients tend to have more functional problems with their stomas than do thinner patients. In contrast, Stryker, Pemberton, and Zinsmeister (1985), found that among elderly patients undergoing Brooke ileostomy, age alone was not a contra-indication to the operation.

Complications

Overall, the morbidity rate following proctolectomy and Brooke ileostomy is reported to be between 19 and 70 per cent (Beauchamp, Beliveau, and Archambault 1981). About 33 per cent of patients experience breakdown of the perineal wound after primary closure of the perineum. Moreover, small bowel obstruction requiring laparotomy occurs in 5–16 per cent of patients (Lyttle and Parks 1977; Sirinek, Tetirick, Thomford, and Pace 1977), which results in a late mortality rate of about 1 per cent per year.

Bladder paresis and sexual dysfunction occur rarely *if an inter-sphincteric proctectomy is performed* (Lee and Dowling 1972; Lyttle and Parks 1977). Sexual dysfunction has been documented previously to occur in 20–30 per cent of men after proctectomy (Watts, de Dombal, and Goligher 1966; Burnham, Lennard-Jones, and Brooke 1977; Grüner, Naas, Fretheim, and Gjone 1977) and in 12 per cent of women.

Complications related to the stoma itself have decreased in frequency since the mucosal eversion technique of Brooke was adapted widely. Problems still occur, however, in 20–30 per cent of patients (Ritchie 1971).

Clinical, functional, and quality of life results

Rapid rehabilitation of patients with an ileostomy is the rule (Morowitz and Kirsner 1981). More recently, we documented the clinical and functional results of a large group of patients with a Brooke ileostomy (Pemberton *et al.* 1985).

All patients who had a Brooke ileostomy constructed between 1966 and 1980 were sent a questionnaire. Of 675 patients responding (81 per cent), the mean follow-up was 8 years. Fifty-seven per cent had the operation for ulcerative colitis while 35 per cent had it for Crohn's disease. The majority (92 per cent) of the patients reported their diet to be satisfactory. Most patients (93 per cent) had no problems managing the stomas, but 11 per cent had to care for the stoma at night. Occasional episodes of peristomal skin excoriation were reported by 40 per cent of the patients. Patients were asked to judge how their ileostomy affected seven categories of daily activity. More patients noted restriction and fewer noted improvements in the more physically demanding categories (sexual function, sports) compared with more socially oriented activities (social interests, work at home, recreation, family relationships, and travel); 30 per cent of patients indicated that their sexual activity had been restricted since their operation, whereas only 15 per cent indicated it had improved. Overall, however, 75 per cent of patients indicated that either the ileostomy had little effect or had affected an improvement in activity status. Overall, 95 per cent of patients were satisfied with their ileostomies.

Although these results were acceptable, it was disturbing that in this most recent group of patients, the quality of life seemed to differ little from that reported previously by Roy, Sauer, Beahrs, and Farrow (1970). It appears, therefore, that the overall outcome of Brooke ileostomy has remained static. If so, the development of alternative procedures seems justified.

Abdominal colectomy and ileal–rectal anastomosis (Fig. 19.2)

The *aim* of the ileal–rectal anastomosis (ileo-rectostomy) is to remove *most* of the diseased colonic mucosa in patients with chronic ulcerative colitis, thereby reducing the risks of haemorrhage, dilation, perforation, and malignant degeneration, while, at the same time, retaining continence for stool and gas.

The *rationale* for ileal–rectal anastomosis for patients with chronic ulcerative colitis is that the operation avoids a permanent stoma, minimizes injury to the pelvic nerves, is easy to perform, and other alternatives are not precluded (Aylett 1966; Watts and Hughes 1977; Grundfest, Fazio, Weiss, Jagelman, Lavery, Weakley, and Turnbull 1981). The rationale *against* the operation, however, is strong; interval proctectomy is required in 6–37 per cent of patients; poor results occur in 50 per cent of patients (Adson, Cooperman, and Farrow 1972), and the risk of developing carcinoma in the retained rectum approaches 17 per cent after 27 years (Johnson, McDermott, Hughes, Pihl, and Milne 1983).

Patient selection

Patients are candidates for the operation if the rectum is distensible and relatively free from disease, and if they are willing to undergo frequent screening examinations for rectal cancer. Basically, patients of any age and of any body habitus may undergo the procedure.

Complications

The operative mortality rate for elective ileal–rectal anastomosis varies between 2 and 8 per cent (Baker, Glass, Ritchie, and Aylett 1978). Nearly all deaths have been caused by anastomotic leakage (Aylett 1963; Parc, Levy, Frileux, and Loygue 1985), which occur in 3–15 per cent of patients

(Baker 1970; Farnell *el al.* 1980). Small bowel obstruction complicates the recovery of 14–20 per cent of patients (Aylett 1960). Sexual function in men is usually preserved after operation, but up to 50 per cent of women experience dyspareunia (Grüner *et al.* 1977).

Clinical outcome

Six months after operation, the mean stool frequency is about five every 24 hours (Parc *et al.* 1985). Incontinence occurs in about 20 per cent of patients (Newton and Baker 1975). Improvement of function occurs steadily over the first 12–18 months and plateaus thereafter.

The best measure of success after ileal–rectal anastomosis is the frequency of interval proctectomy. Interval proctectomy is required for persistence or recurrence of disease and/or the occurrence of rectal cancer. The late proctectomy rate for persistence or recurrence of disease varies between 5 (Aylett 1966) and 58 per cent (Lindham and Lagercrantz 1980); it is 24 per cent at the Mayo clinic (Farnell *et al.* 1980). Furthermore, the chance that a patient will have a good result after operation (no steroids, good health, acceptable stool frequency, and no incontinence) is only 45 per cent (Farnell *et al.* 1980).

In particular, the risk of cancer developing in the retained rectum is about 5 per cent at 15 years after operation; this increases to 15 per cent at 30 years (Baker *et al.* 1978; Lindham and Lagercrantz 1980; Grundfest *et al.* 1981). Unfortunately, these cancers are usually of advanced grade and stage compared with colorectal cancer unassociated with chronic ulcerative colitis (Baker *et al.* 1978).

The quality of life after ileorectal anastomosis has been reported to be good (Mignon and Bonfils 1985); the satisfaction is high and an active, productive lifestyle can be preserved. Overall satisfaction is tempered, however, by the fact that patients often feel they have not been cured because they must undergo frequent follow-up examinations.

Continent ileostomy (Fig. 19.3)

Since Kock described his operation in 1969 more than 1600 continent ileostomy operations have been performed (Fazio and Church 1988).

The *aim* of continent ileostomy is to remove the colon and rectum entirely while concomitantly providing continence for faeces and gas and maintaining a cosmetically acceptable stoma. The *rationale* is that colectomy and proctectomy 'cure' the disease, the ileal pouch functions as a reservoir for gas and stool, and the nipple valve provides continence. By eliminating the necessity of wearing an external appliance, the quality of life theoretically improves.

Patient selection

Patients are candidates for continent ileostomy if they do not have Crohn's disease, are young (< 55 years), thin, and psychologically fit. At present in

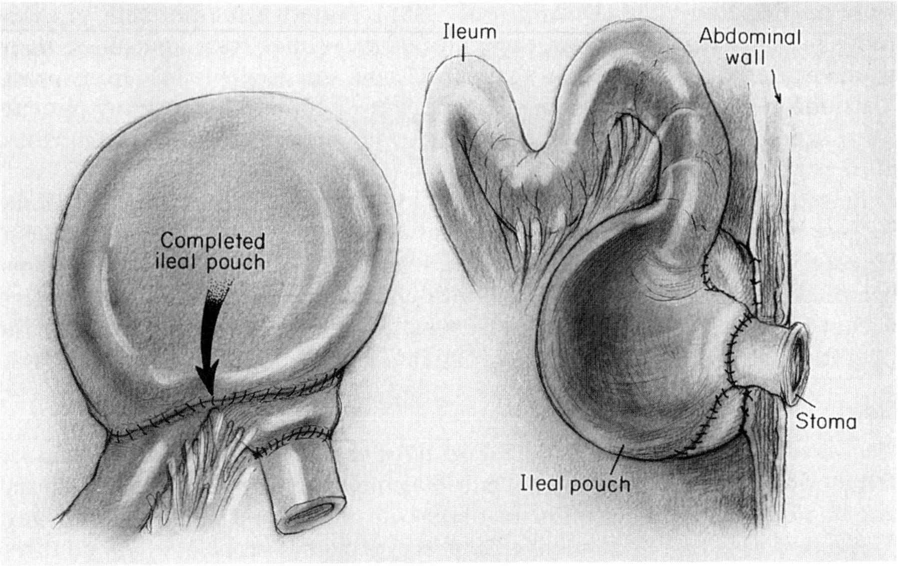

Fig. 19.3. The Koch pouch is anchored to the abdominal wall with the outflow tract flush with the skin. [Reproduced from Kelly and Dozois (1985) by kind permission of Year Book Medical Publishers, Chicago.]

our institution, however, the only candidates for this procedure are patients who have already had a proctocolectomy.

Complications

At Mayo, only one of 460 patients died after continent ileostomy (Dozois, Kelly, Beart, and Beahrs 1985). Fazio and Church (1988) have reported that complications include bowel obstruction (2–17 per cent), haemorrhage (0.5–5 per cent), sepsis (2–11 per cent), and fistula (1–7 per cent). In our series, delayed complications such as valve extrusion usually occurred during the first year after operation. Surgery to revise the valve was required early in 43 per cent of the patients and in 22 per cent later (Dozois *et al.* 1985). 'Pouchitis' occurred in 30 per cent of continent ileostomy patients (Fazio and Church 1988).

Excision of the pouch was required in fewer than 5 per cent of patients over longer term (Dozois *et al.* 1985). The reasons for pouch excision were repeated valve malfunction, recurrent fistula, pouchitis unresponsive to medical management, and unsuspected Crohn's disease.

Clinical, functional and quality of life results

In the Mayo series (mean follow-up 3.5 years), 75 per cent of patients with ileostomy were continent, 23 per cent had occasional leakage, and 3 per cent wore an ileostomy bag (Dozois *et al.* 1985). Ninety-three per cent of ileostomy patients reported their expectations were met fully and all of them would undergo the operation again (McLeod and Fazio 1984). In contrast, Valkamo (1981) found that only 37 per cent of continent ileostomy patients were satisfied after the initial operation, but rates of satisfaction improved after revisional surgery.

In summary, although the complication rate and the rate of revisional surgery seems quite high after continent ileostomy, most patients appear to be satisfied. The rate of late failure (> 10 years) remains unknown. Once again, only rarely would a patient with chronic ulcerative colitis be offered a continent ileostomy primarily, at least at the Mayo clinic. Instead, the operation of choice in appropriate patients is ileal pouch–anal anastomosis.

Ileal pouch anastomosis

The *aim* of the operation is to excise *all* diseased and potentially diseased large bowel and rectal mucosa while concomitantly restoring faecal continence and allowing defaecation to occur via the normal anatomic pathway. The *rationale* is that abdominal colectomy, proximal proctectomy, and distal mucosal rectal resection remove all premalignant mucosa, but preserve the anal sphincter apparatus. The ileal pouch restores reservoir capacity. Moreover, normal bladder and sexual function should be preserved because the distal rectal mucosal resection is performed endorectally. Finally, a perineal wound is avoided.

Selection of patients

The operation is an *elective* one. The best results will not be achieved in patients who require high dose immunosuppressives, have uncontrolled extra-intestinal manifestations, require intensive nutritional support (i.e. have low albumin), or have experienced prolonged growth retardation. In patients such as these, the more straightforward the surgical approach, the better.

Certain patients are better candidates for ileal pouch–anal anastomosis than are others. Younger patients have a superior result when compared with older patients (Metcalf, Dozois, Kelly, Beart, and Wolff 1985; Pemberton, Kelly, Beart, Wolff, and Ilstrup 1987). Moreover, patients experience a better chance of technical success if they are thin. Nearly all of our patients are on low or moderate doses of steroids and, therefore, *steroids per se are not a contra-indication for operation.*

The operation

The technique of ileal pouch–anal anastomosis has been described in detail elsewhere (Pemberton 1987). Figure 19.4 illustrates the final result. We have not as yet performed this operation sparing the anal canal mucosa (anal transition zone) except in a few patients ($n = 7$).

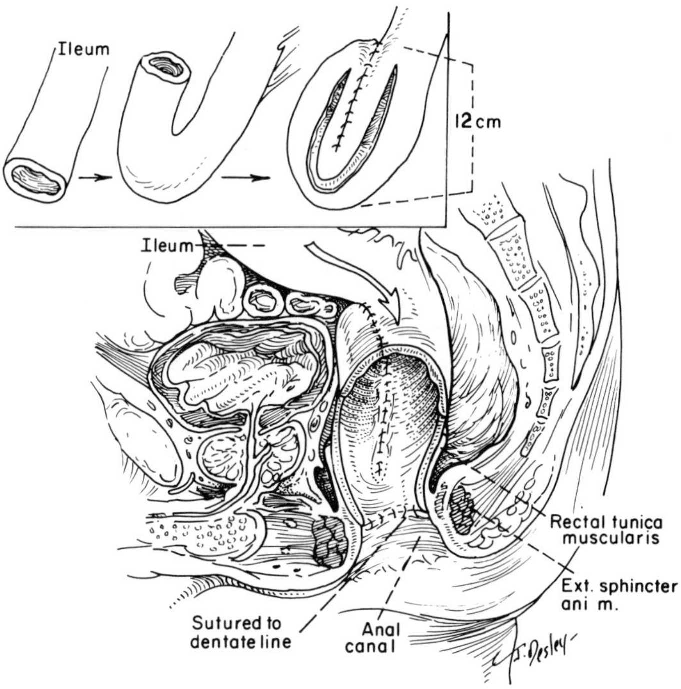

Fig. 19.4. Diagram of the completed ileal pouch–anal anastomosis. [Reproduced from Taylor, Beart, and Dozois (1983) by kind permission.]

Although Johnston *et al.* (1987) found improved sensation and better rates of perfect continence in patients in whom the anal canal transitional zone was spared, Keighley Winslet, Yoshioka, and Lightwood (1987) found no such demonstrable improvement. Moreover, somewhat disturbingly, King, Lubowski, and Cook (1987) found that 14 of 16 patients with chronic ulcerative colitis had inflammation characteristic of colitis in the mucosa of the anal canal. Four patients had moderate dysplasia and one had an unsuspected cancer of the anal canal. This is an interesting controversy and will likely be resolved only by a prospective trial.

Clinical results

At the Mayo clinic, ileal pouch–anal anastomosis has been performed in more than 1100 patients since 1981. The long-term results of ileal pouch–anal anastomosis in a well-defined cohort of patients were reported recently (Pemberton *et al.* 1987). This group consisted of 390 adults with chronic ulcerative colitis who had a 'J' pouch constructed and who were followed up for a mean of 2.3 years (range 6 months to 5 years).

Early results

One patient (0.3 per cent) died. Overall, 29 per cent of patients had a post-operative complication. The most frequent complication was small bowel obstruction, which occurred in 22 per cent. Pelvic sepsis occurred in 5 per cent of the patients; one-third were treated successfully by antibiotic therapy alone, whereas the other two-thirds required operative drainage. Abdominal wound infections occurred in 3 per cent. Urinary retention occurred transiently in 7 per cent but required intermittent catheterization in less than 2 per cent.

After closure of the ileostomy, 9 per cent of patients had a small bowel obstruction, for which operative correction was required in one-half. Anastomotic leakage at the site of ileostomy closure occurred in 2 per cent.

Late results

The principal late complications were anastomotic stricture and 'pouchitis'. Five per cent of the patients had persistent strictures that required dilatation repeatedly.

Pouchitis occurred at variable times after operation. The mean (s.d.) interval from operation to the first occurrence of pouchitis was 16 (14) months. Administration of metronidazole nearly always resulted in prompt subsidence of symptoms. Several patients, however, have required low-dose metronidazole therapy continuously to prevent recurrence of the syndrome.

Sexual dysfunction occurred in 11 per cent of the men and 12 per cent of the women; 1.5 per cent of men were impotent and 4 per cent complained of retrograde ejaculation. Dyspareunia occurred in 7 per cent of the women and was the principal complaint.

Nearly all patients had a favourable outcome over 5 years (Fig. 19.5); only 6 per cent had a failed operation. The causes of failure were recurrent pouchitis, multiple stoods, gross night-time faecal incontinence, and granulomatous ileitis. Of the patients who failed, 75 per cent did so within 1 year. No patient has failed more than 3 years after operation.

Table 19.1 and Figure 19.6 detail the stool frequency, pattern of continence, and ability to discriminate gas from stool, from 6 months to 5 years after ileal pouch–anal anastomosis. The daytime and night-time stool frequency as well as the pattern of daytime continence did not change over time. In contrast, the incidence of nocturnal incontinence and dependency on medication declined.

Quality of life

In order to determine whether there was any difference in the quality of life between patients with a ileal pouch–anal anastomosis and those with a Brooke ileostomy, we surveyed 298 patients with the anastomosis and compared the results with those from 406 patients a Brooke ileostomy operated

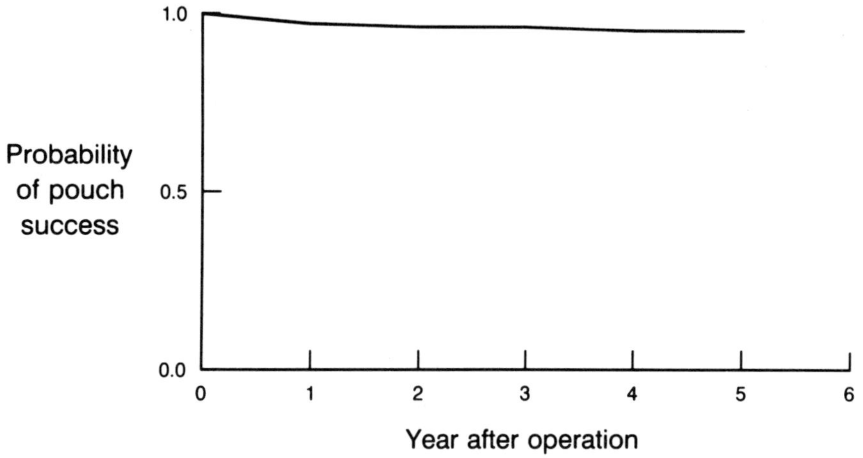

Fig. 19.5. Probability of successful outcome with functioning ileal pouch–anal anastomosis for chronic ulcerative colitis plotted against post-operative year. [Reproduced from Pemberton *et al.* (1987) by kind permission.]

Table 19.1. Functional results of illeal pouch–anal anastomosis from 6 months to 6 years after operation in 389 patients.

Parameter	6 months	1 year	2 years	3 years	4 years	5 years
No. of stools [mean (SD)]						
Day	5 (2)	5 (3)	6 (3)	6 (2)	6 (3)	6 (2)
Night	1 (1)	1 (1)	2 (2)	2 (1)	1 (1)	2 (1)
Able to discriminate gas from stool (%)	69	77	73	84	77	86

on for chronic ulcerative colitis or familial adenomatous polyposis (Pemberton, Phillips, Ready, Zinsmeister, and Beahrs 1989). The mean ages of the patients were similar. The great majority of both groups were satisfied with their operation (anastomosis 95 per cent; ileostomy 93 per cent). After adjusting for age, diagnosis, and reoperation rate, logistic regression analysis of performance scores in seven different categories was used to discriminate between operations. We found that in each performance category, the performance score discriminated between operations, with the probability of having had an ileal pouch–anal anastomosis operation increasing with improvement in performance scores ($p < 0.05$) (Figs 19.7 and 19.8). We concluded that after following ileal pouch–anal anastomosis, patients experience significant advantages in performing daily activities compared with patients with Brooke ileostomy and thus experience a better quality of life.

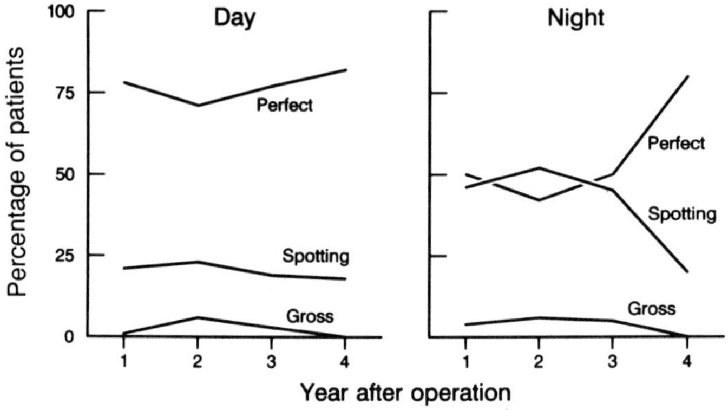

Fig. 19.6. Daytime and night-time continence after ileal pouch-anal anastomosis for chronic ulcerative colitis plotted against post-operative year. Perfect = no faecal leakage; spotting = faecal spotting of underclothes two times or less per week; gross = gross faecal incontinence more than two times per week. Data points are connected for illustrative purposes only. [Reproduced from Pemberton *et al.* (1987) by kind permission.]

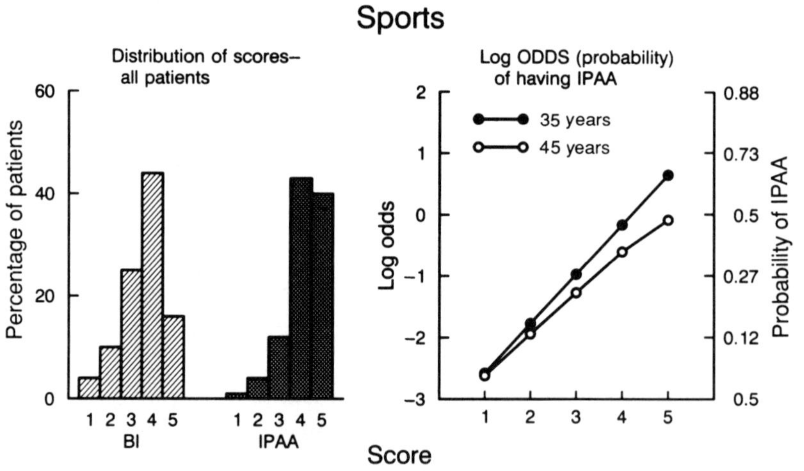

Fig. 19.7. Comparison of performance status; category: Sports. *Left*: Overall distribution of patient performance scores for Brooke ileostomy (BI) and ileal pouch–anal anastomosis (IPAA). The data indicate higher scores among patients with IPAA. *Right*: Plots of estimated log probability of having had the IPAA operation in 35- and 45-year-old patients with chronic ulcerative colitis, and no reoperation. The rising lines ([+] slopes) indicate that an improving performance score is associated with an increased probability of having had the IPAA operation in both age groups ($p \langle 0.05$). [Reproduced from Pemberton *et al.* (1989) by kind permission.]

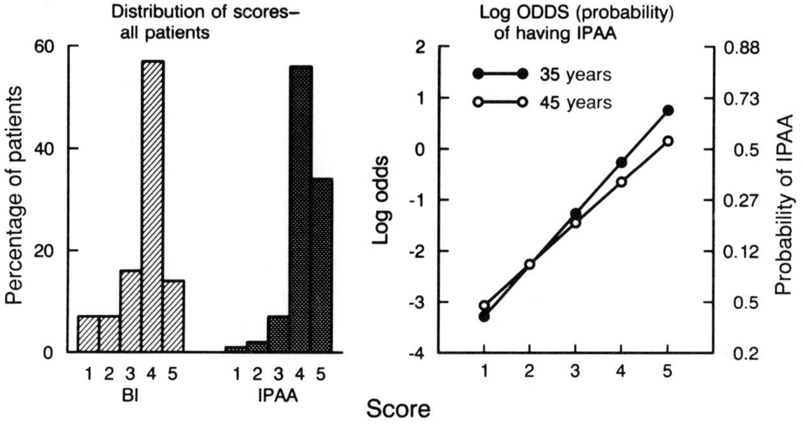

Fig. 19.8. This figure shows that an improving performance score, in the category of sexual activities, is associated with increased probability of having had ileal pouch–anal anastomosis (IPAA). See Figure 19.7 for explanation of graphs. [Reproduced from Pemberton *et al.* (1989) by kind permission.]

Comparing the alternatives

Although the Brooke ileostomy is safe, reliable, and has broad applicability to patients with inflammatory bowel disease, it is *not entirely free from complications*: up to 30 per cent of patients have a septic complication, 20–25 per cent require stomal revision, 15 per cent have recurrent small bowel obstruction, and stomal dysfunction can occur in up to 30 per cent.

Ileal–rectal anastomosis

The primary benefit of ileo-rectostomy is that the rectum is undisturbed by the operative dissection. In most patients, the functional results are good. The major problem with ileal–rectal anastomosis is that diseased mucosa is left *in situ*; in most patients *disease progression continues unabated.* The sequelae of leaving disease include poor anastomotic healing; continued need for steroids; continued bleeding and mucous discharge; incontinence and high stool frequency if disease flares; and the possibility that cancer will occur. Between 20 and 40 per cent of patients with ileal–rectal anastomosis require proctocolectomy for one or several of these complications.

Continent ileostomy

The major benefit is that although a stoma is constructed, discharge is controlled without using an external appliance. The principal problem with continent ileostomy is the impressively high rate of complications requiring reoperation.

Ileal pouch–anal anastomosis

The major benefit of ileal pouch–anal anastomosis is that it restores fecal continence in the great majority of patients, but the major problem is that the complication rate is about 30 per cent. Occasional incontinence occurs in nearly all patients early after operation, particularly at night. Major episodes of daytime incontinence occur in nearly 10 per cent of patients, but this incidence declines to zero by 4 years. As experience with the operation has broadened, however, other complications have decreased in frequency. Despite these problems, the benefits of ileal pouch–anal anastomosis are clear: all disease is removed, the patients do not have a stoma, and defaecation is wilful and controlled.

Conclusions

The one alternative that fulfills the criteria for an ideal alternative to proctocolectomy is ileal pouch–anal anastomosis; ileal–rectal anastomosis falls short because disease is left *in situ*, while the continent ileostomy operation necessitates an abdominal stoma.

Ileal–rectal anastomosis may be the procedure of choice in several specific instances, such as in young people not yet through adolescence. Moreover, patients of any age who are unwilling to accept *any* risk of sexual or bladder dysfunction should be offered ileal–rectal anastomosis.

Continent ileostomy has a minor role in the management of patients with chronic ulcerative colitis; it is an option for patients who have already had a proctocolectomy and who desire control of the stoma.

While no operation restores a patient to normality after colectomy, ileal pouch–anal anastomosis appears to come closest *without leaving residual disease in situ*. Broad clinical experience suggests that in most patients, ileal pouch–anal anastomosis achieves its goals. Ileal pouch–anal anastomosis is an important advance in the management of chronic ulcerative colitis. Although not applicable to everyone, ileal pouch–anal anastomosis should be considered the treatment of choice in nearly all younger patients facing proctocolectomy for chronic ulcerative colitis.

References

Adson, M.A., Cooperman, A.M., and Farrow, G.M. (1972). Ileorectostomy for ulcerative disease of the colon. *Arch. Surg.* **104**, 424–8.

Alexander-Williams, J. (1983). Overview of surgical management and directions of future research. In *Inflammatory bowel disease* (ed. R.N. Allan, M.R.B. Keighley, and J. Alexander-Williams) pp. 496–504. Churchill Livingstone, New York.

Aylett, S.O. (1960). Diffuse ulcerative colitis and its treatment by ileorectal anastomosis. *Ann. R. Coll. Surg. Engl.* **27**, 260–84.

Aylett, S. (1963). Ulcerative colitis treated by total colectomy and ileorectal anastomosis: a ten-year review (abridged). *Proc. R. Soc. Med.* **56**, 183–90.

Aylett, S.O. (1966). Three hundred cases of diffuse ulcerative colitis treated by total colectomy and ileo-rectal anastomosis. *Br. Med. J.* **1**, 1001–5.

Baker, W.N.W. (1970). The results of ileorectal anastomosis at St. Mark's Hospital from 1952 to 1968. *Gut* **11**, 235–9.

Baker, W.N.W., Glass, R.E., Ritchie, J.K., and Aylett, S.O. (1978). Cancer of the rectum following colectomy and ileorectal anastomosis for ulcerative colitis. *Br. J. Surg.* **65**, 862–8.

Beauchamp, G., Beliveau, D., and Archambault, A. (1981). Death and complications after total colectomy for inflammatory bowel disease. *Can. J. Surg.* **24**, 463–6, 484.

Bergman, L. and Krause, U. (1977). Crohn's disease: a long-term study of the clinical course. *Scand. J. Gastroenterol.* **12**, 937–44.

Burnham, W.R., Lennard-Jones, J.E., and Brooke, B.N. (1977). Sexual problems among married ileostomists: survey conducted by the Ileostomy Association of Great Britain and Ireland. *Gut* **18**, 673–7.

de Dombal, F.T., Burton, I.L., and Goligher, J.C. (1971). Recurrence of Crohn's disease after primary excisional surgery. *Gut* **12**, 519–27.

Dozois, R.R., Kelly, K.A., Beart, R.W. Jr., and Beahrs, O.H. (1985). Continent ileostomy: the Mayo Clinic experience. In *Alternatives to conventional ileostomy* (ed. R.R. Dozois) pp. 180–91. Year Book Medical Publishers, Chicago.

Farmer, R.G. and Michener, W.M. (1979). Prognosis of Crohn's disease with onset in childhood or adolescence. *Dig. Dis. Sci.* **24**, 752–7.

Farnell, M.B. and Adson, M.A. (1985). Current results: the Mayo Clinic experience. In *Alternatives to conventional ileostomy* (ed. R.R. Dozois) pp. 100–21. Year Book Medical Publishers, Chicago.

Farnell, M.B., van Heerden, J.A., Beart, R.W. Jr., and Weiland, L.H. (1980). Rectal preservation in nonspecific inflammatory disease of the colon. *Ann. Surg.* **192**, 249–53.

Fazio, V.W. (1990*a*). Conservative surgery for Crohn's disease of the small bowel: the role of strictureplasty. *Med. Clin. North Am.* **74**, 169–81.

Fazio, V.W. (1990*b*). Crohn's disease. In *Surgical treatment of digestive disease* (ed. F.G. Moody) pp. 655–83. Yearbook Medical Publishers, Chicago.

Fazio, V.W. and Church, J.M. (1988). Complications and function of the continent ileostomy at the Cleveland Clinic. *World J. Surg.* **12**, 148–54.

Fazio, V.W. and Galandiuk, S. (1985). Strictureplasty in diffuse Crohn's jejunoileitis. *Dis. Colon Rectum* **28**, 512–18.

Goligher, J.C. (1980). Crohn's disease (granulomatous enteritis). In *Surgery of the anus, rectum and colon* (4th edn.) (ed. J.C. Goligher) pp. 971–1017. Baillière Tindall, London.

Goligher, J.C. (1985). The long-term results of excisional surgery for primary and recurrent Crohn's disease of the large intestine. *Dis. Colon Rectum* **28**, 51–5.

Grundfest, S.F., Fazio, V., Weiss, R.A., Jagelman, D., Lavery, I., Weakley, F.L., and Turnbull, R.B. Jr (1981). The risk of cancer following colectomy and ileorectal anastomosis for extensive mucosal ulcerative colitis. *Ann. Surg.* **193**, 9–14.

Grüner, O.-P.N., Naas, R., Fretheim, B., and Gjone, E. (1977). Marital status and sexual adjustment after colectomy: results in 178 patients operated on for ulcerative colitis. *Scand. J. Gastroenterol.* **12**, 193–7.

Gump, F.E., Sakellariadis, P., Wolff, M., and Broell, J.R. (1972). Clinical pathological investigation of regional enteritis as a guide to prognosis. *Ann. Surg.* **176**, 233–42.

Hellers, G. (1979). Crohn's disease in Stockholm County 1955–1974: a study of epidemiology: results of surgical treatment and long-term prognosis. *Acta Chir. Scand. Suppl.* 490.

Johnson, W.R., McDermott, F.T., Hughes, E.S.R., Pihl, E.A., and Milne, B.J. (1983). The risk of rectal carcinoma following colectomy in ulcerative colitis. *Dis. Colon Rectum* **26**, 44–6.

Johnston, D., Holdsworth, P.J., Nasmyth, D.G., *et al.* (1987). Preservation of the entire anal canal in conservative proctocolectomy for ulcerative colitis: a pilot study comparing end-to-end ileo-anal anastomosis without mucosal resection with mucosal proctectomy and endo-anal anastomosis. *Br. J. Surg.* **74**, 940–4.

Keighley, M.R.B., Winslet, M.C., Yoshioka, K., and Lightwood, R. (1987). Discrimination is not impaired by excision of the anal transition zone after restorative proctocolectomy. *Br. J. Surg.* **74**, 1118–21.

Kelly, K.A. and Dozois, R.R. (1985). Chronic ulcerative colitis. In *Surgical treatment of digestive disease* (ed. F.G. Moody, L.C. Carey, R.S. Jones, K.A. Kelly, D.L. Nahrwold, and D.B. Skinner) pp. 663–46. Year Book Medical Publishers, Chicago.

King, D.W., Lubowski, D.F., and Cook, T.A. (1987). Anal canal mucosa in restorative proctocolectomy for ulcerative colitis. *Br. J. Surg.* **76**, 970–2.

Kock, N.G. (1969). Intra-abdominal 'reservoir' in patients with permanent ileostomy: preliminary observations on a procedure resulting in fecal 'continence' in five ileostomy patients. *Arch. Surg.* **99**, 223–31.

Lee, E.C.G. and Dowling, B.L. (1972). Perimuscular excision of the rectum for Crohn's disease and ulcerative colitis: a conservation technique. *Br. J. Surg.* **59**, 29–32.

Lee, E.C.G. and Papaionnou, N. (1982). Minimal surgery for Crohn's obstruction in patients with extensive or minimal Crohn's disease. *Ann. R. Coll. Surg. Engl.* **64**, 229–33.

Lefton, H.B., Farmer, R.G., and Fazio, V.W. (1975). Ileorectal anastomosis for Crohn's disease of the colon. *Gastroenterology* **69**, 612–17.

Lindham, S. and Lagercrantz, R. (1980). Ulcerative colitis in childhood: should the rectum be preserved at surgery? Long-term results in 50 patients. *Scand. J. Gastroenterol.* **15**, 123–7.

Lock, M.R., Farmer, R.G., Fazio, V.W., Jagelman, D.G., Lavery, I.C., and Weakley, F.L. (1981*a*). Recurrence and reoperation for Crohn's disease: the role of disease location in prognosis. *N. Engl. J. Med.* **304**, 1586–8.

Lock, M.R., Fazio, V.W., Farmer, R.G., Jagelman, D.G., Lavery, I.C., and Weakley, F.L. (1981*b*). Proximal recurrence and the fate of the rectum following excisional surgery for Crohn's disease of the large bowel. *Ann. Surg.* **194**, 754–60.

Lyttle, J.A. and Parks, A.G. (1977). Interspincteric excision of the rectum. *Br. J. Surg.* **64**, 413–16.

McIlrath, D.C. (1971). Diverting ileostomy and colostomy in the management of Crohn's disease of the colon. *Arch. Surg.* **103**, 308–10.

McLeod, R.S. and Fazio, V.W. (1984). Quality of life with the continent ileostomy. *World J. Surg.* **8**, 90–5.

Metcalf, A.M., Dozois, R.R., Kelly, K.A., Beart, R.W. Jr., and Wolff, B.G. (1985). Ilial 'J' pouch–anal anastomosis: clinical outcome. *Ann. Surg.* **202**, 735–9.

Mignon, M. and Bonfils, S. (1985). Altered physiology in ulcerative colitis patients with ileorectal anastomosis. In *Alternatives to conventional ileostomy* (ed. R.R. Dozois) pp. 61–80. Year Book Medical Publishers, Chicago.

Morowitz, D.A. and Kirsner, J.B. (1981). Ileostomy in ulcerative colitis: a questionnaire study of 1803 patients. *Am. J. Surg.* **141**, 370–5.

Newton, C.R. and Baker, W.N.W. (1975). Comparison of bowel function after ileorectal anastomosis for ulcerative colitis and colonic polyposis. *Gut* **16**, 785–91.

Nugent, F.W., Richmond, M., and Park, S.K. (1977). Crohn's disease of the duodenum. *Gut* **18**, 115–20.

Parc, R., Levy, E., Frileux, P., and Loygue, J. (1985). Current result: ileorectal anastomosis after total abdominal colectomy for ulcerative colitis. In *Alternatives to conventional ileostomy* (ed. R.R. Dozois) pp. 81–99. Year Book Medical Publishers, Chicago.

Pemberton, J.H. (1987). Surgery for ulcerative colitis. *Surg. Clin. North Am.* **67**, 633–50.

Pemberton, J.H., Phillips, S.F., Dozois, R.R., and Wendorf, L.J. (1985). Current clinical results. In *Alternatives to conventional ileostomy* (ed. R.R. Dozois) pp. 40–50. Year Book Medical Publishers, Chicago.

Pemberton, J.H., Kelly, K.A., Beart, R.W. Jr., Wolff, B.G., and Ilstrup, D.M. (1987). Ileal pouch–anal anastomosis for chronic ulcerative colitis: long-term results. *Ann. Surg.* **206**, 504–13.

Pemberton, J.H., Phillips, S.F., Ready, R.R. Zinsmeister, A.R., and Beahrs, O.H. (1989). Quality of life after Brooke ileostomy and ileal pouch–anal anastomosis: comparison of performance status. *Ann. Surg.* **209**, 620–8.

Pennington, L., Hamilton, S.R., Bayless, T.M., and Cameron, J.L. (1980). Surgical management of Crohn's disease: influence of disease at margin of resection. *Ann. Surg.* **192**, 311–18.

Pritchard, T.J., Schoetz, D.J., Caushaj, F.P., *et al.* (1990). Strictureplasty of the small bowel in patients with Crohn's disease. An effective surgical option. *Arch. Surg.* **125**, 715–17.

Ritchie, J.K. (1971). Ileostomy and excisional surgery for chronic inflammatory disease of the colon: a survey of one hospital region. Part I. Results and complications of surgery. *Gut* **12**, 528–36.

Ross, T., Fazio, V.W., and Farmer, R.G. (1983). Long-term results of surgical treatment for Crohn's disease of the duodenum. *Ann. Surg.* **197**, 399–406.

Roy, P.H., Sauer, W.G., Beahrs, O.H., and Farrow, G.M. (1970). Experience with ileostomies: evaluation of long-term rehabilitation of 497 patients. *Am. J. Surg.* **119**, 77–86.

Sayfan, J., Wilson, D.A.L., Allan, A., Andrews, H., and Alexander-Williams, J. (1989). Recurrence after strictureplasty or resection for Crohn's disease. *Br. J. Surg.* **76**, 335–8.

Sirinek, K.R., Tetirick, C.E., Thomford, N.R., and Pace, W.G. (1977). Total proctocolectomy and ileostomy: procedure of choice for acute toxic megacolon. *Arch. Surg.* **112**, 518–22.

Stahlgren, L.H. and Ferguson, L.K. (1961). The results of surgical treatment of chronic regional enteritis. *J. A. M. A.* **175**, 986–9.

Stryker, S.J., Pemberton, J.H. and Zinsmeister, A.R. (1985). Long-term results of ileostomy in older patients. *Dis. Colon Rectum* **28**, 844–6.

Taylor, B.M., Beart, R.W. Jr, Dozois, R.R., *et al.* (1983). Straight ileo-anal anastomosis versus ileal pouch–anal anastomosis. *Arch. Surg.* **118**, 696–701.

Valkamo, E. (1981). *Ileostomy in ulcerative colitis: academic dissertation* (thesis). Second Department of Surgery. University Central Hospital, Helsinki Fairbairn.

Watts, J. Mc. K. and Hughes, S.R. (1977). Ulcerative colitis and Crohn's disease: results after colectomy and ileorectal anastomosis. *Br. J. Surg.* **64**, 77–83.
Watts, J. Mc. K., de Dombal, F.T., and Goligher, J.C. (1966). Long-term complications and prognosis following major surgery for ulcerative colitis. *Br. J. Surg.* **53**, 1014–23.
Wolff, B.G. (1990). Crohn's colitis. In *Current therapy in colon and rectal surgery* (ed. V.W. Fazio) pp. 195–8. B.C. Decker, Philadelphia.
Wolff, B.G., Blatt, R.W.P., Frydenberg, H.B., Weiland, L.H., Agrey, M.V., and Ilstrup, D.M. (1983). The importance of disease free margins in resection for Crohn's disease. *Dis. Colon Rectum* **26**, 239–43.
Wolff, B.G., Dozois, R.R. Kelly, K.A. *et al.* (1987). In *Strictureplasty for Crohn's disease*. Proceedings of Symposium — Controversies in Inflammatory Bowel Disease, p. 219. Bologna, Italy.

20. Minor anorectal surgery

Carlos M. Magsanoc

There are significant differences in the approach and methods by which minor anorectal surgery is undertaken in Third World countries and the Philippines, when compared to highly developed countries such as the USA and the UK. In order to understand why this is so requires consideration of economic factors which play an important role in management. Expectations in medical care are high in rich countries and are often taken for granted, whereas care in poorer nations is often inadequate and delayed.

Haemorrhoids

In the Philippines only about 10–15 per cent of the population has access to satisfactory medical attention and it is for this reason that the majority of patients seek consultation for haemorrhoids when they are large and circumferential or when fistulae are already far advanced with multiple openings. Often the ideal management is unobtainable and economics dictate that one has to adapt and improvise in patient care. In Third World countries, a full spectrum of the natural causes of disorders may be observed with appropriate, often original, therapeutic options at different stages of disease. The flap technique for haemorrhoidectomy is herein presented as an alternative procedure in treatment. This procedure was developed following the observation that advanced prolapsed circumferential haemorrhoids were not adequately managed by the standard methods, such as the Milligan–Morgan technique, because the intervening skin bridges between the haemorrhoidectomy sites were still involved with secondary haemorrhoids or redundancy of the skin. These secondary haemorrhoids enlarge with time and become symptomatic.

One of the indications for surgery for haemorrhoids is thrombosis. This usually occurs following a severe bout of diarrhoea, constipation, or severe straining. The patient is usually seen a few days after the acute attack which coincides with the peak period of swelling. Thrombosis may affect a small portion, resulting in a solitary discrete nodule, or an area as large as the whole circumference of the anus, to give rise to a tense, shining, tinned wall. If the thrombus is not evacuated, it takes 2–4 weeks to subside and shrink in size. Immediate pain relief and comfort can be obtained by excision of the thrombus under local anaesthesia. If the thrombus is small it may be easily excised, together with the involved haemorrhoid. If thrombosis is widespread, the swelling is composed of smaller thrombi in a vascular honeycombed matrix requiring extensive electrocauterization for haemostasis.

Pain, bleeding, discomfort, and inconvenience lead patients to accept surgery. Pain may be caused by thrombosis, strangulation, inflammation, infection, and fissure formation, and has been described as itching, burning, and throbbing in nature. If a concomitant fissure is present, a constant ache persists hours after defaecation. Constantly prolapsing haemorrhoids, even on mild straining, can be troublesome and uncomfortable and are as equally inconvenient after when being reduced. Bleeding is, likewise, an inconvenience if slight, but can be alarming and, rarely, life threatening if severe. Unresponsiveness to conservative measures drives patients finally to decide to have surgery.

Two of the most frequently asked questions about the operation concern post-operative pain incontinence. Lay people have the impression that the operation is an extremely painful procedure. Outdated practices of inserting a rectal plug for haemostasis and dilating the anal wound in the immediate post-operative period produce considerable pain. Patients should be assured that fears regarding post-operative pain have been exaggerated in the past.

Incontinence can be caused by an inexperienced operator who inadvertently divides the sphincters when anorectal anatomy is distorted, as in severe oedema, thrombosis, or advanced prolapse of haemorrhoids. Avoidance of this complication is accomplished by careful dissection, demonstration, and isolation of the muscles before any division is commenced. The patient should be informed that incontinence is not a natural consequence but a complication of an incorrectly performed haemorrhoidectomy.

Basic requirements for haemorrhoidectomy include gentle handling of structures, complete removal of diseased tissues, leaving generous islands of skin between the sites of excision, preserving the continuity of the sphincters, and adequate wound drainage.

There are numerous techniques for haemorrhoidectomy and as long as basic principles are followed, these are of equal merit. Surgical preferences are obviously dependent on individual familiarity with techniques acquired during formative training.

The Milligan–Morgan operation involves isolation and dissection of the three major haemorrhoidal vessels with ligation of the bases. The wounds at the site of excision are left open. In the Ferguson technique, the wounds which result, in a similar dissection and ligation procedure, are closed. The authors claim that such closure produces less discomfort and leads to faster healing time. In a similar operation, Parks described a plastic incision in the anorectal mucosa with dissection of the haemorrhoids submucosally, after which the incision is closed. Since no anoderm is removed, the risk of stenosis is minimal. All other operations in use at present are variations of the three operations mentioned.

I personally advocate the Milligan–Morgan technique in ordinary uncomplicated haemorrhoids. In the Philippines, however, a majority of haemorrhoids tend to be large, circumferential, and prolapsed [Fig. 20.1(A)]. In such instances, the Milligan–Morgan procedure alone leaves a large residue of secondary haemorrhoids and redundant tissue in the intervening islands of skin. Thrombosis and oedema may convert these into a large, unsightly, vascular mass in the immediate post-operative period, eliciting comments that after surgery the haemorrhoids were bigger than before the operation. These residual haemorrhoids later enlarge and give rise to the same symptoms which made treatment necessary.

A technique was devised to remove the primary and secondary haemorrhoids completely without the pitfalls of the Whitehead operation, namely stenosis and mucosal prolapse. Stenosis may be avoided or at least reduced by using the anoderm or peri-anal skin as intervening islands of skin between the open wound from which epithelialization can originate. Ideally, the anoderm should, if possible, be retained in its original position in order not to disturb afferent receptors responsible for continence. In severely prolapsed haemorrhoids, however, the anoderm or even the dentate line becomes extruded outside the anal verge so that the receptors are already displaced at the outset. Replacement of the excised pile-bearing anoderm, with a flap composed of anal and peri-anal epithelium, may temporarily disrupt the reflex arc involved in defaecation and continence but, in due course, the new lining will adapt and bowel habit can return to normal in a few weeks.

Prevention of 'wet anus', which is an unwelcome complication of the Whitehead operation, may be accomplished by suturing the anal and peri-anal skin flaps above the level of the dentate line. In this way no rectal mucosa will protrude beyond the anal verge.

Surgical technique for flap reconstruction

Under spinal anaesthesia the patient is placed in the jackknife position with the buttocks retracted laterally using adhesive tapes, the ends of which are attached to the side of the operating table.

Using a large Hill–Ferguson retractor, primary haemorrhoids are identified and isolated with clamps. Usually haemorrhoids are located at the right anterior, right posterior, and left lateral positions [Fig. 20.1(B)]. Nevertheless, it is not uncommon for haemorrhoids not to be located in their standard positions so that the distance between each is unequal. In such cases clamps should be placed in the usual positions where the haemorrhoids are most often situated (i.e. equidistant from each other, even if the intervening tissue between clamps, usually on the right anterior phase, is a primary haemorrhoid). This irregularly sited haemorrhoid, after being divested of its vascular components, may eventually be incorporated into a skin flap.

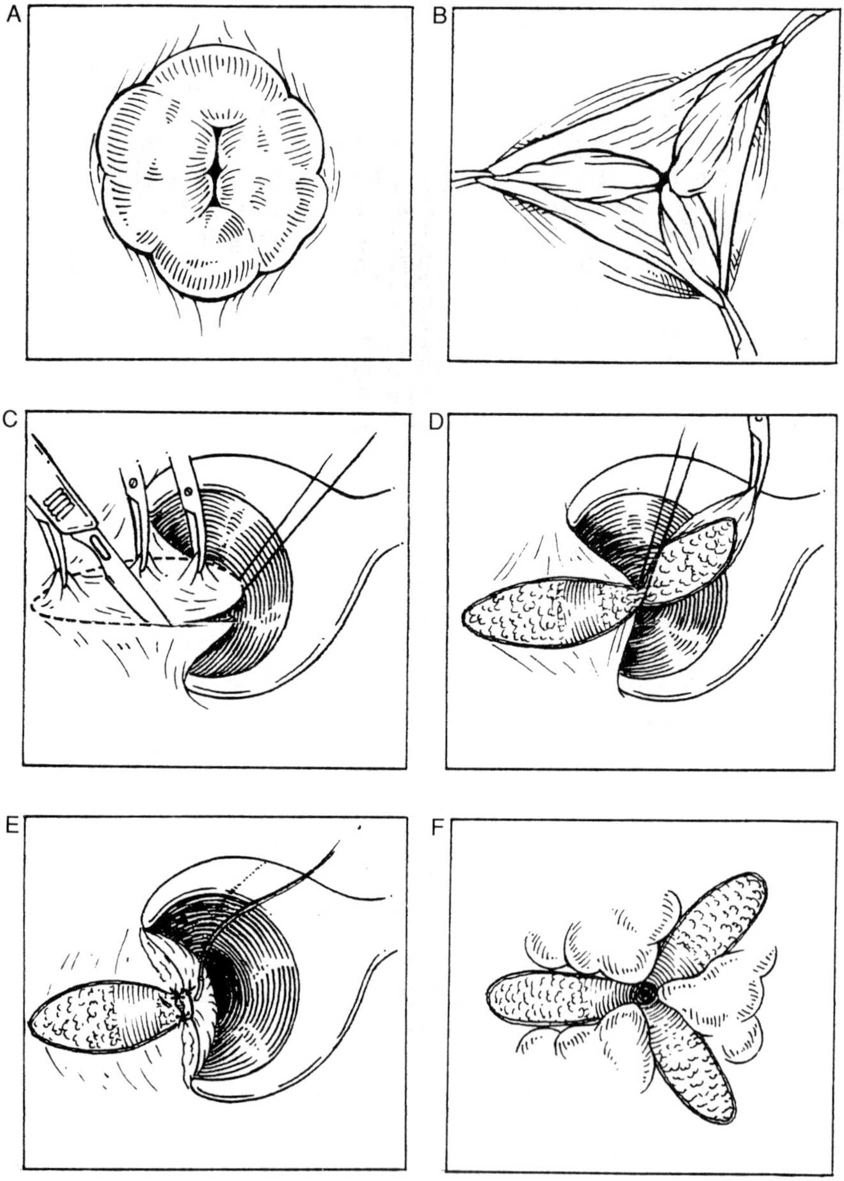
A
B
C
D
E
F

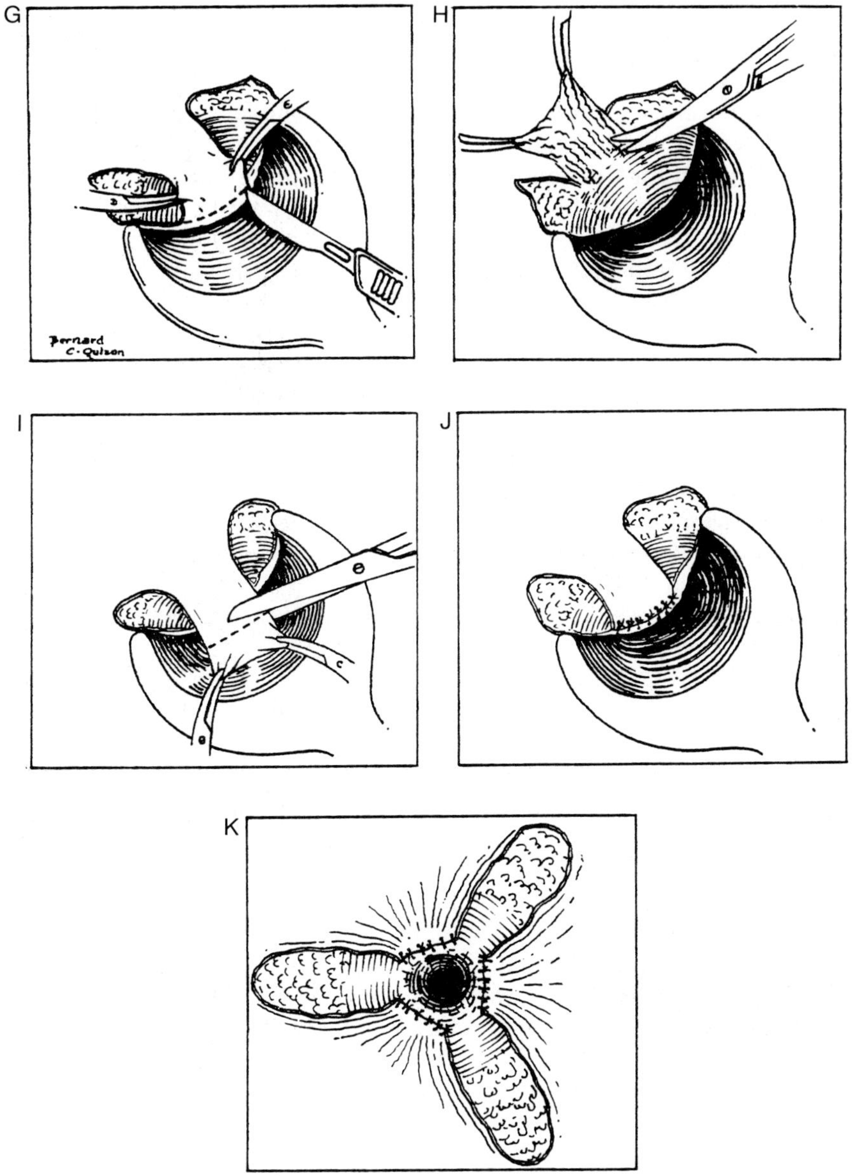

Fig. 20.1. Haemorrhoids. (A) Large circumferential prolpased haemorrhoids; (B) right anterior and posterior and left lateral positions; (C) clamps placed on haemorrhoids for traction; (D) elliptical skin incision; (E) stump suture; (F) redundant skin overflow; (G) horizontal incision above stump; (H–J) flap technique of haemorrhoidectomy; (K) completed operation.

Equidistant positioning of the clamps is important in order that the width of the intervening islands of anoderm and peri-anal skin, which will eventually become flaps, is uniform.

The left lateral haemorrhoid is the first to be removed. Clamps are placed over the haemorrhoid just above the dentate line, at the anal verge, and on the peri-anal skin for traction [Fig. 20.1(C)]. A suture ligature of 0 Dexon® is placed at the base of the haemorrhoid, superior to the dentate line, just above the first traction clamp. An elliptical skin incision is made around the haemorrhoid and the related skin and dissected upward, taking care to avoid the external sphincters [Fig. 20.1(D)]. The dissection is extended to the base of the haemorrhoid where it is excised. The stump is then sutured to the superficial external sphincter muscle for fixation [Fig. 20.1(E)]. The same haemorrhoidectomy procedure is carried out for the two remaining haemorrhoids.

If the haemorrhoids are large and circumferential, redundant skin overflows into the wounds where primary haemorrhoids were removed [Fig. 20.1(F)]. Obviously, haemorrhoidectomy is inadequate and further measures have to be considered to remove the excess haemorrhoid-bearing anal and peri-anal skin.

A horizontal incision just above the level of the haemorrhoidal stump is made at the base of the intervening island of anorectal tissue on the left lateral side [Fig. 20.1(G)]. The dissection, which creates a flap, is carried downwards, avoiding the internal sphincter, the superficial, and subcutaneous external sphincter muscles [Fig. 20.1(H)]. This must be a full-thickness flap in order for it to be viable, with its length not more than twice its width. The flap is then trimmed [Fig. 20.1(I)], removing redundant skin and haemorrhoidal tissue. The flap must be long enough to avoid tension when sutured back to the rectal mucosa, using 3–0 Dexon® interrupted sutures [Fig. 20.1(J)]. To ensure immobility of the flap at the suture line, the sutures should pass through the sphincter muscles to attach the flap to its corresponding rectal component.

The same procedure is performed for the two other islands of intervening skin on the opposite sides. Figure 20.1(K) shows the completed operation. Eversion of the anal canal is exaggerated to show the flaps and their attachment to the rectal mucosa above the dentate line. Usually the suture line cannot be seen. After operation, two fingers are inserted into the rectum to ensure adequate patency of the anus. No rectal plugs of any kind are introduced and the wound is simply dressed.

Anal stenosis and flap detachment are two complications of this technique. The incidence of complications is inversely proportional to the experience of the surgeon. Flap detachment is minimized by taking care with blood supply and avoidance of tension where it is attached to the rectal mucosa. A full-thickness flap must be utilized at all times. Large tissue bites, taken to ligate the base of the haemorrhoids, can reduce the circumference of the anus considerably and are to be avoided. Due to the circumferential arrangement of the suture lines in the anal canal, fibrosis of the scar can lead to a possible purse-string effect leading to tightness or, at most, a stenosis. The use of a large Ferguson–Hill rectal retractor can minimize this effect by stretching the anal canal and, at the same time, provides a larger exposure of the operative field. Large tissue bites must not be taken to ligate the base of the haemorrhoids as these can reduce the circumference of the anal canal. The width of the intervening islands of skin must be adequate and viable, to act as bridges for epithelization, rather than fibrotic scar tissue which can contract and narrow the anal opening. The anus must admit at least two fingers at the conclusion of the operation.

Gentle anal dilatation is performed weekly to counteract any muscle spasm and break any fibrous adhesions that may form. Stenosis is most likely to be widened by the fourth week after surgery. Before this time, prophylactic measures may be encouraged to prevent stenosis because, after the fourth week, the scar will have matured and further dilatation will be painful and futile. The use of antibiotics may reduce the risk of infection, which can lead to flap disruption or fibrosis of the anal wounds.

The most obvious feature of this technique is the improved cosmetic appearance of the wound immediately after surgery, and complete wound healing. Since all the haemorrhoid-bearing tissues have been removed, and all redundant skin and connective tissue eliminated, there are no unsightly skin tags or residual haemorrhoids to contend with. The likelihood of further haemorrhoids is reduced to a minimum if the operation is correctly performed, with no skin tags which patients can mistake for haemorrhoids, nor residual haemorrhoids which may enlarge.

Anorectal abscess and fistula-*in-ano*

The surgical treatment of fistula-*in-ano* may be extremely simple or one of the most complex of all anorectal procedures to perform. An ill-informed surgeon may venture into complicated fistulotomy, oblivious of the pitfalls that may be encountered, or withhold fistulotomy when an unexpectedly deep and tortuous tract penetrating the sphincter muscles is seen.

A high incidence of recurrence attests to deficiences in understanding, regarding the classification and appropriate management for complicated fistulae. There is, as yet, no universally accepted classification of fistula-*in-ano*, nor a standard nomenclature of anorectal anatomy. The classification of fistulae is based on the assumption that the majority originate from an infection of the inter-sphincteric anal glands and that classification of fistulae is based on the direction of the tract in relation to the external sphincter.

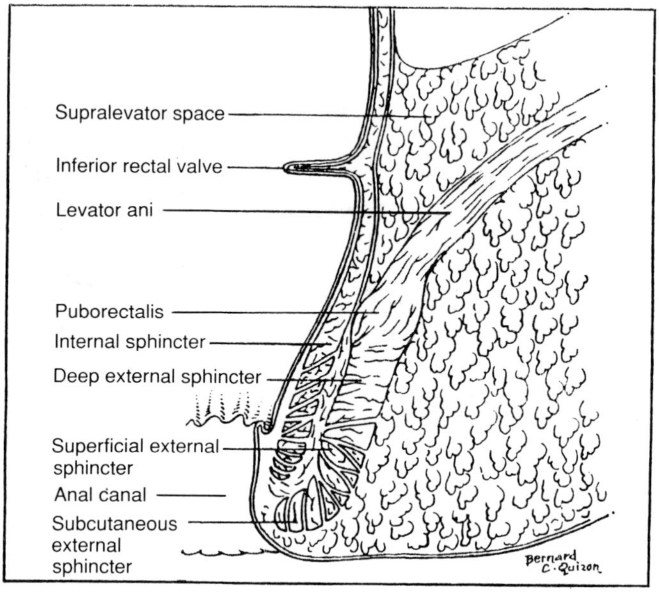

Fig. 20.2. Anorectal anatomy.

The anatomy of the anorectal region showing pertinent structures is presented in Fig. 20.2. This shows the interrelationships of the sphincter muscles and potential spaces where abscesses and fistulae can occur. There are four main types of fistulae, namely: inter-sphincteric, trans-sphincteric, supra-sphincteric and extra-sphincteric.

Inter-sphincteric fistula The internal opening, located in the anal crypt in the upper anal canal, and the external opening, situated in the region of the peri-anal area, are joined by a tract running between the internal and external sphincter muscles. This is the most common type of fistula [Fig. 20.3(A)].

Trans-sphincteric fistula The internal opening in the anal canal is joined to the external opening, located more than about 2–3 cm from the anal verge, by a tract which penetrates the external and internal sphincters along the same plane into the ischiorectal space. This is the next most frequent type of fistula [see Fig. 20.5(A)].

Supra-sphincteric fistula The internal opening in the anal canal is joined to the external opening, located at least 3 cm from the anal verge, by a tract which penetrates the internal sphincter and then arcs over the puborectalis muscle into the supra-levator space, penetrating the levator muscle inferiorly into the ischiorectal fossa [see Fig. 20.5(F)].

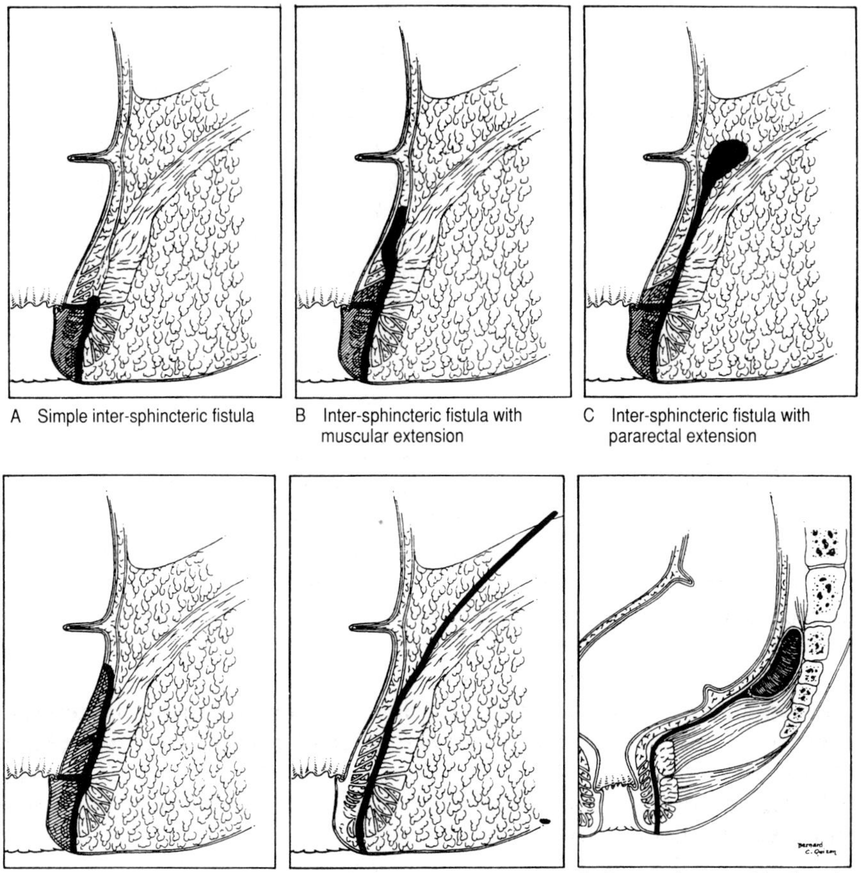

A Simple inter-sphincteric fistula

B Inter-sphincteric fistula with muscular extension

C Inter-sphincteric fistula with pararectal extension

D Inter-sphincteric fistula with secondary internal opening in rectum

E Inter-sphincteric fistula from pelvic disease

F Pre-sacral cyst emptying through an inter-sphincteric tract

Fig. 20.3. Fistulae with external openings within 3 cm from the anal verge.

Extra-sphincteric fistula The internal opening which is located high in the rectum, or from a hollow organ in the pelvis, is connected to an external opening far from the anal verge by a tract which passes through the levators into the ischiorectal space. The aetiology of this condition is usually due to foreign bodies, Crohn's disease, ulcerative colitis, tuberculous diverticulitis, or pelvic infection [see Figs 20.5(D), (G), and (H)].

There are numerous variations in each group and each will be dealt with in the appropriate sections below.

A methodical approach in essential if treatment of a fistula is to be successful. An intimate knowledge of the anatomy of the anorectal region, coupled with anticipation of the possibilities that one may encounter, are needed for confident management of this intriguing disease.

Before one evaluates a fistula, the presence of concomitant pathological colorectal disorders must be considered, since such fistulae do not behave in the same way as isolated fistulous disease so that local treatment for fistulae alone may result in failure. Often therapy directed to pre-existing disease will also help eradicate anorectal pathology.

The location of the external opening gives a clue to the type of fistula present. Openings less than 3 cm from the anal verge are usually associated with inter-sphincteric fistulae. Openings situated beyond 3 cm from the anal verge are most often caused by trans-sphincteric fistulae and rarely by the supra-sphincteric or extra-sphincteric varieties. According to Goodsall's rule, openings situated above a transverse line across the anus with the patient in the jackknife position have their internal openings in the posterior mid-line, while external openings below this line have their internal openings situated radially. However, occasional exceptions occur.

Multiple external openings on one side are usually interconnected with a common internal opening. In the case of two openings, one above and one below a line drawn across the anus, the internal opening is usually situated in the posterior mid-line. Symmetrically situated openings on both sides may indicate a horseshoe fistula, with an internal opening likewise in the posterior commissure. External openings may be located in the inner thigh or, not uncommonly, in the scrotum. A clear watery or viscous mucoid discharge from an external opening posterior to the anal verge most likely originates from a pre-sacral cystic tumour.

Initial localization of the internal opening, even before probing, may be suggested by palpation of induration in a tract, noting its direction with regard to the anal opening. A definite tract will have an internal opening at its termination. Tugging on the tract may produce a dimpling in the anal canal, revealing the location of the internal opening. Pressure on the perianal skin or an abcess may lead to extrusion of a spot of pus from an anal crypt.

The use of a dye (e.g. methylene blue) in locating a tract can be very helpful if properly employed. Sloppy infusion of a dye into a tract or abcess cavity can indiscriminately discolour the surrounding tissues, thus defeating the purpose of delineating the tract. Dye injection must be done slowly and deliberately, if possible via a watertight entry point, to prevent the dye from extravasating into the surrounding skin. The volume of the injected dye required gives an idea of the size of the tract or abscess cavity. One notable feature of methylene blue is that it heavily stains granulation tissue lining a tract, so enabling visualization of the complicated twists and turns of a fistula, which a probe cannot possibly follow (as in a supra-sphincteric fistula, for example). Even less than 1 ml of dye can stain the urine blue, and the patient must be forewarned to prevent alarm. If the dye can be introduced without much pain, a pre-operative injection of methylene blue the night before exploration will help to isolate a tract more clearly; excess dye will have been eliminated by the time the operation is performed.

Pre-operative fistulography is not routinely recommended unless one anticipates a complex fistula, which dye injection and probing may not delineate. Fistulography, however, is very helpful in recurrent fistulae, where the anatomy has been distorted and the predicted routes of a tract have been disturbed. Visualization of the tract can be achieved using oil-based or water-soluble radio-opaque solutions. Demonstration of the mucosal folds of the bowel wall on fistulography indicates that the dye has exited via an internal opening into the bowel lumen. If the operating room is well equipped and prepared, intra-operative fistulography is of great help in locating a complicated fistulous tract.

It is important that an abscess felt inside the rectum by a palpating finger can be differentiated from: (a) an inter-sphincteric muscular abscess in the rectal wall [Fig. 20.3(B)]; (b) a high infra-levator ischiorectal abscess [see Figs. 20.5(B)]; or (c) a pararectal abscess caused by inter-sphincteric, trans-sphincteric, and supra-sphincteric fistulae [see Fig. 20.3(C), 20.5(C), and 20.5(E), respectively]. Accurate differentiation is imperative for appropriate management. An incorrectly placed incision to drain an abcess produces an iatrogenic extra-sphincteric fistula which, needless to say, is catastrophic.

Probing remains the paramount procedure in the diagnosis of fistulae and one must be thoroughly acquainted with the classification of fistulae in order to anticipate the numerous possible directions a tract may take. In differentiating the aetiology of rectal abscesses, errors in diagnosis can be minimized by noting the direction in which the probe travels in relation to the rectal wall and the distance between the probe and the palpating finger. The tract of an inter-sphincteric rectal abscess [Fig. 20.3(B)] travels intimately close to the internal sphincter, and a probe inside it may be felt just beneath the bowel wall. A probe inside a pararectal abscess caused by an inter-sphincteric, trans-sphincteric, or supra-sphincteric fistula can be felt outside the rectal wall [Figs 20.3(C), 20.5(C), and 20.5(E)]. Discrimination between these three entities lies with their external openings. The inter-sphincteric abscess has its opening in the peri-anal area, the trans-sphincteric abscess has an external opening more than 3 cm from the anal verge, and the supra-sphincteric abscess, while having an external opening similar to the trans-sphincteric abscess, has no short trans-sphincteric tract which opens into an internal opening. A probed infra-levator trans-sphincteric ischiorectal abscess [see Fig. 20.5(B)] feels lower and further away from the palpating finger due to the intervening levator ani muscle.

Gentle but deliberate and decisive probing is to be practised at all times. Ignorance and an over-aggressive approach can create iatrogenic openings with dire consequences. Appropriate instruments are essential with thin, pliable, silver probes, long probes, grooved probes, angled tip probes, blunt tip needles used for injecting dyes, and crypt hooks being the basic minimum.

A seton is used when there is the possibility that incontinence might be produced by cutting a muscle bundle. Its usage is practically indispensable when treating a supra-sphincteric or trans-sphincteric fistula whose tract has penetrated high into the deep external sphincter muscle. Setons are currently manufactured in polypropylene, silastic, and silk.

Transection of the subcutaneous external sphincter and the internal sphincter have no effect on continence. Even the superficial external sphincter, when severed, does not, in practice, result in incontinence.

The puborectalis plays an essential role in continence and it must be identified and protected before a questionable muscle bundle is divided. In some patients continence may be unaffected, or slight incontinence may be caused by deep external sphincter division.

An approach to the management of fistulae

External opening located within 3 cm of the anal verge

Almost all solitary external openings located in the peri-anal area within 2–3 cm from the anal verge are due to inter-sphincteric fistulae, with two rare exceptions. The first is an inter-sphincteric sinus or fistula arising from pelvic infection due to Crohn's disease, diverticulitis, ulcerative colitis, or tuberculosis [Fig. 20.3(E)]. The second is related to a sinus draining from a pre-sacral hollow tumour [Fig. 20.3(F)]. The aetiology of the former may be determined by diagnosing the presence of inflammatory bowel disease which gives rise to the fistula. In the latter, the sinus of a draining pre-sacral tumour usually exudes a clear or viscous mucoid material from an external opening located in the mid-line posterior to the opening [Fig. 20.3(F)]. A rectal examination may simultaneously reveal a pre-sacral tumour.

There are four possible types of inter-sphincteric fistula which can be encountered [Fig. 20.3(A–D)], almost all having an internal opening located radially toward the anus. A systematic method to arrive at diagnosis can be made by the following procedure.

Insert a probe into the external opening, directing it towards the anus to look for a possible internal opening, which is usually located in the region of an anal crypt. If the probe negotiates an internal opening in the anus, with no evidence of any other tract, then one is dealing with a simple inter-sphincteric fistula [Fig. 20.3(A)]. The direction of the probe is usually radial and slightly upward. However, if, apart from the internal opening, an upward tract is discovered, one must verify whether the tract ends blindly upwards (Fig. 20.3(B) and (C)] or emerges from the rectum at a higher level as a secondary internal opening [Fig. 20.3(D)].

A tract leading upward and ending blindly may be either an inter-sphincteric fistula with an upward extension into the rectal wall [Fig. 20.3(B)] or an inter-sphincteric fistula with an upward extension into the pararectal space [Fig. 20.3(C)]. Differentiation between the two can be made by noting by palpation the proximity of the tip of the probe to the finger, and whether the rectal wall moves in an identical fashion to the probe when it is manipulated. In an intramuscular tract, the probe is almost underneath the mucosa so the probe is practically felt bare, whereas the probe in a pararectal abscess feels distant because of the intervening rectal wall and pararectal fat. Movement of a probe embedded in the rectal musculature, as in an intramuscular abscess, will elicit the same movement in the wall itself. The movement of a probe in a pararectal abscess will not produce a similar movement in the rectal wall.

An external opening with an indeterminate upward tract makes one suspect the possibility of pelvic pathology (diverticulitis, Crohn's disease, or ulcerative colitis), while a posteriorly located external opening with a blind upward tract, coupled with a palpable retrorectal mass, suggests a pre-sacral hollow tumour.

Surgical treatment The management of each type of fistula is illustrated with shaded areas representing muscle bundles which have to be divided [Fig. 20.3(A–F)]. Note that abscesses in the rectal wall and the pararectal space are treated similarly, namely, division of the subcutaneous and superficial external sphincter together with the lower part of the internal sphincter to promote adequate drainage. In the case of the fistula with two internal openings [Fig. 20.3(D)], fistulotomy of the tract between the openings must be performed.

Pre-sacral tumours are excised either via a perineal or abdominal approach. Fistulae caused by inflammatory bowel pathology usually heal when the primary disease is treated; a diverting colostomy is indicated in intractable cases.

No external opening present

Two entities will be described. In the first, obvious inflammation of the peri-anal or perineal area is present, and in the second no inflammation is seen but pus extrudes from the anus.

The pathogenesis of a fistula is such that an abscess is but the first phase in its formation. It follows that abscesses located around the peri-anal area, drained either spontaneously or iatrogenically, eventually give rise to an inter-sphincteric fistula as previously described [Fig. 20.4(A)]. In the same manner, abscesses located more than 3 cm from the anal verge, when drained, become trans-sphincteric fistulae [Fig. 20.4(B)] or rarely, supra- or extra-spincteric fistulae.

In a majority of cases, anorectal abscesses progress to fistula formation, but in a significant minority of patients drained abscesses close spontaneously following healing of their internal openings.

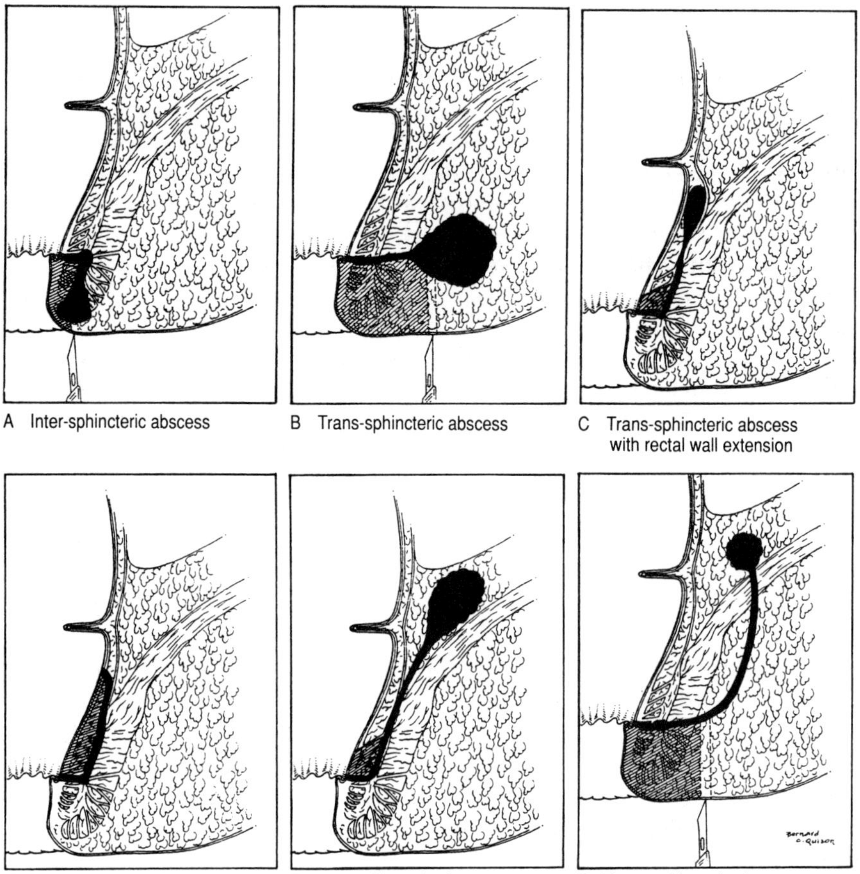

A Inter-sphincteric abscess

B Trans-sphincteric abscess

C Trans-sphincteric abscess with rectal wall extension

D Inter-sphincteric abscess with internal opening in rectum

E Inter-sphincteric abscess with pararectal extension

F Trans-sphincteric abscess with supra-levator extension

Fig. 20.4. Fistulae and abscesses without external opening.

My preference in the management of abscesses is to attempt to do a one-stage procedure, namely, drain the abscess and undertake fistulotomy if the internal opening is obvious. If, however, the internal opening is not seen, its presence is doubtful, or the tract is deep and involves either the deep external sphincter or the puborectalis, fistulotomy is deferred for a more definitive elective operation in the future. In the latter case, where the deep muscles are affected, a seton is placed.

There are patients who complain of anorectal discomfort and pain suggestive of anorectal infection but upon examination do not show evidence of any external opening in the peri-anal region. Occasionally, the patients complain of pus spontaneously exuding out of the anus or accompanying the stools.

A detailed examination reveals purulent material arising from an internal opening in the region of the anal crypts. The different types of sinus or fistulae that can produce this kind of suppuration are illustrated in Fig. 20.4 and are enumerated below.

There are four such possibilities, three of which are of the inter-sphincteric variety [Fig. 20.4(C–E)]; the other is a trans-sphincteric fistula with an ischiorectal component which penetrates the levators to end as an abscess cavity in the pararectal space (Fig. 20.4(F)].

Insert a probe into the internal opening from which the purulent exudate originates. An upward trajectory of the probe parallel to and intimately close to the inner rectal wall indicates an inter-sphincteric tract. This can lead to either a rectal wall abscess [Fig. 20.4(C)] or a pararectal abscess [Fig. 20.4(E)]. Distinctions between these have been discussed above. If, alternatively, the probe, which is pushed upward, exits from the upper rectum [Fig. 20.4(D)], an internal fistula exists with a secondary internal opening high in the rectum.

Returning to the initial exploration, if the probe, which is inserted into the internal opening, penetrates the external sphincter in a transverse direction and traverses the ischiorectal space to curve upwards through the levator ani muscle, one is dealing with a supra-levator trans-sphincteric sinus [Fig. 20.4(F)].

Sinus treatment The surgical management of fistulae and sinuses under this heading is transection of the shaded muscles as illustrated [Fig. 20.4(A–F)]. For those sinuses and fistulae of inter-sphincteric origin, adequate division of shaded muscles is a must, in order that complete and continuous drainage is obtained. Obliteration of the tracts resulting from adequate drainage subsequently occurs.

There are two other types of abscess in this category which require differentiation. Both are manifest as pararectal abscess but their management is entirely different. An inter-sphincteric abscess with a pararectal extension [Fig. 20.4(E)] should not be drained through the anal region as this would result in a supra-sphincteric fistula, whereas a trans-sphincteric abscess with a supra-levator extension [Fig. 20.4(F)] must not be drained via the rectum, or else an extra-sphincteric fistula will be created. Both complications are catastrophic. The key to differentiating between the two lesions is to note the relationship of the tracts to the puborectalis muscle, and this can be done by meticulous probing and careful palpation of the position of the probe in relation to the rectal wall.

External opening located more than 3 cm from the anal verge

The fistulae and sinuses which manifest themselves through these external openings (Fig. 20.5) are more difficult to diagnose and treat. Before exploration of the tract, inquiry must be made for a history of Crohn's disease,

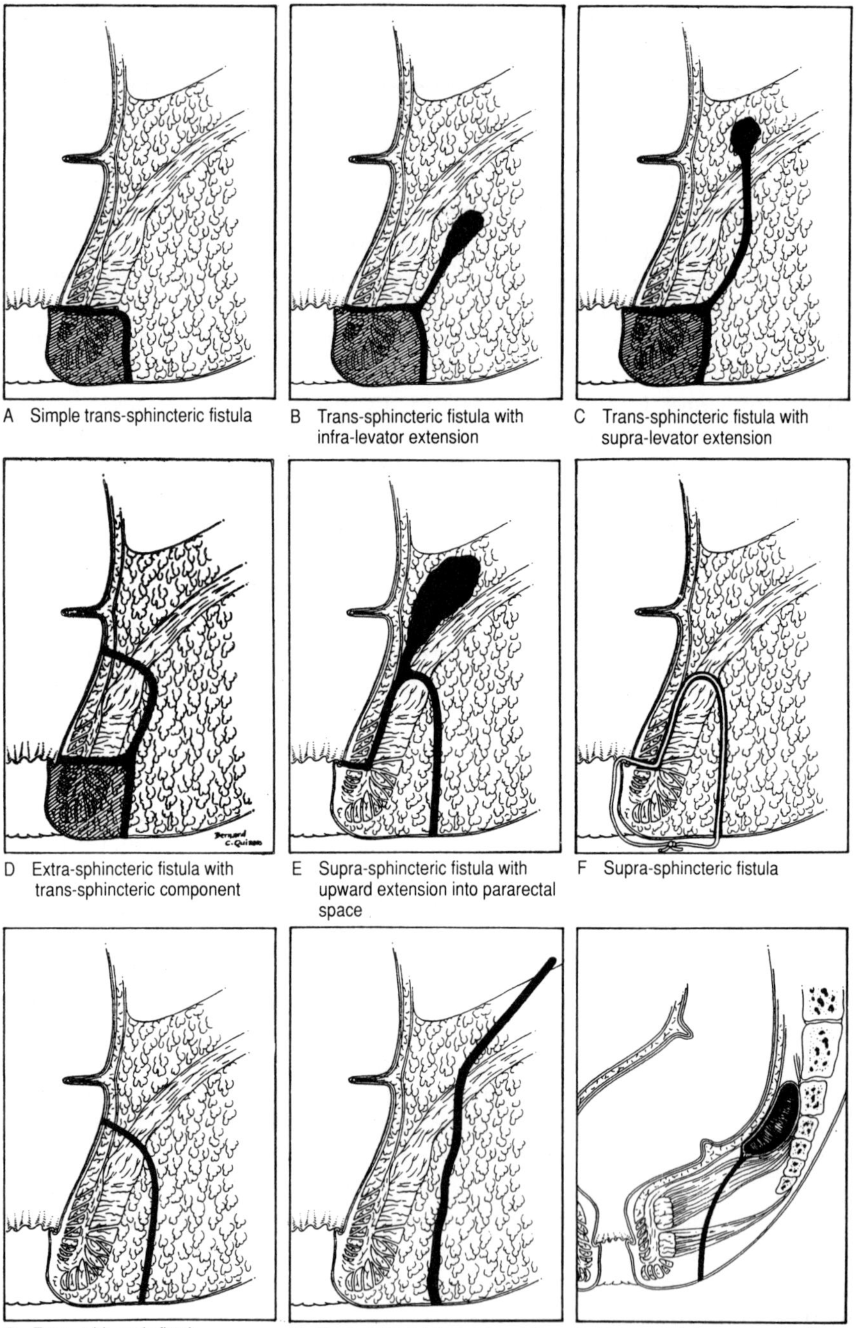

A Simple trans-sphincteric fistula

B Trans-sphincteric fistula with infra-levator extension

C Trans-sphincteric fistula with supra-levator extension

D Extra-sphincteric fistula with trans-sphincteric component

E Supra-sphincteric fistula with upward extension into pararectal space

F Supra-sphincteric fistula

G Extra-sphincteric fistula

H Extra-rectal fistula due to pelvic disease

I Extra-rectal sinus secondary to a draining pre-sacral hollow tumour

Fig. 20.5. Fistulae beyond 3 cm from the anal verge.

ulcerative colitis, or diverticulitis. A fistula with a seemingly endless tract is usually associated with pelvic disease and one of the above disorders. Even the openings produced by the above diseases take on distinctive appearances, which are quite different from those found in their absence.

An investigation should be made of the history of previous fistula surgery, especially of attempted drainage of a pararectal abscess. An iatrogenic opening may have been made in a trans-sphincteric fistula with a supra-levator extension creating an intractable extra-rectal fistula [Fig. 20.5(D)]. In complicated cases with multiple operations from recurrent fistulae, preliminary fistulography may be helpful in tracing a problematic tract.

Goodsall's rule is a very helpful guide and although most fistulae predictably follow the standard routes, a number of fistulous tracts do not conform to the rule.

A helpful hint to remember is that multiple openings located on one side are usually interconnected to each other and end as a single tract. Multiple openings on both sides may imply an underlying horseshoe fistula with a common opening in the posterior mid-line.

Awareness of the possibility that internal openings may exit at different levels may help to explain why openings are found at the level of the peri-anal area, the ischiorectal fossa, or above the puborectalis, especially in those associated with horseshoe fistulae. In contemplating a fistulotomy, it is important to determine accurately the exit point of the internal opening and at what level it emerges. Any internal opening which is located above the puborectalis should not be managed by cutting the muscles below it, but, alternatively, by inserting a seton, or in intractable cases fashioning a diverting colostomy. Divisions of the deep external sphincter may or may not produce incontinence depending on many factors, but if one is in doubt insertion of a seton is the safest option.

There are nine possible types of fistula or sinus which can be encountered in this category (Fig. 20.5(A–I)]. A simple systematic process of elimination is presented to arrive at their diagnosis.

After all preliminary examinations and observations have been completed, proceed by inserting a finger in the rectum to rule out the presence of a retrorectal tumour. This, together with an external opening posterior to the anus, which exudes a watery or a viscous mucoid discharge, is suggestive of a hollow pre-sacral tumour, which has drained through the perineum [Fig. 20.5(I)]. If a patient suffering from Crohn's disease, ulcerative colitis, tuberculosis, or diverticulitis has a fistula, it is likely that it is related to the primary disease, especially if the tract does not heal after surgery or is very high, traversing the pelvic cavity [Fig. 20.5(H)].

Of the seven possibilities which have still to be considered, four belong to the trans-sphincteric category [Fig. 20.5(A–D)], two to the supra-sphincteric variety [Fig. 20.5(E) and (F)], and the last is an extra-sphincteric type [Fig. 20.5(G)].

Proceed by inserting a probe in the external opening. If the probe travels more or less in a horizontal direction and comes out of an internal opening in the anal canal, a simple trans-sphincteric fistula is present [Fig. 20.5(A)]. If, however, aside from the transverse tract leading to the internal opening, an upward vertical tract is encountered, three alterations are possible: (a) the tract is an upward extension within the ischiorectal fossa below the levator ani [Fig. 20.5(B)]: this tract is approximately 4–6 cm in length and a probe within is felt not to be in close proximity to an examining finger in the rectum; (b) the tract goes further upward and penetrates the levator ani muscle to end in the pararectal space [Fig. 20.5(C)]; the length of this tract varies from 7 to 12 cm: an infection, if present at the end of the tract, manifests itself as pararectal abscess; (c) the tract, which has already reached the pararectal space, exits from another internal opening in the rectum [Fig. 20.5(D)]: this type can also be considered an extra-sphincteric fistula with a trans-sphincteric component; this type of fistula is most likely iatrogenic, due to a transrectal drainage of a pararectal abscess.

Fistulae with external openings directly leading to internal openings in the anus, with or without upward extensions, have been discussed. Investigation will now focus on fistulae where the probe, when inserted into the external opening, passes directly upward without any trans-sphincteric extension leading to an internal opening.

When the probe is inserted into the external opening and the tract traverses vertically upward, note carefully with a palpating finger whether the probe exits high in the upper rectum. If it does, an extra-sphincteric fistula is present [Fig. 20.5(G)]. The absence of an internal opening high in the rectum leaves two remaining possibilities: a supra-sphincteric fistula [Fig. 20.5(F)] or a supra-sphincteric fistula with an abscess in the pararectal space [Fig. 20.5(E)]. The two are basically identical, the abscess being an extension of the fistula itself. Diagnosis differs between the two in that, with an abscess, the probe goes deeper upward and rectal examination demonstrates a pararectal abscess. Nevertheless, it is still very important to inject a dye such as methylene blue into the tract, not only to verify the diagnosis arrived at by elimination, but also to demonstrate positively the fistulous tract as it arcs over the puborectalis and passes inferiorly between the internal and external sphincter to end as an internal opening in the anal canal. Diagnosis can be difficult at this stage and simple probing alone may not demonstrate the convoluted course of a supra-sphincteric fistula, unless a dye is introduced.

Surgical treatment The treatment of a trans-sphincteric fistula, with its numerous variants, is division of the internal and external sphincters as shown in the shaded areas of Figure 20.5(A–C). Provided that drainage is adequate, the extensions will close. In the case of a trans-sphincteric fistula, whose superior extension through the levator has penetrated the rectum

[Fig. 20.5(D)], resulting in an extra-sphincteric fistula, closure of the internal opening, complemented with a diverting colostomy, may be necessary. Similar management may be instituted for extra-rectal fistulae due to pelvic disorders or inflammatory bowel disease. Pre-sacral tumours producing perineal fistulae may be approached either trans-abdominally or via the perineal route, depending on the accessibility of the tumour.

A supra-sphincteric fistula is best managed by a seton [Fig. 20.5(F)].

Finally, there is the problem of what to do when no internal opening is seen in a fistula-*in-ano*, and inflammatory bowel, pelvic diseases, and pre-sacral tumours have already been eliminated. The failure to demonstrate an internal opening using dye injection does not mean that an internal opening is not present. The tract may be filled with debris, which is a hindrance to the passage of the dye, or the internal opening may have healed over and be obstructed. In either case, gentle repeated probings may dislodge whatever obstruction may be present. Tracing a dye-stained tract may require serial incisions and multiple dye applications before the internal opening is found. If, however, this procedure does not yield positive results, examine closely the anal canal and the areas immediately around it. By applying Goodsall's rule, look for possible elevations of rectal mucosa, an infected crypt, or a hypertrophied papilla in the area where the internal opening is supposed to be. With a crypt hook, explore for deep crypts forming 'pockets' which may conceal an internal opening at the base. If the tract travels transversely and radially, suggestive of a trans-sphincteric tract, push the probe gently toward the anal opening and note whether the probe encounters little resistance as it reaches the anal crypts. A thin membrane of rectal mucosa at the end of a probe which practically protudes inside the anal canal suggests that the probe has exited the internal opening, covered only by a diaphanous membrane of mucosa.

If the fistulous tract passes transversely toward the anus yet no obvious internal opening is demonstrated despite inquisitive probing, a sliding flap is made over the suspected crypt or crypts in the hope that any potential internal opening may be covered by the flap. The frequency of infection is high when such a flap is used, so adequate antibiotic coverage is strongly recommended.

For those cases where there is no indication at all as to the site of an internal opening, notably for a tract which is directed vertically, ensure that the possibility of a high internal opening due to an extra-rectal fistula is eliminated at proctosigmoidoscopy and carry out careful inspection for emergence of the tip of a probe or extravasated dye inside the rectum.

When exploration is negative it is tempting, out of frustration, to proceed with reckless abandon and desperately seek an opening during the process of which a false passage is created. Prudence dictates that one should tactically retreat and hope for a more successful attempt at a later date. After all, complicated fistulae are seldom cured after the first operation.

21. New techniques in the management of urinary calculus

Stephen T.K. Lim

The last decade has witnessed a great revolution in the treatment of urinary stones. Conventional open surgery for stones has now been virtually replaced by non-invasive, or minimally invasive, surgery. The indication for open surgery for both renal and ureteric stones has dropped to less than 1 per cent in many centres (Drach, *et al.* 1986; Lingeman *et al.* 1986; Dretler, Fair, Finlayson, Gillenwater, Griffith, Lingeman, and Newman 1986; Lingeman, Newman, Mertz, Mosbaugh, Steele, Kahnoski, Coury, and Woods 1986; Dretler 1990).

In 1981, the percutaneous approach to the pelvi-calyceal system for stone removal was improved and successfully reported by Wickham and Kellett (1981) and Alken, Hutschenreiter, Gunther, and Marberger (1981). At the same time there was rapid progress in development of nephroscopes, grasping forceps, and guide-wires and catheters, together with auxiliary devices for stone fragmentation using ultrasonic and electrohydraulic technology. More recently laser appliances have been improved and added to the armamentarium. The biggest breakthrough in technology came, however, when a completely non-invasive method of stone fragmentation using extra-corporeal shock waves was reported by Chaussy, Brendel, and Schmiedt (1980). Extra-corporeal shock wave lithotripsy (ESWL) was initially designed for renal stone fragmentation but its indications have widened to include both upper (Tung, Tan, and Foo 1990) and lower ureteric stones (Jenkins and Gillenwater 1988).

Extra-corporeal shock wave lithotripsy

The first generation lithotripter, the HM-3 model, is manufactured by Dornier of West Germany. Shock waves are generated by an underwater spark discharge and are reflected by a semi-ellipsoid reflector to a fixed focus. The anaesthetized patient, supported on a cradle in a water bath, is then moved until the stone is positioned exactly at the site of the focal point. Localization of the stone is by means of biplanar fluoroscopy. Depending on the size and number of stones, about 800–2500 shock waves can be delivered at one treatment session. The stones should be fragmented into sand-like particles of less than 4 mm in diameter, which can pass spontaneously via the ureter.

The HM-3 lithotripter has stood the test of time and its success and reliability in fragmentation has been regarded as the hallmark of standard in ESWL treatment.

However, the HM-3 lithotripter has inherent drawbacks. It requires the use of anaesthesia, either general or epidural, as well as a water-bath system to permit effective transmission of shock waves. The localization of stones by fluoroscopy allows only the treatment of radiopaque stones. In addition, irradiation received during lithotripter therapy average 20 cGy, which is high when compared to the 3 cGy received during a routine intravenous urogram (van Swearingen, McCullough, Dyer, and Appel 1987). Its expensive initial outlay and high maintenance costs have limited its availability in many urological centres and, therefore, prompted competitive manufacturers to seek alternative systems.

A second generation lithotripter, the LT-01 manufactured by EDAP of France, uses a generator consisting of 360 piezo-electric disks arranged around a hemisphere to generate the synchronous shock waves. Ultrasonic imaging allows localization of even radiolucent stones and eliminates irradiation exposure. A water-filled balloon replaces the water bath of the original Dornier system. The piezo-electric energy is relatively painless and therefore eliminates the need for anaesthesia. Unfortunately 50 per cent of the patients still require intravenous analeptics during treatment (Tung *et al.* 1990). Treatment with this machine has been performed on an out-patient basis (Miller, Collins, Turbow, Turbow, Beall, Berger, Lebowitz, Young, Kahn, Korol, Collins, and Getson 1989).

Initially urologists were sceptical with regard to the ultrasonic localization and monitoring capabilities of the EDAP LT-01. The stones, either radiopaque or radiolucent, appear as a bright image with a strong acoustic shadow. Fragmentation of the stone can be continuously monitored on the screen and fine adjustment to the focus of the shock waves on to the stone can be made continuously without interruption of treatment. During treatment the stone can be seen to swell, change its shape, and become a cloud of dust. The USA co-operative group concluded that ultrasonic localization and monitoring proved surprisingly easy to learn and were increasingly less of a problem as experience was gained (Miller *et al.* 1989).

Other second-generation lithotripters such as Piezolith (West Germany), Sonolith (France), Lithostar (West Germany), and the new Dornier MPL 9000 also do not require anaesthesia for treatment. The HM-3 model can be modified to use ultrasound for imaging as well as to avoid anaesthesia (Graff, Pastor, Herberhold, Hankemeier, and Senge 1987).

The selection of stones suitable for ESWL treatment has widened ever since its inception in 1981. Initially, only renal stones less than 2 cm were selected. Stones that were larger tended to have higher complication rates, such as severe ureteric colic, urosepsis, and obstruction by 'steinstrasse' (stone street) (Eisenberger, Fuchs, Miller, Bub, and Rassweiler 1985).

With double-pigtail ureteric stents and the development of auxiliary ureteroscopic procedures, larger stones and even staghorn calculi can be safely treated. The lumen of the double-pigtail stent (6 or 7 Fr) permits free drainage of urine while stone fragments pass down the ureter alongside the stent (Libby, Meacham, and Griffith 1988; Constantinides, Recker, Jaeger, and Hauri 1989). When all the fragments are discharged, the stent can then be removed endoscopically or withdrawn by pulling on a thread which has been pretied to the distal catheter tip. However, these stents can cause troublesome symptoms such as loin pain, dysuria, bladder pain, haematuria, and frequency (Pollard and MacFarlane 1988); Pryor and Jenkins 1990). Early removal of stents was required in 27 per cent of patients because of severe irritation, early migration, or accidental removal.

For staghorn renal calculi, monotherapy using ESWL has its advocates. With pre-treatment stenting and multiple ESWL sessions, 85 per cent of patients with partial staghorn calculi were free of stones after 6 months (Constantinides *et al.* 1989). Patients with partial staghorn calculi require 1.6 ESWL sessions (range 1–4), in which a total of 2912 shocks (range 1000–8400) were used. With complete staghorn calculi, 1.8 ESWL sessions (range 1–3) with 3341 shocks (range 1450–5100) were required (Winfield, Clayman, Chaussy, Weyman, Fuchs, and Lupu 1988).

Initial debulking of a staghorn stone (removing more than 90 per cent of the stone burden) by percutaneous nephrolithotripsy, followed by ESWL for the remaining fragments, can hasten the whole treatment process (Schulze, Hestle, Graff, Funke, and Senge 1986). A 67 per cent stone-free status at 3 months was reported by these latter authors. With this combined method at least 90 per cent of all staghorn calculi can be successfully and safely treated.

Shock wave therapy to the kidney has proven to be safe, even in patients with a solitary kidney (Kulb Lingeman, Coury, Steele, Newman, Mertz, Mosbaugh, and Knapp 1986). Transient macroscopic haematuria lasting for 1–2 days invariably occurs after treatment. Only 3 of 68 patients with a solitary kidney had transient serum creatinine elevations greater than 2 mg/100 ml, and they were caused by obstruction from stone fragments (Kulb *et al.* 1986). Transient, nephrotic-range proteinuria has been observed immediately after treatment, but this returned to normal within 3–6 months (Gilbert, Riehle, and Vaughan 1988). Quantitive radionuclide renography showed a statistically significant decrease in the percentage of effective renal plasma flow to kidneys which were treated by ESWL (Williams, Kaude, Newman, Peterson, and Thomas 1988). Hypertension following ESWL has been reported (Lingeman and Kulb 1987; Williams *et al.* 1988) but further controlled studies are required to confirm, or refute, this finding.

The most adverse and alarming complication is the development of a haematoma, which may be subcapsular or peri-renal. A drop in haemoglobin level of up to 7.4 g/100 ml can occur after treatment. Fortunately this complication is infrequent: its occurrence in fewer than 1 per cent of patients was reported by Knapp, Kulb, Lingeman, Newman, Mertz, Mosbaugh, and Steele (1988), but with hypertensive patients an incidence of 2.5 per cent was noted which increased to 3.8 per cent in patients with unsatisfactory control of hypertension. The incidence of peri-nephric haematoma is also increased in patients with pretreatment urinary tract infections and those undergoing simultaneous bilateral treatment. Management is mainly conservative with a third of patients requiring transfusion. Nephrectomy has not been necessary (Knapp *et al.* 1988).

A peri-nephric haematoma can cause severe flank pain, with 90 per cent of patients requiring narcotic analgesics. The pain is often mistaken for ureteric colic from passage of stone fragments, and unless the urologist is vigilant this complication can be easily overlooked. Any patient with a drop in haemoglobin of more than 2 g/100 ml the day after ESWL should be investigated for peri-nephric haematoma with ultrasonography and a computed tomography scan. Ultrasonography alone may miss massive retroperitoneal hemorrhage (of 2–3 litres blood) which can be fatal (Stoller, Litt, and Salazar 1989). Ironically, the majority of patients (54 per cent) who develop a peri-nephric haematoma have a pelvic stone of 1 cm or less in diameter, and 64 per cent have received 1000 or fewer shock waves (Knapp *et al.* 1988). A normal pre-treatment coagulation profile does not eliminate the possibility of this complication.

In a co-operative study in the USA (Drach *et al.* 1986) involving 2501 treatments in 2112 patients, 77.4 per cent of patients with single stones remained stone free at 3 months. With stones larger than 1 cm, or multiple stones, the risk of obstruction, increased post-operative pain, and need for additional urological operations was higher. Adjunctive urological surgical management was required in 9 per cent of patients before operation and in 8 per cent after operation. Only 0.6 per cent of patients required some type of open incisional operation to clear residual stone complications after ESWL. Similarly, Lingeman and associates (1986) reported that 70 per cent of their 982 patients were stone free at 3 months, with only 1 per cent of the patients requiring surgical removal of calculi.

There is still some concern over the significance of residual fragments (smaller than 3 mm in diameter) in the kidney. Graff, Diederichs, and Schulze (1988), in their series of 1003 patients, reported that 60 per cent of patients who were discharged from hospital with residual fragments (650 patients) eventually became free of stones. In 17 per cent, regrowth of stone particles occurred, and in another 22 per cent no change was observed. True recurrences were encountered in 6.2 per cent of their patients. Stones located in the lower calyces, as well as multiple stones, have a higher incidence of residual fragments. Longer follow-up is required to resolve the issue of residual stones.

In the report of the USA co-operative study, four deaths within 6 weeks after operation were recorded (Drach *et al.* 1986). Two deaths were related to cerebrovascular accidents and hypertension, while the other two deaths occurred because of unrelated diseases. In another large series of 982 patients (Lingeman *et al.* 1986), the only significant intra-operative complication was in a patient who suffered a myocardial infarction following a hypotensive episode during epidural anaesthesia. No deaths were noted in 461 patients treated with the EDAP LT-01 (Miller *et al.* 1989).

Prophylactic treatment with antibiotics during ESWL treatment was shown to be unnecessary in a randomized clinical study unless an infective element was evident (Petterson and Tiselius 1989). In all the 149 patients who were studied, the occurrence of bacteriuria was low (6.7 per cent), despite the fact that almost 30 per cent of patients had a ureteric catheter.

Stones that have been impacted in the ureter for more than 6 weeks do not disintegrate easily when treated *in situ* by ESWL. The lack of an expansion chamber around the stone has been incrimated, and thus a push–bang technique has been advocated. The ureteric stone is flushed (using either saline, lidocaine viscous solution, or dilute surgical lubricant) back into the pelvi-calyceal system by means of a retrograde uteteric catheter, inserted under fluoroscopic control (Evans, Wingfield, Morollo, and Jenkins 1988). The dislodged stone is then treated by ESWL as for a renal stone with the expected success of fragmentation. Even if an impacted ureteric stone fails to be dislodged, the mere presence of an ureteric catheter alongside the stone could improve the success of fragmentation, since it creates an artificial expansion chamber. Such stones have a 88.9 per cent success rate of fragmentation (Nuzzarello, Rubenstein, and Norris 1990).

For those ureteric stones which can not be bypassed by a catheter, a new technique using an ureteral stone brush has been described (Nuzzarello *et al.* 1990). The brush is constructed of Nylon bristles on a 0.038-inch stainless steel wire. The outside diameter of the brush ranges from 0.098 to 0.138 inches, with an average bristle length of 0.05 inch. This brush can be inserted through an open-ended 6 Fr ureteric catheter which is placed just below the stone. After delivery of 750–1000 shocks, the stone is brushed 7–10 times under fluoroscopic control. At this point the stone can usually be bypassed by the catheter. This procedure is repeated after every 200–400 shocks until complete dispersion of all the stone fragments is evident. The rationale behind the brushing technique is to counteract the ineffective absorption of shock wave energy within the multiple interfaces of the fragmented outer shell which, in effect, eliminates adequate shock wave application to the core of the stone. Thus, the brush effectively removes the fragmented outer shell after each bout of shocks. With this technique, complete fragmentation was achieved in 84.6 per cent of casts.

Disimpaction of ureteric stones can also be achieved by various manoeuvres such as high pressure irrigation, carbon dioxide flushing with a venting nephrostomy tube (Hulbert, Reddy, Hunter, Young, Castaneda-Zuniga, Amplatz, and Lange 1985), pushing the stone with a rigid ureteroscope under direct vision, or placing an occlusion balloon below the stone to allow for hydrodilatation of the ureter (Beckmann and Roth 1985). More recently, pulse-dye laser has been used successfully for disimpaction (Dretler 1990).

Not only does second-generation lithotriptsy avoid the need for anaesthesia, it also permits cheaper retreatment sessions whenever necessary. With these two advantages, *in-situ* ESWL treatment, for ureteric stones, has become an acceptable first choice of treatment (Tung *et al.* 1990). The push–bang technique is advocated only when stones fail to disintegrate.

When ureteric stones are treated *in-situ*, the success rate is significantly lower (80.8 per cent) compared with stones that are successfully manipulated into the kidney (98.2 per cent) (Fetner, Preminger, Seger, and Lea 1988).

Bladder stones have also been successfully treated. Using a second-generation Lithostar lithotripter, patients were placed prone on the machine. All 10 patients with bladder stones (range 8–30 mm in diameter) had complete disintegration of their stones (Vandeursen and Baert 1990). Minute fragmentation was achieved and uncomplicated evacuation occurred without the need for adjuvant procedures, even in the presence of prostatic hypertrophy or neurogenic bladder dysfunction.

Stones of varying composition respond differently to shock wave fragmentation and vary in the following order from greatest to least fragility: calcium oxalate dihydrate, uric acid, calcium oxalate monohydrate, struvite, and cystine (Dretler 1988).

For evaluation of asymptomatic patients after ESWL, a combination of abdominal radiography and ultrasonography is as good or better than intravenous urography in identifying residual stone fragments and intrarenal or peri-renal abnormalities. It is recommended that these are carried out 1 month after treatment and, if abnormalities of the collecting system are visualized, intravenous urography is then performed since ultrasonography is less specific in identifying dilatation of part or all of the collecting system (Coughlin, Risius, Streem, Lorig, and Siegel 1989). An intravenous urogram at 3 months post-treatment would be valuable because it provides information regrading the function of the kidney as well as providing a view of the whole length of the ureter.

Percutaneous Nephrolithotripsy (PCNL)

To gain access to the renal stone, a nephrocutaneous track has to be created. This is first achieved by locating the calyx (usually the lower pole calyx) with a fine-puncture needle under fluoroscopic control. A floppy-tip guide-wire is then inserted and manoeuvred down the ureter. By means of a series of Teflon or metal 'telescopic' dilators, the track is gradually dilated in one or two stages to accept either a 26 Fr nephroscope or a 30 Fr Amplatz sheath.

Smaller renal and upper ureteric stones (less than 1.0 cm in diameter) are extracted intact, under endoscopic or fluoroscopic control, with grasping forceps or Dormia baskets. Larger stones, including staghorn calculi, require additional devices for fragmentation before removal of the pieces can be achieved.

The ultrasonic probe, with its drilling-like action, will break down a stone gradually into small particles of less than 2–3 mm in diameter. These fine fragments are constantly aspirated along the lumen of the probe during the procedure. The larger pieces can be removed with grasping forceps or further fragmented and aspirated.

Alternatively an electrohydraulic probe sends out explosive charges and will cause the stone to fragment into several pieces suitable for removal with forceps, thus enabling a more rapid surgical clearance of stones. A nephrostomy catheter is left via the nephrocutaneous track after the procedure. Besides providing post-operative drainage for the pelvi-calyceal system, it allows antegrade radiological studies of the upper tracts. If a further endoscopic procedure is required, the track may be reused. Patients are discharged on the third or fourth post-operative day, after removal of the nephrostomy catheter, with a return to work after a week.

In a comparative study between percutaneous and open surgery, Preminger, Clayman, Hardeman, Franklin, Curry, and Peters (1986) reported that in patients with calculi that were 2.5 cm or less in diameter, the percutaneous procedure resulted in a lower post-operative morbidity rate, more rapid convalescence, less hospital cost, and greater patient satisfaction. Even with stones larger than 2.5 cm, percutaneous surgery offered a markedly shortened convalescent period with patients returning to work and resuming vigorous activity between 8.5 and 20 days, respectively. Success rates of up to 97 per cent in the complete removal of targeted calculi has been reported (Brannen, Bush, and Lewis 1986).

In the past, non-obstructive but symptomatic calyceal stones received a more conservative approach since open surgery may result in a 20 per cent risk of prolonged wound discomfort in exchange for resolution of renal pain, which may be caused by a small calculi (Brannen *et al.* 1986). Furthermore, intra-operative localization of a small calyceal stone may be difficult and the risk of failure to achieve stone removal is high. But in the present era of advances in technology, stones that are causing pain, infection, and haematuria, or are progressively enlarging in size should be considered for removal. The percutaneous approach to these calculi was successful in 96 per cent of cases in a series of 51 patients, and in more than 90 per cent it resulted in resolution of associated discomfort (Brannen *et al.* 1986). Alternatively, calyceal stones can be treated successfully by ESWL (Drach *et al.* 1986). Mee and Thuroff (1988) felt that it was justifiable to treat small calyceal stones (less than 1 cm in diameter) by ESWL when correlation with persistent flank pain was indeterminable. These authors reported that 91 per cent of their 22 patients had achieved complete or significant relief of pain after treatment.

Complications are not serious and no kidneys were lost after PCNL (Brannen *et al.* 1986; Preminger *et al.* 1986). Extravasation of fluid and urine following perforation of the renal pelvis is common but healing occurs spontaneously within 2 days after the procedure. However, a death from hyponatraemia and cardiac arrhythmia has been recorded (Preminger *et al.* 1986). Blood transfusion was required in 2 per cent of the patients following percutaneous surgery, compared with 22 per cent for open surgery. Arterio-venous fistulae can occur and may require embolization via a percutaneous trans-femoral approach.

Hypertension following percutaneous surgery has not been noted, and the procedure has been shown to be safe and effective, with minimal late morbidity (Merberger, Stackl, Hruby, and Kroiss 1985), with no significant change in creatinine clearances of the operated kidneys (Mayo, Krieger, and Rudd 1985). In fact, there is significant improvement in the function of kidneys containing infected stones following percutaneous removal of the calculi.

Ureteroscopic Lithotripsy

With the development of fine-calibre instruments (7–12.5 Fr), stones in the lower and mid-ureter can be reached easily with either flexible semi-rigid or rigid ureterscopes. With instruments larger than 8 Fr in size, prior dilatation of the ureteric orifice has to be performed before introduction of the scope. This is achieved by balloon dilatation, or with a series of metal or Teflon dilators passed over a guide-wire under fluoroscopic control.

Smaller stones can be engaged in a wire basket under direct vision at endoscopy, and both the basket and ureterscope gently withdrawn (Tolley 1987). With larger stones, ultrasonic probes or electrohydraulic probes (5 Fr) are required to fragment the stones into smaller particles before removal with a basket (Huffman, Bagley, Schoenberg, and Lyon 1983). Success rates of 91 per cent (Denstedt and Clayman 1990) and 97 per cent (Tolley 1987) have been documented.

Both ultrasonic and electrohydraulic probes require larger ureteroscopes (more than 10.5 Fr) but with the development of lasers in the armamentarium, a new era of lasertripsy has emerged. The laser fibre measures only 0.25 mm in diameter and can be passed through the operating channel of a 7.2 Fr semi-rigid or a 7 Fr flexible ureterscope. The pulse dye laser is the current solution to the problem of finding a laser with a stone-fragmenting ability, which has the advantage of small size (250 μm) and a pulse width short enough to prevent thermal damage and long enough (1 μs) to cause stone fragmentation (Dretler 1990).

Laser lithotripsy does not require the ureteric stone to be trapped in a basket, as the risk of proximal migration of the stone is less likely when compared with ultrasonic lithotripsy. In a series of 225 patients, the laser failed in 8 per cent of the patients treated (Dretler 1990). The laser has also been shown to be useful for disimpaction of impacted ureteric stones prior to ESWL treatment.

Calculi that are 100 per cent calcium oxalate monohydrate may be resistant to laser treatment unless they are mixtures of calcium oxalate monohydrate and calcium oxalate dihydrate or of calcium oxalate monohydrate and apatite (Dretler 1990).

A new electrohydraulic probe (3 Fr) is available for use with the flexible ureterscope (Huffman *et al.* 1983). Electrohydraulic lithotripsy is more cost effective when compared with expensive laser machines and has been proven to be safe. It is generally agreed that complications of ureterscopic lithotripsy are related primarily to the ureterscopes, regardless of which method of stone fragmentation is chosen.

Therapeutic Options

With a wide choice of methods now available, it has become even more challenging for urologists to decide on the best modality of treatment for their patients.

In developed countries where all modalities of treatment are easily available, ESWL treatment alone or combined with percutaneous surgery is strongly favoured for renal stones, because it is a non-invasive and yet effective procedure. More than 500 000 patients world-wide have already been treated with ESWL. Approximately 70 per cent of patients, either with renal or ureteric stones, can benefit from ESWL alone. The remaining 25–30 per cent require combined treatment with endourological techniques, leaving fewer than 1 per cent needing open surgery. For bigger stones, pre-ESWL stenting with a double-pigtail catheter may reduce complications of the large stone burden. Ureteroscopic expertise and facilities should be made available when such stones are being treated.

As anaesthesia is no longer required with the second-generation lithotripters, upper-third stones as well as distal stones can be treated *in situ* initially, even if they are impacted. Thus, it is only in the 10–20 per cent ESWL failures that more invasive ureterscopic procedures, either manipulation or lithotripsy, is necessary. For mid-ureteric stones, ureteroscopic lithotripsy or the push–bang method can be offered.

In centres without ESWL facilities, as in less developed countries, endourology has to be developed so that the need for open surgery is kept below

3–5 per cent of cases. The cost to set up an endo-urological service, even with laser lithotripsy, is still well below the cost of a lithotripter machine.

Patients with large renal stones, who travel long distances to a urological centre for treatment, may well benefit from percutaneous surgery rather than ESWL as its outcome is more predictable. The initial aftercare of patients following ESWL treatment is just as important as the success of fragmentation itself and thus close urological supervision, until complete clearance of steinstrasse, is mandatory. Few symptoms are present in a large percentage of patients with steinstrasse despite urinary obstruction, decreased renal function, infection, and even impending sepsis (Weinerth, Flatt, and Carson 1989).

While the long-term side-effects and risks associated with shock waves are not yet fully understood and precisely defined, it is imperative that the indications for removal of stones should not be expanded yet, just because of the simplicity of performance of ESWL.

References

Alken, P., Hutschenreiter, G., Gunther, R., and Marberger, M. (1981). Percutaneous stone manipulation. *J. Urol.* **125**, 463–6.

Beckmann, C.F. and Roth, R.A. (1985). Use of retrograde occlusion balloon catheters in percutaneous removal of renal calculi. *Urology* **25**, 277–283.

Brannen, G.E., Bush, W.H., Correa, R.J., Gibbons, R.P., and Elder, J.S. (1985). Kidney stone removal: percutaneous versus surgical lithotomy. *J. Urol.* **133**, 6–12.

Chaussy, C., Brendel, W., and Schmiedt, E. (1980). Extracorporeally induced destruction of kidney stones by shock waves. *Lancet* **ii**, 1265–8.

Coughlin, B.F., Risius, B., Streem, S.B., Lorig, R.J., and Siegel, S.W. (1989). Abdominal radiograph and renal ultrasound versus excretory urography in the evaluation of asymptomatic patients after extracorporeal shock wave lithotripsy. *J. Urol.* **142**, 1419–24.

Constantinides, C., Recker, F., Jaeger, P., and Hauri, D. (1989). Extracorporeal shock wave lithotripsy as monotherapy of staghorn renal calculi: 3 years of experience *J. Urol.* **142**, 1415–18.

Denstedt, J.D. and Clayman, R.V. (1990). Electrohydraulic lithotripsy of renal and ureteral calculi. *J. Urol.* **143**, 13–17.

Drach, G.W., Dretler, S., Fair, W., Finlayson, B., Gillenwater, J., Griffith, D., Lingeman, J., and Newman, D. (1986). Report of the United States cooperative study of extracorporeal shock wave lithotripsy. *J. Urol.* **135**, 1127–33.

Dretler, S.P. (1988). Stone fragility: a new therapeutic distinction. *J. Urol.* **139**, 1124–7.

Dretler, S.P. (1990). An Evaluation of ureteral laser lithotripsy: 225 consecutive patients. *J. Urol.* **143**, 267–72.

Eisenberger, F., Fuchs, G., Miller, K., Bub, P., and Rassweiler, J. (1985). Extracorporeal shock wave lithotripsy (ESWL) and endourology: an ideal combination for the treatment of kidney stones. *World J. Urol.* **3**, 41–50.

Evans, R.J., Wingfield, D.D., Morollo, B.A., and Jenkins, A.D. (1988). Ureteral stone manipulation before extracorporeal shock wave lithotripsy. *J. Urol.* **139**, 33–6.

Fetner, C.D., Preminger, G.M., Seger, J., and Lea, T.A. (1988). Treatment of ureteral calculi by extracorporeal shock wave lithotripsy at a multi-use center. *J. Urol.* **139**, 1192–4.

Gilbert, B.R., Riehle, R.A., and Vaughan, E.D. Jr. (1988). Extracorporeal shock wave lithotripsy and its effects on renal function. *J Urol.* **139**, 482–5.

Graff, J., Diederichs, W., and Schulze, H. (1988). Long-term followup in 1003 extracorporeal shock wave lithotripsy patients. *J. Urol.* **140**, 479–83.

Graff, J., Pastor, J., Herberhold, D., Hankemeier, U., and Senge, Th. (1987). Technical modifications of the Dornier HM-3 lithotriptor with an improved anesthesia technique. *World J. Urol.* **5**, 202–7.

Huffman, J.L., Bagley, D.H., Schoenberg, H.W., and Lyon, E.S. (1983). Transurethral removal of large ureteral and renal pelvic calculi using ureteroscopic ultrasonic lithotripsy. *J. Urol.* **130**, 31–4.

Hulbert, J.C., Reddy, P.K., Hunter, D.W., Young, A.T., Castaneda-Zuniga, W.R., Amplatz, K., and Lange, P.H. (1985). Percutaneous management of ureteral calculi facilitated by retrograde flushing with carbon dioxide or diluted radiopaque dye. *J. Urol.* **134**, 29–32.

Jenkins, A.D. and Gillenwater, J.Y. (1988). Extracorporeal shock wave lithotripsy in prone position: treatment of stones in distal ureter or anomalous kidney. *J. Urol.* **139**, 911–15.

Knapp, P.M., Kulb, T.B., Lingeman, J.E., Newman, D.M., Mertz, J.H.O., Mosbaugh, P.G., and Steele, R.E. (1988). Extracorporeal shock wave lithotripsy-induced perirenal hematomas. *J. Urol.* **139**, 700–3.

Kulb, T.B., Lingeman, J.E., Coury, T.A., Steele, R.E., Newman, D.M., Mertz, J.M.O., Mosbaugh, P.G., and Knapp, P. (1986). Extracorporeal shock wave lithotripsy in patients with a solitary kidney, *J. Urol.* **136**, 786–8.

Libby, J.M., Meacham, R.B., and Griffith, D.P. (1988). The role of silicone ureteral stents in extracorporeal shock wave lithotripsy of large renal calculi. *J. Urol.* **139**, 15–17.

Lingeman, J.E. and Kulb, T.B. (1987). Hypertension following extracorporeal shock wave lithotripsy. *J. Urol.* **137**, 142A (Abstract).

Lingeman, J.E., Newman, D., Mertz, J.H.O., Mosbaugh, P.G., Steele, R.E., Kahnoski, R.J., Coury, T.A., and Woods, J.R. (1986). Extracorporeal shock wave lithotripsy: the Methodist Hospital of Indiana Experience. *J. Urol.* **135**, 1134–7.

Marberger, M., Stackl, W., Hruby, W., and Kroiss, A. (1985). Late sequelae of ultrasonic lithotripsy of renal calculi *J. Urol.* **133**, 170–4.

Mayo, M.E., Krieger, J.N., and Rudd, T.G. (1985). Effect of percutaneous nephrostolithotomy on renal function. *J. Urol.* **133**, 167–9.

Mee, S.L. and Thuroff, J.W. (1988). Small caliceal stones: is extracorporeal shock wave lithotripsy justified? *J. Urol.* **139**, 908–10.

Miller, H.C., Collins, L.A., Turbow, A.M., Turbow, B.A., Beall, M.E., Berger, R.M., Lebowitz, J.M., Young, I.S., Kahn, R.I., Karol, J.B., Collins, E.J., and Getson, P.R. (1989). Initial EDAP LT-01 lithotripsy group experience in the United States. *J. Urol.* **142**, 1412–14.

Nuzzarello, J., Rubenstein, M.A., and Norris, D.M. (1990). Extracorporeal shock wave lithotripsy and the ureteral stone brush: initial results. *J. Urol.* **143**, 261–2.

Pettersson, B. and Tuselius, H.G. (1989). Are prophylactic antibiotics necessary during extracorporeal shock wave lithotripsy? *Br. J. Urol.* **63**, 449–52.

Pollard, S.G. and MacFarlane, R. (1988). Symptoms arising from double-J ureteral stents. *J. Urol.* **139**, 37–8.

Preminger, G.M., Clayman, R.V., Hardeman, S.W., Franklin, J., Curry, T., and Peters, P.C. (1986). Percutaneous nephrostolithotomy vs open surgery for renal calculi: a comparative study *J.A.M.A.* **254**, 1054–8.

Pryor, J.L. and Jenkins, A.D. (1990). Use of double-pigtail stents in extracorporeal shock wave lithotripsy. *J. Urol.* **143**, 475–8.

Schulze, H., Hestle, L., Graff, J., Funke, P., and Senger, T. (1986). Combined treatment of branched calculi by percutaneous nephrolithotomy and extracorporeal shock wave lithotripsy. *J. Urol.* **135**, 1138–41.

Stoller, M.L., Litt, L., and Salazar, R.G. (1989). Severe hemorrhage after extracorporeal shock wave lithotripsy. *Ann. Intern. Med.* **111**, 612–13.

Tolley, D.A. (1987). Endoscopic ureteric stone extraction. Experience with the short ureteroscope. *Br. J. Urol.* **59**, 401–4.

Tung, K.H., Tan, E.C., and Foo, K.T. (1990). *In situ* extracorporeal shock wave lithotripsy for upper ureteral stones using the EDAP LT-01 lithotriptor. *J. Urol.* **143**, 481–2.

Vandeursen, H. and Baert, L. (1990). Extracorporeal shock wave lithotripsy monotherapy for bladder stones with the second generation lithotriptors. *J. Urol.* **143**, 18–19.

van Swearingen, F.L., McCullough, D.L., Dyer, R., and Appel, B. (1987). Radiation exposure to patients during extracorporeal shock wave lithotripsy. *J. Urol.* **138**, 18–20.

Weinerth, J.L., Flatt, J.A., and Carson, C.C. (1989). Lessons learned in patients with large steinstrasse. *J. Urol.* **142**, 1425–7.

Wickham, J.E.A. and Kellett, M.J. (1981). Percutaneous nephrolithotomy. *Br. J. Urol.* **53**, 297–9.

Williams, C.M., Kaude, J.V., Newman, R.C., Peterson, J.C., and Thomas, W.C. (1988). Extracorporeal shock-wave lithotripsy: long-term complications. *A.J.R.* **150**, 311–15.

Winfield, H.N., Clayman, R.V., Chaussy, C.G., Weyman, P.J., Fuchs, G.J., and Lupu, A.N. (1988). Monotherapy of staghorn renal calculi: comparative study between percutaneous nephrolithotomy and extracorporeal shock wave lithotripsy. *J. Urol.* **139**, 895–9.

Index